CHRONICLES OF DRUG DISCOVERY

CHRONICLES
OF
DRUG DISCOVERY

Volume 1

Edited by

JASJIT S. BINDRA
Pfizer Inc.
Groton, Connecticut

DANIEL LEDNICER
Adria Laboratories Inc.
Columbus, Ohio

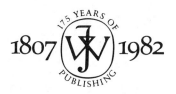

1807 1982

A Wiley-Interscience Publication
John Wiley & Sons

New York • Chichester • Brisbane • Toronto • Singapore

Library of Congress Cataloging in Publication Data
Main entry under title:

Chronicles in drug discovery.

   "A Wiley-Interscience publication."
   Includes index.
      1. Pharmaceutical research—History—Addresses, essays,
lectures. 2. Drugs—History—Addresses, essays, lectures. I.
Bindra, Jasjit S. II. Lednicer, Daniel, 1929-   . [DNLM: 1.
Drugs—Personal narratives. 2. Research—Personal
narratives. 3. Technology, Pharmaceutical—Personal
narratives. QV 55 C553]

RS122.C48   615′.1′09047   81-11471
ISBN 0-471-06516-1   AACR2

Printed in the United States of America

10 9 8 7 6 5 4 3 2 1

To
Ranjna and Beryle

Preface

That the advent of modern drug therapy has profoundly altered the outlook and expectations of humanity is no longer a subject for debate. The availability of effective drugs has permitted control of many once dreaded diseases, and has changed the mission of discovery medicine in many diseases from alleviating pain to curing disease.

The early stages of modern drug development were highly dramatic, since each advance helped conquer disease and led to rapid, miraculous recovery from diseases which were visibly distressing or frequently fatal. In recent years, public attention — except for the war on cancer — has been considerably muted. Past successes may have led the public to expect even greater achievements. Recent successes, while still significant medical advances, have been less spectacular, and the increasing scientific complexity of current research has made these advances more difficult to explain to the public. It is far easier to generate excitement for an antibiotic which rapidly arrests infection and saves lives than for an antiarrhythmic agent with an effect that is less obvious and whose mode of action needs to be explained in the arcane language of electrophysiology. Increased regulatory control and drugs targeted for chronic versus acute diseases have played a role as well by lengthening the period between the time a new drug is discovered in the laboratory and the date it becomes available to the general public. Dramatic or not, it cannot however be overlooked that the flow of discoveries from drug research laboratories has continued, though at a perhaps attenuated pace. An increasing number of diseases can now be at least partially managed by drug therapy.

In spite of some five decades of success, the process of drug discovery has not yet been reduced to a system which can be applied by rote. In spite of enormous advances in the sciences which provide the basis for the development of new medicinals, serendipity, inspired hunches, hard work and plain luck continue to play an important role in the development of a new therapeutic entity.

Attempts have been made to systematize the process and make it more predictable. However, successes achieved by these more systematic — sometimes called rational — approaches are still few.

The practitioners in the diverse disciplines involved in drug research — be they chemists, biochemists, pharmacologists, or clinicians — know that the chances of developing a successful drug are statistically very low. The scientist who can point with pride to a drug first synthesized in his laboratory is a rare individual. Accounts of successful discovery are thus of continual interest.

Though the story of the development of specific drugs has been recorded in various places, this has seldom been done from the point of view of the individual most closely connected with the initial discovery. Such accounts as exist are almost universally couched in the formal language of scientific journals.

This volume attempts to highlight the discovery process, or processes, which have led to new drugs. The discoverers have been chosen as narrators since they speak with the most authoritative voice on just what transpired in their minds and laboratories. In order to make a livelier story, they have been encouraged to be candid and depart from the arid language of their journals.

The choice of compounds discussed was deliberately narrowed to marketed drugs; premarketing candidates have been included if these seem unusually novel, or have shown sufficient clinical promise so that their commercialization is but a matter of time. Only drugs developed in the past one and a half decades have been included in the interest of making this account relatively up-to-date.

Jasjit S. Bindra
Daniel Lednicer

Groton, Connecticut
Columbus, Ohio
October 1981

Contents

Contributors
to Volume 1

B.G. Christensen, Merck Sharp & Dohme Research Laboratories, Rahway, New Jersey

D.J. LeCount, Imperial Chemical Industries Limited, Macclesfield, U.K.

E. Eichenberger, Wander Research Institute, Berne, Switzerland

Peter W. Feit, Leo Pharmaceutical Products, DK-2750 Ballerup, Denmark

C. Robin Ganellin, Smith Kline & French Research Limited, Welwyn Garden City, England

D.R. Hoff, Merck Sharp & Dohme Research Laboratories, Rahway, New Jersey

L.G. Humber, Ayerst Research Laboratories, Montreal, Canada

Joseph G. Lombardino, Pfizer Central Research Laboratories, Groton, Connecticut

John S. Nicholson, The Boots Company Ltd., Nottingham, U.K.

H.C. Richards, Pfizer Central Research, Sandwich, England

J. Schmutz, Wander Research Institute, Berne, Switzerland

P. Sensi, Lepetit Research Laboratories, Milan, Italy

Helmut Stähle, C.H. Boehringer Sohn, Ingleheim am Rhein, West Germany

Edward H. Wiseman, Pfizer Central Research, Groton, Connecticut

Acknowledgments

It is a pleasure to thank our many colleagues for helpful discussions which shaped this book. Special thanks are due to Drs. H. -J. Hess and C. A. Harbert of Pfizer Central Research, and Dr. Stanley Kudzin of John Wiley & Sons for their valuable comments, continued encouragement and support which nurtured this project from the start. We are indebted to Dr. E. H. Wiseman who made available the facilities for production of the camera-ready manuscript at Pfizer; to John Stratton and B. F. Bell for editorial assistance; to the ever cheerful Charles J. Kenney and his group, especially Phil Grzymkowski and Heike Holley, and the wizardry of Carol Milne for artwork and structural drawings; to Tony Russo's Duplicating Services Group, especially Mike Foley; and to Anita Parker and her magic fingers, which effortlessly and expertly phototypeset the manuscript.

CHRONICLES OF DRUG DISCOVERY

Cimetidine

C. Robin Ganellin

1

The idea that hormones and transmitter substances act at specific sites that we call receptors has been extremely valuable in the development of new drugs. These substances have a chemical individuality that is specifically recognized at the receptor sites; that is, the sites discriminate among different hormones. Thus hormonal control is a highly selective process. It follows that the design of compounds to act in competition with the hormone for occupation of these sites is a potential way of attaining specificity of drug action. It also appears that the receptor sites for a particular hormone are not necessarily homogeneous. Drugs have been discovered that appear to differentiate among sites for the same hormone, suggesting different populations of drug receptors. This allows further scope for introducing selectivity of drug action.

1. HISTAMINE RECEPTORS

Histamine [2-(imidazol-4-yl)ethylamine] appears to be a locally acting transmitter substance (it has been called an "autocoid") that has very specific actions. In 1910 Dale and Laidlaw, working at the Wellcome Physiological Research Laboratories, published the first of a series of papers describing the pharmacological effects of histamine[1]; in particular, they noted the powerful effect of histamine in stimulating contractions of smooth muscle and its potent action in lowering blood pressure. The early studies on histamine indicated a similarity in some of its effects with the symptoms that appear during inflammation and with symptoms characteristic of shock produced by trauma or allergic reactions. It became widely assumed that histamine was a principle mediator of inflammation and shock and this stimulated a search by Bovet in Paris for substances capable of counteracting these apparent injurious effects. Initial

1

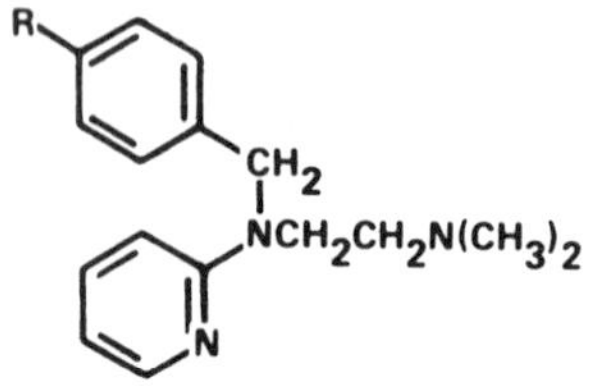

1a, R = OCH$_3$, Mepyramine

1b, R = H, Tripelennamine

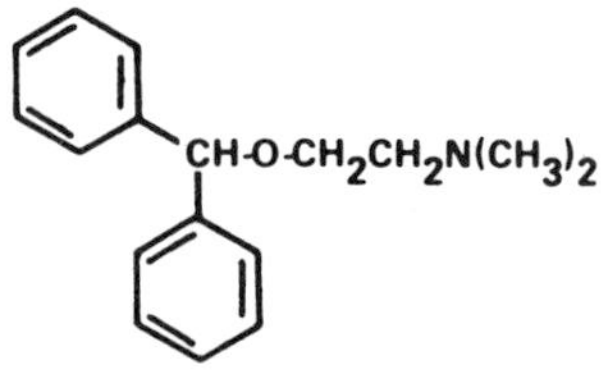

2
Diphenhydramine

findings were published in 1937[2] and led to the development of the anti-histamine drugs in the 1940s and to their introduction for the treatment of allergic conditions such as urticaria and hay fever.[3] Drugs such as mepyramine (pyrilamine, **1a**), tripelennamine (**1b**), and diphenhydramine (**2**) were found to be very selective in blocking certain actions of histamine. Quantitative dose-response analysis from studies on blood pressure[4] or on isolated smooth muscle[5] suggested that the mode of antagonism was competitive and, in 1947, Schild[6] introduced pA_x values to characterize the antagonism. Two typical compounds, mepyramine (**1a**, Neonantergan) and diphenhydramine (**2**, Benadryl) were thereby shown to be specific in antagonizing histamine-stimulated contractions of the isolated ileum of the guinea pig relative to other stimulants; they were effective at low concentrations and the antagonism they produced was surmountable and reversible. These antagonists came to be regarded as acting in competition with histamine for occupation of its specific receptor sites. Subsequently, they were also shown to antagonize actions of histamine on the vascular system, namely, the histamine-induced increase in capillary permeability and certain vasoconstrictor actions; however, it was also found that these antagonists reduced the intensity of, but did not abolish, vasodilator actions, and in 1948 it was suggested that there may be "two types of receptors sensitive to histamine only one of which can be blocked by Benadryl and related compounds".[7]

These antihistamines were used to compare receptors in different tissues and species[8,9]; for example, mepyramine gave similar pA_2 values when tested against histamine on the perfused lung of the guinea pig, on the isolated ileum and trachea of the guinea pig, and on human bronchi; the results indicated a homogeneity for the histamine receptors in these tissues.

Several actions of histamine had been noted that could not be specifically antagonized by these drugs; for example, stimulation of gastric acid secretion,[10] stimulation of isolated atria,[11] inhibition of rat uterus contractions,[12] and the vasodilator effects of large doses of histamine.[7] Various workers suggested that these nonantagonizable actions of histamine might involve other histamine receptors but proof was lacking. Some pointers to the differentiation of histamine receptors had been obtained by considering the selectivity of action of agonists on different tissue systems. For example, Grossman et al.[13] compared the histamine-like activities of some 60 compounds chemically related to histamine on gastric secretion in the dog, guinea pig intestinal strip, and cat blood pressure. A more extensive list was compiled by Jones.[14] Ash and Schild[15] made quantitative estimates of the relative activities of different histamine congeners on the isolated guinea pig ileum, on the isolated rat uterus, and *in vivo* as stimulants of rat gastric acid secretion; they obtained a correlation in activity ratios suggesting that a common receptor mechanism might be involved in rat gastric acid secretion and rat uterus inhibition. Such considerations led Ash and Schild to propose in 1966 that the actions of histamine blocked by the antihistamine drugs characterized one type of histamine receptor, which they named the H_1-receptor. Other actions of histamine not specifically antagonized were probably mediated by other histamine receptors, but the characterization of these receptors awaited the discovery of specific antagonists; in the meantime they were to be regarded as non-H_1.

2. THE SEARCH FOR AN ANTAGONIST

The inability of the antihistaminic drugs (H_1-receptor antagonists) to inhibit histamine-stimulated gastric acid secretion has been known for many years[3] and there have been a few published reports of concerted efforts to discover a specific antagonist to this action of histamine. Robertson and Grossman[16] screened compounds in a search for inhibitors of gastric acid secretion, and Grossman et al.[13] reported on an extensive study of compounds, chemically related to histamine, that were examined for their action on acid secretion and also tested as possible inhibitors of histamine stimulation. Lin et al.,[17] Ash and Schild,[15] and van den Brink[18] also examined close analogues of histamine for possible antagonism of histamine-stimulated acid secretion. However, none of these studies uncovered a histamine antagonist.

A similar analysis by Dr. James Black at our laboratories led him to establish in 1964 the test procedures needed to detect antagonists of these other effects of histamine. It was hoped that the work would lead to a new type of pharmacologic agent with possible clinical utility. It was argued that at the very least, such an agent ought to provide a valuable scientific tool that would assist investigation of the physiological role of histamine. But the prize, seen at the outset, was a possible means for selective pharmacological control of gastric acid secretion with the potential for treating peptic ulcer disease. This was a radically different approach from most of the investigations then being conducted in the pharmaceutical industry, where it was more usual to screen for "antiulcer" compounds in a less specified way either as inhibitors of gastric acid secretion (e.g., in the Shay rat preparation) or as inhibitors of ulcer formation, produced by various means.

In our laboratories, compounds were tested for ability to inhibit histamine-stimulated gastric acid secretion in anesthetized rats on the assumption that if non-H_1 receptor antagonists were to be found it seemed reasonable to expect the inhibition. Routinely, gastric acid secretion was measured by the pH of the lumen perfusate from the stomach of an anesthetized rat using a preparation developed by Parsons[19] and based on that described by Ghosh and Schild.[20] Initially, compounds were administered as a constant intravenous infusion in the middle of a train of fixed-dose histamine responses (given by rapid intravenous injection). Subsequently, the system was modified and a plateau of gastric acid secretion was established by continuous intravenous infusion of histamine (at a dose high enough to produce a near maximal response) and potential inhibitors were then given by rapid intravenous injection. Since other types of inhibitors of gastric secretion could also be picked up by this test, compounds found to be active were also tested on isolated tissue systems to provide additional criteria for specific antagonism to histamine. Two *in vitro* test systems were set up, namely, histamine-induced stimulation of the guinea pig right atrium (which continues to beat spontaneously *in vitro* because it contains the pacemaker and histamine increases the rate of beating) and inhibition by histamine of evoked contractions of the rat uterus.

It is worth recording that the atmosphere prevailing in gastroenterological science at that time was far from conducive to the search for a histamine antagonist as a means of controlling gastric acid secretion. In the 1960s the polypeptide hormone gastrin was isolated,[21] its chemical structure was sequenced and proved,[22] and many researchers turned their attention to seeking specific inhibitors of gastrin-induced acid secretion. The import of histamine was difficult to prove[23] and there was a widely held view, typified by an article published in 1971,[24] that histamine had no place in the physiological maintenance of gastric acid secretion. The concerted but unsuccessful effort by researchers at Eli Lilly in the 1950s to find an antagonist of histamine-stimulated acid secretion[14,16,17] added further to the feeling that the approach was "played-out." However, there were still some adherents to the view that histamine played a key role in gastric acid secretion, although they were very much in a minority.[25]

Once the problem of obtaining a competitive antagonist was posed in biological terms it was then necessary to consider how to approach it chemically. How could one obtain such a compound? Where should one start, given no obvious "lead" compound? Nothing was known chemically about the physiological site of action of histamine and, returning to first principles, the structure of histamine (Figure 1a) was used as a chemical starting point. The

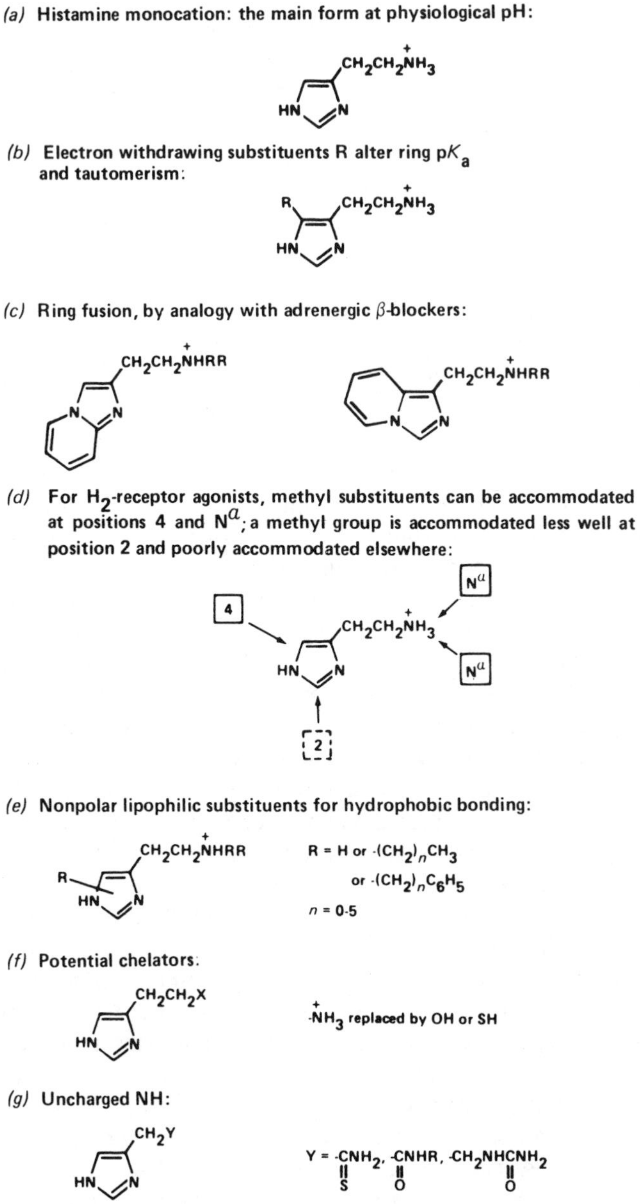

(a) Histamine monocation: the main form at physiological pH:

$$CH_2CH_2\overset{+}{N}H_3$$

(b) Electron withdrawing substituents R alter ring pK_a and tautomerism:

(c) Ring fusion, by analogy with adrenergic β-blockers:

(d) For H_2-receptor agonists, methyl substituents can be accommodated at positions 4 and N^α; a methyl group is accommodated less well at position 2 and poorly accommodated elsewhere:

(e) Nonpolar lipophilic substituents for hydrophobic bonding:

$$R = H \text{ or } -(CH_2)_nCH_3$$
$$\text{or } -(CH_2)_nC_6H_5$$
$$n = 0\text{-}5$$

(f) Potential chelators:

$-\overset{+}{N}H_3$ replaced by OH or SH

(g) Uncharged NH:

$$Y = -\underset{\underset{S}{\parallel}}{C}NH_2, -\underset{\underset{O}{\parallel}}{C}NHR, -CH_2NH\underset{\underset{O}{\parallel}}{C}NH_2$$

Figure 1. Some attempts to design a histamine antagonist

simple minded view was taken that since the search was for a molecule that would compete with histamine for its receptor site, such a molecule would have to be recognized by the receptor and then bind more strongly than histamine, but not trigger the usual response. It therefore seemed worthwhile to retain in potential antagonist structures some chemical features of histamine to aid receptor recognition, and to include chemical groups that might assist binding.

Many different approaches were tried, including the use of analogies derived from known examples of chemical-biological relationships between other types of receptor agonists and antagonists, or enzyme substrates and inhibitors, or antimetabolites. The structure of histamine was modified to deliberately alter its chemical properties, while retaining some definite aspect of its structure or chemistry. Some examples, summarized in Figure 1, have also been discussed elsewhere.[26] Modifications were made to the imidazole ring of histamine to change ionization properties (pK_a and tautomerism), for example, electronegative substituents were introduced into the 4-position (Figure 1b) and other heterocyclic analogues were examined; an analogy with the adrenergic β-blockers led to fusion of a benzene ring to the imidazole ring of histamine (Figure 1c), as in the relationship between the β-adrenergic agonist isoprenaline (isoproterenol) and its antagonist pronethalol.[27]

In another approach, nonpolar lipophilic substituents were introduced at various positions in histamine, since many competitive antagonist drugs contain such groups, which are thought to contribute to drug-receptor association through hydrophobic interaction at nonpolar regions of the receptor at the active site or its immediate vicinity (see reference 28). A range of alkyl and arylalkyl substituted histamines was examined since it was not possible to know in advance which groups might match molecular requirements. The problem was to find appropriate groups and the correct substitution position [see Baker[29] in his pioneering design of active-site-directed enzyme inhibitors]. Methyl was used as a model group to see where substituents in histamine could be tolerated, and all the possible monomethylhistamines were made and tested.[30] It was found that for stimulating acid secretion, a methyl group was tolerated well only at the 4-position of the ring or on the amino nitrogen atom of the side chain (Figure 1d) and to a lesser extent at the 2-position. Various alkyl and aralkyl substituents were then introduced into histamine, either singly or in combination, as in Figure 1e.

Many compounds of the above types were made, but none was active as an antagonist. The problem is that even small modifications of the natural stimulant histamine introduce many variables. Even when most of the structure was specified there were still numerous aspects to investigate and many of the avenues explored turned out to be blind alleys.

By this time, after numerous failures to achieve antagonism, grave doubts arose about the feasibility of obtaining such an antagonist. However, evidence giving further hints of two types of receptors had come from selectively acting agonists (stimulants). It had been found that 2-methylhistamine was active in stimulating the ileum (17% the potency of histamine), the H_1 site, but was only slightly active as a stimulant of gastric acid secretion in the rat, the putative H_2-site. 4-Methylhistamine showed the reverse type of selectivity, and to a remarkable degree, having only 0.2% of the potency of histamine on the ileum yet having nearly half the potency of histamine as a stimulant of gastric acid secretion: a separation of over 200-fold.[31] These results bolstered our confidence to continue.

The above approaches were concerned mainly with modifications to the imidazole ring of histamine or with making the molecule lipophilic, but none of the compounds was found to antagonize the non-H_1 actions of histamine. Attention was also directed to compounds in which the imidazole ring was unaltered and the side chain was modified. For example (Figure 1*f*), the $-N^+$ group was replaced by $-SH$ or $-OH$ to see whether an alteration of potential chelating properties might provide an antagonist. A number of other polar-substituted imidazoles resembling histamine were also examined; some amidic derivatives (shown in Figure 1*g*) differ from histamine in having side-chain nitrogen atoms uncharged.

Many compounds were made, based on histamine. In the first four years some 200 compounds were synthesized and tested, without providing a blocking drug. Toward the end of this time many doubts were expressed about whether it really would prove possible to block the action of histamine on gastric acid secretion and, indeed, there was considerable pressure within the Company to abandon this approach (see reference 96). The scientists involved in the project were, however, firmly resolved to continue, and during this period the test system was refined and chemical ideas began to crystallize. A most important aspect of research is to conduct the work in such a way as to learn from negative results. Even a list of inactive compounds is informative if they have been selected for particular reasons. Having tested many compounds with lipophilic substituents without seeing antagonism, the pharmacologists re-examined some of the early hydrophilic compounds, one of which showed some blocking activity. It was very weak but provided the vital lead. It was missed originally because this compound also acted as a stimulant; in fact it is a partial agonist. The compound is a histamine derivative in which a guanidine group replaces the amino group in the side chain, namely, N^α-guanylhistamine (Table 1). It was originally selected for synthesis based on an analogy with guanidine structures, which have a high affinity for catecholamine storage sites.[32]

Table 1
Structures and Antagonist Activities of Some Key Compounds in the Development of H_2-Receptor Antagonists

Compound	Structure	Antagonist activity in vitro[a] ($K_B \times 10^{-6}$)	Antagonist activity in vivo[b] (ID_{50} μmol/kg)	Reference
N^α-**Guanylhistamine:** The "lead"; a weakly active partial agonist	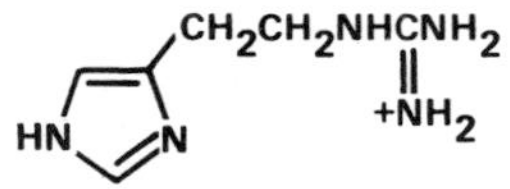	130	800	32
SK&F 91486 Lengthening the side chain increases activity; it is still a partial agonist	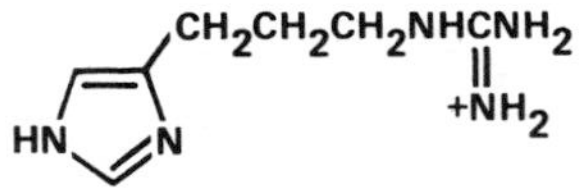	22	100	34
SK&F 91581 Thiourea analogue is much less active as an antagonist, but is not an agonist	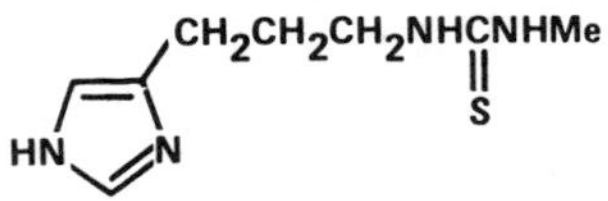	115[c]	d	35
Burimamide Lengthening the side chain again dramatically increases antagonist activity	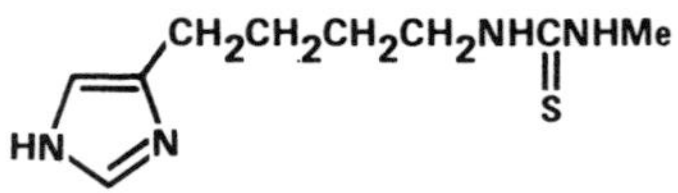	7.8	6.1	31

8

	Structure		
Metiamide Introducing —S— in the side chain and CH$_3$ in the ring alters imidazole tautomerism and increases activity	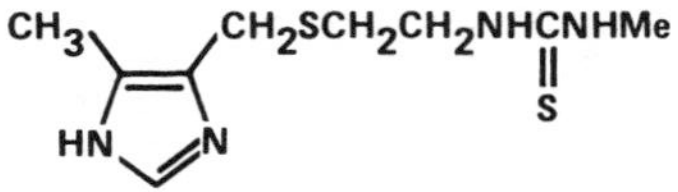 CH$_3$ / HN N / CH$_2$SCH$_2$CH$_2$NHCNHMe $\parallel$ S	0.92	1.6	57
SK&F 92408 (Guanidine Isostere) Replacing C=S by C=NH gives a basic side chain and reduces activity	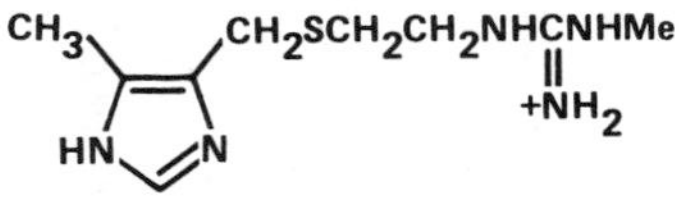 CH$_3$ / HN N / CH$_2$SCH$_2$CH$_2$NHCNHMe $\parallel$ +NH$_2$	16	12	64
Cimetidine Introducing a CN substituent reduces basicity and increases activity	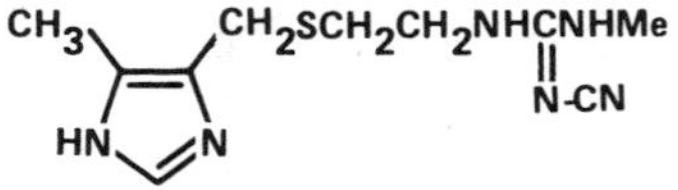 CH$_3$ / HN N / CH$_2$SCH$_2$CH$_2$NHCNHMe $\parallel$ N-CN	0.79	1.4	65

9

---

[a]*In vitro*, determined against histamine stimulation of spontaneously beating isolated guinea-pig right atrium. The dissociation constant (K_B) was calculated from the equation $K_B = B/(x - 1)$, where x is the respective ratio of concentrations of histamine needed to produce half maximal responses in the presence and absence of different concentrations (B) of antagonist, and -log K_B = pA_2.

[b]Activity as an antagonist of histamine-stimulated gastric acid secretion in the anesthetized rat using a lumen-perfused preparation.[19] Compounds given by rapid intravenous injection during a near maximal plateau of histamine-stimulated gastric acid secretion. The ID$_{50}$ is the dose required to produce 50% of inhibition and was estimated from the linear regression of log $[I/(100 - I)]$ on log dose where I = percentage inhibition (R. C. Blakemore and M. E. Parsons, The Research Institute, Smith Kline and French Research Limited, Welwyn Garden City, England).

[c]Data refined since initial report of 350 x 10^6 *M*.

[d]No antagonism seen up to an intravenous dose of 256 μmol/kg.

N^α-Guanylhistamine, tested *in vivo* on gastric acid secretion using the lumen perfused stomach of the anesthetized rat preparation, was found to be a stimulant at doses in the range 16-512 μmol/kg given by rapid i.v. injection. The maximal response obtained with guanylhistamine was between 50 and 60% of that obtainable with histamine. Agonist potency, which was assessed by comparison of the doses of guanylhistamine and histamine required to produce equal acid secretory responses, was found to be less than 0.5% of the potency of histamine ($n = 9$), that is, guanylhistamine is a weak agonist on gastric acid secretion.[32]

To test for antagonist activity, guanylhistamine was injected i.v. after a plateau of secretion had been established to an i.v. infusion of histamine. When first tested the rate of histamine infusion used (0.05 mol/kg/min) produced a secretory response that was less than 50% of maximal and guanylhistamine caused either no effect or a slight further increase in acid secretion. However, when guanylhistamine was retested at a later date, a near-maximal secretory response to histamine was used (infusion rate 0.25 μmol/kg/min) and inhibition was detected at doses of 256 μmol/kg and greater. The approximate i.v. ID_{50} (that is the dose to produce 50% inhibition of near-maximal secretion) was calculated to be 800 μmol/kg ($n = 15$). Guanylhistamine thus appeared to be acting as a partial agonist on gastric acid secretion and its antagonist activity went undetected initially because the secretory response to the histamine infusion did not exceed the maximal agonist activity of guanylhistamine. Antagonism could only be demonstrated when the rate of histamine infusion was increased so that the secretory response exceeded the maximum response to guanylhistamine. Although these studies indicated that guanylhistamine acted as a partial agonist on gastric acid secretion, further evidence was necessary to establish that this action was the result of interaction with histamine receptors. The compound was therefore investigated on isolated guinea-pig atrium *in vitro*. By use of cumulative dose-response curves guanylhistamine was found to have agonist activity at high concentrations up to 5 μM but only achieved 60 $\pm$ 5% ($n = 7$) of the maximal response obtainable with histamine and the dose-response curves were not parallel. This behavior is typical of a partial agonist and, therefore, because of nonparallelism, only an approximate activity relative to histamine of 0.7% could be estimated. Antagonist activity was demonstrated by comparing control cumulative dose-response curves for histamine (Figure 2) with those obtained after equilibration with a series of different concentrations of guanylhistamine. The apparent dissociation constant (K_B) was estimated to be 1.3 x $10^{-4}M$ (0.44-4.6, $n = 8$), which corresponds to an empirical pA_2 value of 3.9 (3.3-4.4). Partial agonist activity could also be demonstrated by superimposing a cumulative dose-response curve to guanylhistamine on top of a sustained maximal tachycardia to histamine. As seen in the gastric secretion studies the maximal inhibitory effect of guanylhistamine (34.5 $\pm$ 8.3%, $n = 6$)

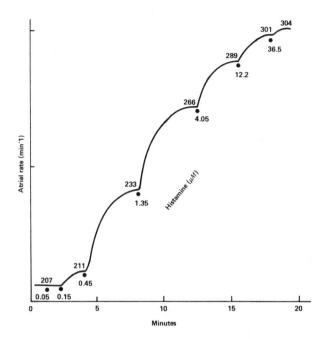

Figure 2. Cumulative response of the rate of beating of the guinea pig right atrium *in vitro* to successive increases in histamine concentration. As shown on the left hand side of the curves the rate of beating increases from the resting level of 207 beats/min to a near maximum value of 304 (vertical axis). The micromolar concentration of histamine, shown on the right hand side of the curves, is increased stepwise in a geometric sequence, the next dose being introduced when the response to the preceding one has reached a steady value. The horizontal axis provides the time scale (minutes). Studies by Dr. M. E. Parsons, Smith Kline and French Research Limited. Reproduced with permission from Ganellin.[35]

did not exceed the maximal agonist activity seen with the compound alone.[32] Ironically, N^α-guanylhistamine was first synthesized by van der Merwe[33] and was reported to be "devoid of interesting physiological activity." Clearly, biological activity may be present, but its discovery depends on the way one looks for it!

The appearance of antagonism, albeit weak, provided a much needed lead and within a few days an analogous compound was retested and found to be more active, namely, S-[2-(imidazol-4-yl)ethyl]-isothiourea (Figure 3a, $x = 2$, R = H). However, a much more active compound was required. An immediate question to be answered was whether activity was due to the presence of the guanidine or isothiourea groups (amidines) *per se* or to the resemblance to histamine. Structure-activity studies suggested that the imidazole ring was important; antagonism did not appear to be a property of amidines in general. This suggested that the imidazole and amidine groups probably acted cooperatively, and it allowed a limiting selection to be made, for example, to retain the imidazole ring and concentrate attention on the amidine part of the molecule. It was also necessary to identify the particular chemical properties that conferred antagonist activity in order to make analogues of increased potency. The amidine groups are strong bases and are protonated and positively charged at physiological pH. Thus the molecules resemble histamine monocation, but also differ in several ways; the amidinium group is planar (whereas the ammonium group of histamine is tetrahedral) and the positive charge is distributed over three hetero atoms. It was noted that the distance between ring and terminal N is potentially greater than in histamine, and there are several N sites for potential interactions instead of one. Various structural features were examined, for example, to determine whether all three hetero atoms were needed and also to see what happened on extending the chain, that is, on increasing the distance from the ring.

2.1 The Discovery of Burimamide

Many analogues were made and it was found that the guanidine homologue 3-[4(5)-imidazolyl]propylguanidine, SK&F 91486 (Table 1) was a more active antagonist.[34] Although antagonist potency of SK&F 91486 was increased by a factor of six- to eight-fold over N^α-guanylhistamine, the stimulant activity was also increased, that is, N^α-guanylhistamine was also a *partial agonist*.[35] At this stage it became desirable to increase the side chain length still further, but problems of chemical synthesis were experienced and new synthetic routes were required. Meanwhile, there was an investigation of which nitrogen atoms of the guanidine group were required for antagonist activity. Various related amidinium and isothiouronium structures (Figure 3) having only two of the nitrogen atoms were found to have activity as antagonists and are described in several patents;[36] it was also shown that substituents could be accommodated on the nitrogen atoms. Many of these compounds were also found to be partial agonists, which appeared to impose a limitation on the potential of this type of structure for providing antagonists and seemed to be hindering progress. Although the compounds antagonized the action of histamine, they were not sufficiently effective inhibitors of gastric acid secretion because of interference from their inherent stimulatory activity.

Thus a critical stage was reached in the need for selectivity: it was necessary to achieve a separation between agonist and antagonist activities. It seemed that these compounds might act as agonists by mimicking histamine chemically,

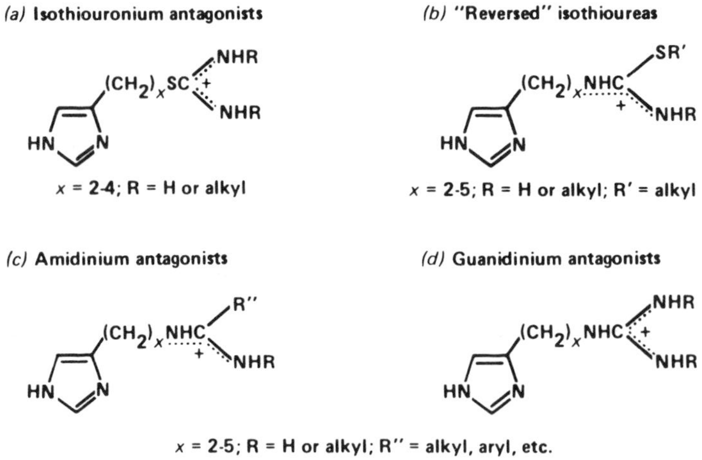

(a) Isothiouronium antagonists

$x = 2\text{-}4$; R = H or alkyl

(b) "Reversed" isothioureas

$x = 2\text{-}5$; R = H or alkyl; R' = alkyl

(c) Amidinium antagonists

(d) Guanidinium antagonists

$x = 2\text{-}5$; R = H or alkyl; R'' = alkyl, aryl, etc.

Figure 3. Isothiouronium, amidinium, and guanidinium structures compared with histamine. All form side-chain cations at pH 7.4.

since like histamine, they have an imidazole ring and, being basic amidines, the side chain at physiological pH is protonated and carries a positive charge (Figure 3). It also seemed likely that these features would permit receptor recognition and provide binding for a competitive antagonist but would allow the molecule to mimic histamine and act as an agonist. This posed a considerable dilemma because the chemical groups that appeared to be required for antagonist activity were the same groups that seemed to confer the agonist effect.

In an attempt to separate these activities, the strongly basic guanidine group was replaced by nonbasic groups that, though polar, were not charged. Such an approach furnished analogues that indeed were not active as agonists; however, they were also not active as antagonists. Fortunately, one example, the thiourea derivative (SK&F 91581) that did not act as a partial agonist exhibited weak activity as an antagonist (Table 1). Thioureas are essentially neutral in water because of the electron-withdrawing thiocarbonyl group. Conjugation forces the nitrogen atoms into a planar form and limits the availability of the lone electron pairs, as in amides. At this time the higher homologous amine (with the four carbon atom chain length) was synthesized and further exploration revealed that with this type of structure, extension of the alkylene side chain resulted in a marked increase in antagonist potency, exemplified by the compound burimamide, *N*-methyl-*N*´-[4-(imidazol-4-yl)butyl]thiourea (Table 1).

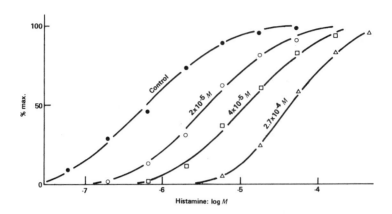

Figure 4. Histamine cumulative log-dose response curves from isolated guinea pig atrium: without antagonist (•) and after equilibration with burimamide 2 x 10⁻⁵ M) (o), 4 x 10⁻⁵ M (□), and 2.7 x 10⁻⁴ M (Δ). The percentage of the maximal histamine response is plotted vertically against log molar concentration of histamine (horizontal axis). Burimamide produces a dose-related displacement of the curves without significantly affecting their slope or maximum. Reproduced with permission from Black et al.[31]

In 1972 Black et al.[31] were able to announce the discovery as a specific competitive antagonist of histamine on non-H₁ tissue systems, thereby defining histamine H₂-receptors.

2.2   Burimamide, and the Characterization of a Histamine H₂-Receptor Antagonist

Burimamide was an important breakthrough. It was highly selective, showed no agonist activity, and antagonized the action of histamine in a competitive manner on the two *in vitro* systems, namely, guinea-pig atrium and rat uterus. It allowed these to be defined as H₂-receptor systems, and thereby burimamide was defined as an H₂-receptor antagonist.[31] The main pieces of evidence for the pharmacological characterization of burimamide are:

1. On the spontaneously beating isolated guinea-pig right atrium, burimamide produces a dose-related displacement of the cumulative histamine dose-response curve without significantly affecting the slope or maximum (Figure 4).

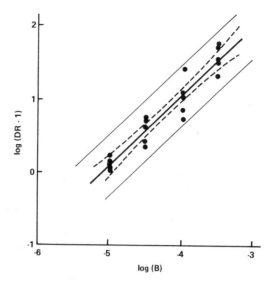

Figure 5. Antagonism of histamine by burimamide on guinea pig atrium *in vitro*. Antagonism is expressed by histamine dose ratios (DR) needed for equal responses before and after burimamide (B) equilibration. If burimamide and histamine compete for a common site (and certain assumptions hold), then log (DR - 1) = log (B) - log K_B, where K_B = (apparent) dissociation constant for the antagonist-receptor interaction; the data are plotted to test this relationship. Concentrations of burimamide were 1×10^{-5}, 3×10^{-5}, 1×10^{-4}, and 3×10^{-4} M. Regression of log (DR - 1) on log (B) was calculated by the method of least squares, and 95% confidence limits for the regression (- - - -) and for a single estimation (————) are shown. K_B (apparent) = 7.8×10^{-6} M (6.4-9.6); pA_2 = 5.11 (5.02-5.19). Slope = 0.98 (0.90-1.06). Reproduced with permission from Black et al.[31]

2. The regression of log (histamine dose ratio − 1) on log (concentration of antagonist) is linear with a slope not significantly different from unity, that is, the Schild plot[9] (Figure 5). This behavior indicates that the interaction between histamine and burimamide is consistent with competition and enables the dissociation constant (K_B) to be calculated (Tables 2 and 3).
3. The estimated K_B value was shown to be independent of the agonist used as a stimulant. Thus the values obtained for K_B using 2-methylhistamine or 4-methylhistamine were not significantly different from that obtained using histamine (Table 2).[31]

4. Similar results were obtained when burimamide was tested against histamine on the rat uterus preparation. The histamine dose-response curves were displaced without change in maximum or slope. The regression between log (DR - 1) and log (B) was found to be linear, and the slope and estimated K_B were not significantly different[31] from that found using the guinea pig atrium preparation (Table 3). This supports the argument that the histamine receptors on these two tissues are homogeneous.

5. The specificity of this histamine antagonism was examined by testing for an interaction between burimamide and isoprenaline (isoproterenol). Like histamine, isoprenaline stimulates guinea pig atrium and inhibits rat uterus, but it does so by acting on catecholamine β-receptors. Burimamide, in concentrations up to $8 \times 10^{-4}M$, failed to displace isoprenaline dose-response curves significantly on either tissue. The specificity of burimamide antagonism was also examined on guinea pig ileum where the histamine responses are mediated by H_1-receptors. When large enough doses of burimamide were used, the ileal contractions produced by histamine could be suppressed. A similar result was obtained using carbachol (Table 3) as stimulant, which acts on cholinergic muscarinic receptors. The apparent K_B values estimated for both histamine and carbachol with each agonist were very much larger than that found in the H_2-receptor systems and in each case the antagonism appeared to be noncompetitive.

The above results indicate that burimamide is pharmacologically very selective, and it fulfills the criteria required for characterizing the existence of another set of histamine receptors, the H_2-receptors. Burimamide also antagonized the action of histamine as a stimulant of gastric acid secretion in the rat, cat, and dog.[31] It is about 20-100 times as active as N^α-guanylhistamine, the original guanidine lead, and it was the first H_2-receptor antagonist to be investigated in man.[37] Given intravenously, it blocked the action of histamine as a stimulant of gastric acid secretion, thereby confirming that burimamide behaves in humans as it does in animals. However, its one drawback was that it was not sufficiently active to be given orally. Thus, although burimamide was selective enough to define H_2-receptors, it was not active enough to permit proper drug development.

2.3   Sulfur-Methylene Isosterism, Imidazole Tautomerism, and the Development of Metiamide

Various ways to alter the structure of burimamide were examined in an attempt to increase potency. One approach that proved successful resulted from two

Table 2

Dissociation Constant (K_B) for Burimamide Estimated *in vitro* on Guinea-Pig Atrium Using Three Agonists [31]

Agonist	Agonist $(ED_{50} \times 10^{-6} M)^a$	Burimamide $(K_B \times 10^{-6} M)^a$
Histamine	1.1 (0.9 – 1.4)	7.8 (6.4 – 9.6)
4-Methylhistamine	3.1 (2.0 – 4.3)	7.2 (5.2 – 9.2)
2-Methylhistamine	19.8 (9.7 – 29.9)	6.9 (5.7 – 8.2)

^{a}with 95% confidence limits.

Table 3

The Antagonist Activity of Burimamide on Isolated Tissues [31]

Tissue	Agonist	Burimamide $(K_B \times 10^{-6} M)^a$	Slope of log $[(DR - 1)$ on log $(B)]^a$
Atrium	Histamine	7.8 (6.4 – 9.6)	0.98 (0.90 – 1.06)
Uterus	Histamine	6.6 (4.9 – 8.3)	0.96 (0.80 – 1.12)
Ileum	Histamine	288 (95 – 870)	1.32 (1.11 – 1.54)
Ileum	Carbachol	174 (60 – 500)	1.44 (1.16 – 1.72)

^{a}with 95% confidence limits.

lines of exploration that merged. On one hand, attempts were being made to overcome the problem of synthesizing the side chains by inserting a thioether link. Meanwhile, a study was being made of the pK_a characteristics of burimamide, since it was realized that burimamide in aqueous solution is a

Table 4
Apparent pK_a Values[a] of Substituted Imidazole Cations at 37°C and Their Mole Percentages at pH 7.4[38]

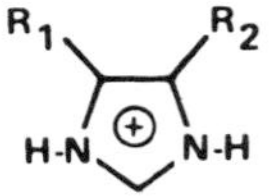

Compound	R_1	R_2	pK_a'	Preferred tautomer[b]	Mol % of cation at pH 7.4
Methylburimamide	CH$_3$	—(CH$_2$)$_4$NHCSNHCH$_3$	7.80		72
4(5)-Methylimidazole	H	—CH$_3$	7.40	1,5	50
Burimamide	H	—(CH$_2$)$_4$NHCSNHCH$_3$	7.25	1,5	40
Imidazole	H	—H	6.80		20
Metiamide	CH$_3$	—CH$_2$SCH$_2$CH$_2$NHCSNHCH$_3$	6.80	1,4	20
4(5)-Methylthio-methylimidazole	H	—CH$_2$SCH$_3$	6.35[c]	1,4	8
Thiaburimamide	H	—CH$_2$SCH$_2$CH$_2$NHCSNHCH$_3$	6.25	1,4	7
4(5)-Methoxymethyl-imidazole	H	—CH$_2$OCH$_3$	6.00[c]	1,4	4
Histamine	H	—CH$_2$CH$_2$NH$_3^+$	5.90	1,4	3

[a]The pK_a values were determined potentiometrically at 25°C on 0.05 M solutions in 0.1 M KCl by titration against HCl, corrected to 37°C by subtracting 0.0225 units per degree rise for values in the range 7.5 = 7.0, and 0.02 for the range 6.5 – 6.0, and rounded off to the nearest 0.05 unit.

[b]Structures in Figure 6; R$_2$ = R.

[c]Reference 41.

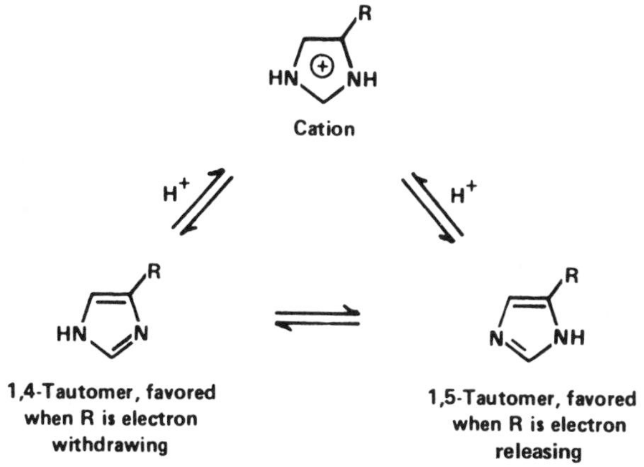

Cation

1,4-Tautomer, favored when R is electron withdrawing

1,5-Tautomer, favored when R is electron releasing

Figure 6. Equilibria between imidazole species: substituents R in the 4(5)-position of the imidazole ring alter tautomerism.[39]

mixture of many chemical species in equilibrium.[38] For example, at physiological pH there are three main forms of the imidazole ring, namely, the cation and two uncharged tautomers [1,4] and [1,5] as shown in Figure 6; these do not interconvert instantaneously, but probably require a water-mediated proton transfer. It was argued that if only one of these forms were active its relative population might determine the amount of drug required for a given effect. The populations of these species were estimated from the electronic influence of the side chain using pK_a data since the substituent R in the 4(5)-position of imidazole alters the electron densities at the ring nitrogen atoms and affects proton acidity. As indicated by Charton,[39] the substituent effect is more marked at the nearer nitrogen atom so that if R is an electron-withdrawing group, the 1,4-tautomer should predominate; if R is electron releasing the 1,5-tautomer should predominate. The fraction present as cation is determined by the ring pK_a and the pH of the medium. The electronic influence of the side chain was assessed from the measured ring pK_a using the Hammett equation (see reference 66): $pK_a(R) = pK_a(H) + \varrho\sigma_m$. The pK_a values of relevant compounds are given in Table 4. For burimamide the ring pK_a is 7.25, which is greater than that of imidazole itself; it was argued that the side chain [R = $-(CH_2)_4NHCSNHCH_3$] must therefore be electron releasing and should favor the 1,5-tautomer. Electronically, the side chain appears to resemble a methyl group, since the pK_a is close to that of 4(5)-methylimidazole. At pH 7.4 the cation is one of the main species for burimamide (40 mol%) and the 1,4-tautomer

Table 5
Comparison of Methylene (—CH$_2$—), Thioether (—S—), and Ether (—O—) Linkages

RCH$_2$—X—CH$_2$R

	Units	X = CH$_2$	X = S	X = O	Reference
C—X bond length	Å	1.54	1.81	1.43	42
CXC bond angle, R = H	°	109	105	111	42
C···C interatomic distances between centers	Å	2.51	2.87	2.37	a
Van der Waals radius of X	Å	2.0	1.85	1.40	42
Group contribution of X to van der Waals volume	cm^3/mol	10.2	10.8	3.7	43
Molar volume increment of X	cm^3/mol	16.6	10.8	6.7	44
Log P (octanol – H$_2$O), R = CH$_3$		3.39[b]	1.95	0.77	45 – 47
Hydrophobic fragmental constant, f of group X		+ 0.53	– 0.51	– 1.54	48
		+ 0.54	– 0.79	– 1.81	45
Basicity (pK_a), R = CH$_3$			– 6.8	– 2.4	49

[a] By inspection of molecular geometry.
[b] Previously reported value, 2.50.[50]

is the least favored. For histamine the ammonium-ethyl side chain (R = $CH_2CH_2\overset{+}{N}H_2$) lowers the p$K_a$ of the imidazole ring, that is, it withdraws electrons and favors the 1,4-tautomer; there is only a small proportion of cation present at pH 7.4 (about 3%), and the main species is the 1,4-tautomer to the extent that nearly 80% of histamine molecules are in this form.[40]

Thus, although both histamine and burimamide are monosubstituted imidazoles, the structural similarity is misleading in that the properties of the respective imidazole rings are chemically different. If the active form of the antagonist were the 1,4-species, the form most preferred for histamine, then increasing its relative population might increase activity. To effect this increase it was necessary to incorporate an electronegative atom in the antagonist side chain to convert it into an electron-withdrawing group, while attempting to minimize disturbance to other biologically important molecular properties such as stereochemistry and lipid-water partition. In this sense, the methylene group (-CH$_2$-) is isosteric with a thioether linkage (-S-) as the data in Table 5 show. The groups have similar van der Waals radii and give rise to similar bond angles, although the C-S bond is somewhat longer than a C-C bond.

Making the substitution of S for CH$_2$ in burimamide at the carbon atom next but one to the ring gave the compound "thiaburimamide" (R = -CH$_2$SCH$_2$CH$_2$NHCSNHCH$_3$), reduced ring pK_a (to 6.25), thereby altering the tautomerism, and increased activity.[38] To obtain a further increase in this tautomer, it seemed that an electron-releasing substituent might be required in the vacant 4(5)-position of the ring, since electron-releasing groups favor the form with the hydrogen atom on the adjacent nitrogen. There are very few possibilities, and a methyl group was selected because it seemed likely that it would not interfere with receptor interaction since 4-methylhistamine was known to be an effective H$_2$-receptor stimulant. Incorporating methyl into the ring of thiaburimamide indeed gave a more active compound, namely, the drug metiamide, N-methyl-N'-[2-(5-methylimidazol-4-yl)methylthioethyl] thiourea.[38,51] The two ring substituents are seen to have electronic effects of equal magnitude but of opposite direction. They should combine to favor the 1,4-tautomer but should have opposing effects on ring pK_a; indeed, they must exactly cancel since the pK_a's of metiamide and imidazole are identical (Table 4). This means that at pH 7.4 the main species of metiamide would be the 1,4-tautomer, as for histamine, although there would still be a substantial proportion of cation present (20%). For metiamide, in comparison with burimamide, the ratio of tautomers is reversed and the population of cation is decreased.

The pharmacological consequences of these manipulations are shown in Table 6. The effectiveness of each compound as an H$_2$-receptor histamine antagonist was compared by estimating the dissociation constant K_B (with 95% confidence limits) for the drug-receptor complex. The reliability of these

Table 6

H$_2$-Receptor Antagonist Activities^a of Burimamide and Analogues, Determined *in vitro* on Guinea-Pig Atrium and Rat Uterus^{b38}

Compound^c	Atrium (x 10^{-6} *M*)	Uterus (x 10^{-6} *M*)
Metiamide	0.92 (0.74 − 1.15)	0.75 (0.40 − 1.36)
Thiaburimamide	3.2 (2.5 − 4.5)	3.2 (2.5 − 4.5)
Burimamide	7.8 (6.4 − 9.6)	6.6 (4.9 − 8.3)
Methylburimamide	8.9 (5.6 − 15)	10.7 (4.5 − 31)
Oxaburimamide^d	28 (13 − 69)	

^{a}The dissociation constant (K_B) was calculated as indicated in Table 1, footnote *a*.

^{b}Values represent the K_B (95% limits).

^{c}Structures in Table 4.

^{d}Oxaburimamide is N-{2[(imidazol-4-yl)methoxy]ethyl}-N'-methylthiourea; R$_1$ = H, R$_2$ = CH$_2$OCH$_2$CH$_2$NHCSNHCH$_3$ tested by R. C. Blakemore.[52]

estimates was tested by making separate measurements on two tissues, heart muscle and uterine muscle, that came from different animal species and that responded to histamine in different ways; heart muscle is stimulated and uterine muscle is inhibited. The results obtained on the two tissues are in good agreement and, taken together, show that metiamide *in vitro* is three to four times as active as thiaburimamide and eight to nine times as active as burimamide. By contrast, analogous methyl substitution of burimamide to give "methylburimamide" does not increase activity. In this compound, the two ring substituents have nearly equal electronic effects in the same direction; the methyl group counterbalances the electronic influence of the side chain on tautomerism, but it raises the pK_a to 7.80 so that at pH 7.4 over 70% of the molecules are present as the imidazolium cation (Table 4).

These results illustrate one of the problems of attempting to manipulate the biological properties of drug molecules through altering chemical structure. The changes in chemical properties accompanying structural modifications often impose their own inherent limitations. Methyl was introduced to alter tautomerism, but it also raises the pK_a and increases the cation population; these are opposing influences and an optimum balance must be determined empirically.

Another example of the sensitivity of the system to changes in drug structure is illustrated by the use of an -O- ether linkage in place of -CH_2- or -S-. Although the oxygen linkage is electronically similar to that of sulfur (with respect to pK_a, see Table 4), oxaburimamide is less active than burimamide. The O has a geometry similar to that of CH_2, but is substantially smaller in size and is a powerful H-bond acceptor. Thus, in this series, CH_2 and S are bioisosteres, whereas O is only a partial bioisostere. The ether oxygen atom is also more basic and hydrophilic than sulfur or methylene (Table 5). These differences may explain why oxygen is less successful than sulfur as an isosteric replacement for CH_2 in the H_2-receptor antagonist series. The question has been considered in greater detail elsewhere,[53] particularly with regard to conformation and possible intramolecular hydrogen-bonding interactions. Table 5 compares CH_2, S, and O linkages in terms of stereochemistry and octanol-water partition coefficients (log P). Figure 9 compares CPK space filling molecular models of burimamide and metiamide and shows the isosterism between CH_2 and S linkages.

Although special consideration was given to studies of the chemistry of the imidazole ring, not all antagonists had to possess an imidazole structure, and other ring systems were found to be effective alternatives, for example, thiazole and pyridine.[54] The corollary still stands, however, namely, for compounds that incorporate a tautomeric imidazole ring, the state of the ring and its particular chemical properties may influence activity. Subsequent to these developments, other researchers have found replacements for imidazole that appear to provide antagonists of even greater potency.[55,56]

Metiamide represented a major improvement. Not only was it 10 times as active *in vitro,* but, more importantly, it was sufficiently active in man to be useful orally.[38,57] Metiamide was shown to be a potent inhibitor of stimulated acid secretion in man[58] and was investigated for its potential use in peptic ulcer therapy. It produced a significant increase in the healing rate of duodenal ulcers and marked symptomatic relief.[59] However, of 700 patients treated, there were a few cases of granulocytopenia which, although reversible, imposed a limitation to clinical work.[60,61]

2.4 Isosteres of Thiourea, Guanidine Equilibria, and the Development of Cimetidine

The possibility existed that the granulocytopenia associated with metiamide was caused by the thiourea group in the molecule and this led to the need to examine another compound. Fortunately, exploration of other possible structures had continued and had been directed in particular toward alternatives to the thiourea group, the latter having been considered a potential disadvantage since some thioureas are known to have antithyroid activity. One approach taken was to examine isosteric replacement of the thiourea sulfur atom (=S) of

Table 7

Structures and H$_2$-Receptor Antagonist Activities[a,b,c] of Metiamide, Cimetidine, and Isosteres[63,64]

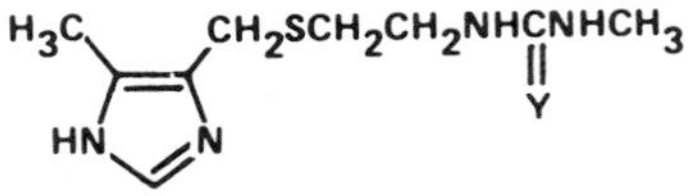

$$H_3C \diagdown \text{imidazole ring} \diagup CH_2SCH_2CH_2NHCNHCH_3 \quad (Y)$$

| Compound | Y | H$_2$-antagonist activity | | in vivo[c] |
		Atrium[a] K_B (95% limits) (x 10^{-6} M)	Uterus[b] K_B (95% limits) (x 10^{-6} M)	ID$_{50}$ (μmol/kg)
Metiamide (thiourea)	S	0.92 (0.74 – 1.15)	0.75 (0.40 – 1.38)	1.6
Urea isostere	O	22 (8.9 – 65)	7.1 (1.6 – 30)	27
Guanidine isostere	NH	16 (8.1 – 32)	5.5 (2.8 – 13)	12
Guanylurea derivative	N·CONH$_2$	7.1 (4.0 – 14)	6.9 (4.1 – 12)	7.7
Nitroguanidine isostere	N·NO$_2$	1.4 (0.79 – 2.8)	1.4 (0.72 – 3.2)	2.1
Cimetidine (cyanoguanidine)	N·CN	0.79 (0.68 – 0.92)	0.81 (0.54 – 1.2)	1.4

[a]Activities determined against histamine stimulation of guinea-pig right atrium in vitro. The dissociation constant (K_B) was calculated as indicated in Table 1, footnote a.

[b]Activities determined against histamine inhibition of electrically evoked contractions of rat uterus in vitro.

[c]Activities as antagonists of histamine-stimulated gastric acid secretion in the anesthetized rat as indicated in Table 1, footnote b.

24

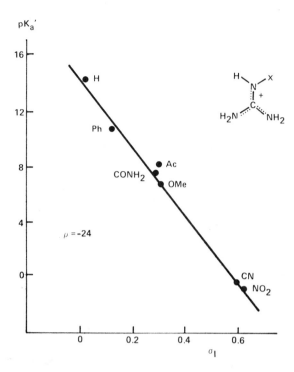

Figure 7. Apparent pK_a values at 25 °C of N-substituted guanidinium cations versus σ_I substituent constants. Data from Charton.[62] The line corresponds to the equation $pK_a' = 14.20-24.1\sigma_I$. Reproduced with permission from Durant et al.[63]

metiamide. Replacement of carbonyl oxygen ($=O$) gave the urea analogue, which was much less active (Table 7). Returning to the idea of guanidine derivatives, which had provided the original breakthrough, led to replacement by imino nitrogen ($=NH$) and afforded the guanidine isostere shown in Table 7; interestingly, this guanidine was not a partial agonist but a fairly active antagonist. However, the K_B values determined *in vitro* on the atrium indicate that the urea and guanidine isosteres were both about 20 times less potent than metiamide, and other ways of removing the positive charge were investigated.

The guanidine is charged because it acquires a proton and, being very basic, exists almost exclusively in the protonated form at physiological pH. Fortunately, basicity can be markedly reduced by electron-withdrawing substituents. Figure 7 shows the relationship[62] between the pK_a of monosubstituted

Table 8
Comparison of Thiourea, Urea, Cyanoguanidine, and Nitroguanidine

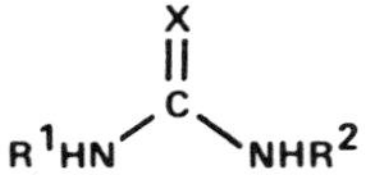

$$R^1HN-\overset{\underset{\|}{X}}{C}-NHR^2$$

		$Y = S$	$Y = O$	$Y = NCN$	$Y = NNO_2$
$R^1 = R^2 = H$					
Geometry:	C–N bond length (Å)	1.34^a	$1.35,^b 1.34^c$	$1.34,^d 1.32^e$	1.34^f
	N–C–N bond angle (°)	119^a	$117,^b 118^c$	$124,^d 120^e$	118^f
Basicity (pK_a):	proton gained at 25°C	-1.2^g	-0.15^h	-0.4^i	-0.9^j
Acidity:	proton lost at 25°C	15^k	13.7^l	14^m	12.2^n
Hydrophilicity:	$P = \dfrac{C_{oct}}{C_{H_2O}}$ at 37°C	0.09^p	0.02^p	0.07^p	0.13^p
	Dipole moment, μ, dioxane (D)	4.89^q(25°C)	4.56^q(25°C)	8.16^r(35°C)	6.95^s(30°C)
$R^1 = R^2 = CH_3$					
Partition, P (octanol-H_2O) 37°C		0.58^p	$\sim 0.11^p$	0.40^p	0.20^p
$\Delta G^\ddagger$ for interconversion between conformers (kcal/mol)		11.8^t	$\sim 7.5^t$	12.4^u	—
$R^1 = CH_3$ $\quad CH_2SCH_2CH_2$ $\quad R^2 = CH_3$ HN—N					
Partit	Partition, P (octanol-H_2O) 37°C	3.2^p	0.87^p	2.5^p	1.5^p

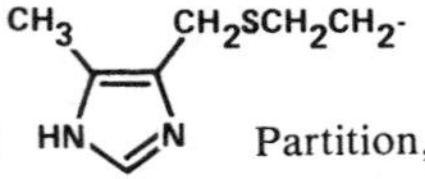

References: [a]67 [b]68 [c]69 [d]70 [e]71 [f]72 [g]73 [h]74 [i]75 [j]76 [k]77 [l]78 [m]79 [n]80 [p]81 [q]82 [r]83 [s]84 [t]85 [u]86.

26

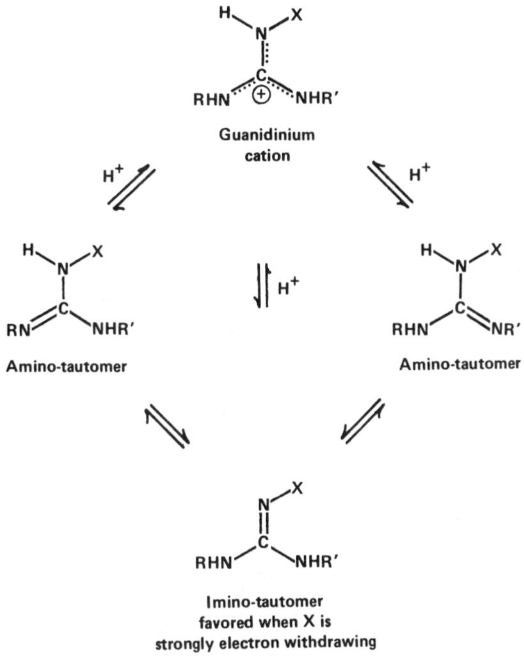

Figure 8. Equilibria between guanidinium cation and the three conjugate bases.

guanidines and the electronic influence of the substituent, represented by the inductive substituent constant σ_I. The ϱ value of -24 indicates the extreme sensitivity of pK_a to substituent effects in guanidines. The cyano and nitro groups are sufficiently electron withdrawing to reduce pK_a by over 14 units, to values <0; indeed, the ionization constants of cyanoguanidine (pK_a -0.4) and nitroguanidine (pK_a-0.9) approach that of thiourea (-1.2). The nitroguanidine and cyanoguanidine analogues of metiamide were synthesized and were found to be active antagonists (Table 7), comparable with metiamide.[63] Of these two compounds, the cyanoguanidine (cimetidine) was slightly more potent and was selected for development. [64,65]

As shown in Figure 8, the guanidinium cation may lose a proton from each of the three nitrogen atoms to give three different forms of the conjugate base. Powerful electron-withdrawing substituents X favor the imino tautomer over the amino tautomers since the proton on the adjacent nitrogen in the cation is more acidic than the protons on the more distant terminal nitrogen atoms. Thus cyanoguanidines exist predominantly in the cyanoimino form, and in cimetidine the cyanoimino group (=NCN) replaces the thione (=S) sulfur atom of metiamide. In cyanoguanidines and thioureas the cyanoimino and thione functionalities have a similar effect in reducing the electron density on the amino groups in the 1,1-diaminomethylene [$(H_2N)_2C =$] system. Cyanoguanidine and thiourea have many chemical properties in common (Table 8): they are planar structures of similar geometries (Figure 9), they are weakly amphoteric (very weakly basic and acidic) so that in the pH range 2-12 they are unionized, and they are very polar and hydrophilic.

The similar behavior of cimetidine and metiamide as histamine H_2-receptor antagonists and the close similarity in physicochemical characteristics of thiourea and cyanoguanidine permit the description of the thiourea and cyanoguanidine groups in the present context as bioisosteres.[64] The equi-effectiveness of cyanoguanidine and thiourea groups in H_2-receptor antagonists was also illustrated for a series of imidazole derivatives in which the thioureas and corresponding cyanoguanidine antagonists were compared.[64]

The similarity in many physico-chemical properties of cyanoguanidine and thiourea has been discussed.[63-65] Table 8 indicates some properties of cyanoguanidine, thiourea, nitroguanidine, and urea. All these molecules are planar π electron systems with similar geometries, for example, equal C-N bond distances and bond angles. They are also weakly amphoteric, that is, both weakly acidic and weakly basic with similar pK_a's. These molecules are all polar and hydrophilic with high dipole moments (μ) and low octanol/water partition coefficients (P). However, the partition coefficient of urea is even lower than that of thiourea, cyanoguanidine, or nitroguanidine. Nitro-guanidine may also be considered to be a bioisostere of thiourea, whereas urea must be regarded as being only a "partial bioisostere" of thiourea in H_2-receptor antagonists. Differences in polarizability and in partition of thiourea and urea groups may contribute to the quantitative differences in antagonist potency between metiamide and its urea analogue. Another important factor may be the difference in conformational behavior between these groups. Four conformations of the thiourea group in metiamide are theoretically possible (Figure 10, X = S), but only three have been observed by low temperature nuclear magnetic resonance spectroscopy in solution (CD$_3$OD), namely, the Z,Z and staggered E,Z and Z,E forms.[87,88] The E,E form is not observed, presumably being disfavored by steric interactions between the groups R and R '. Corresponding cyanoguanidines such as cimetidine exhibit only the two staggered conformations, namely, E,Z and Z,E (Figure 10, X = NCN),[87,88] the Z,Z form probably being sterically disfavored by inter-actions between the cyano group and the R and R ' substituents; the E,E form would be unfavorable for the reasons indicated for the analogous thiourea. For the urea, nuclear magnetic resonance studies[87] indicate that it exists predominantly as the Z,Z conformation (Figure 10, X = 0),[87] and it may be

Burimamide

Metiamide

Cimetidine

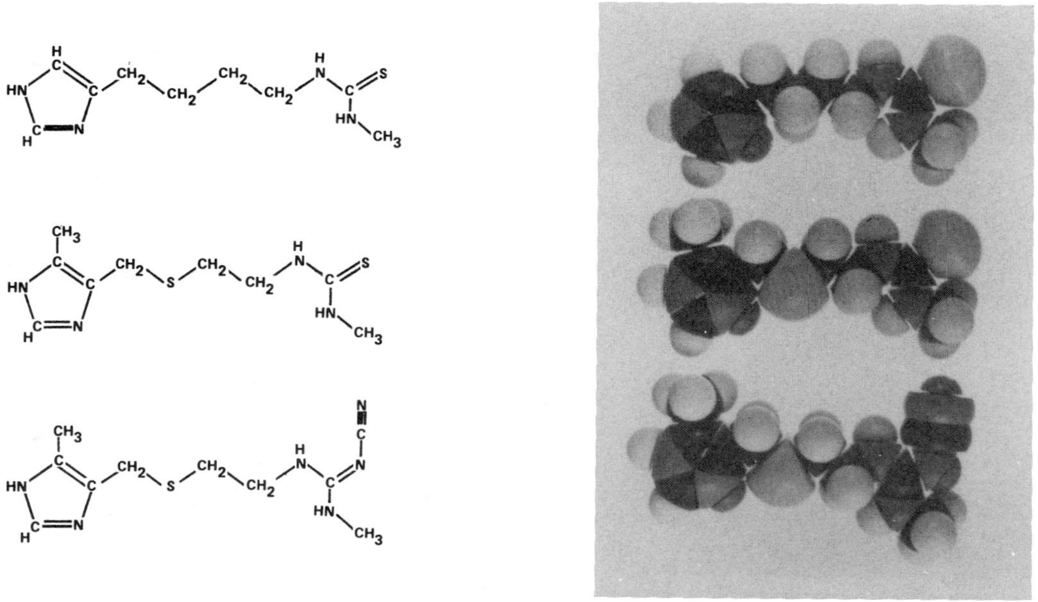

Figure 9. CPK space-filling molecular models of burimamide (top), metiamide (middle), and cimetidine (bottom), illustrating the isosterism between the S and CH_2 side-chain linkages, and thiourea and cyanoguanidine groups. For simplicity, the models are shown in a planar, all-*trans* (extended) conformation. Reproduced with permission from Ganellin.[66]

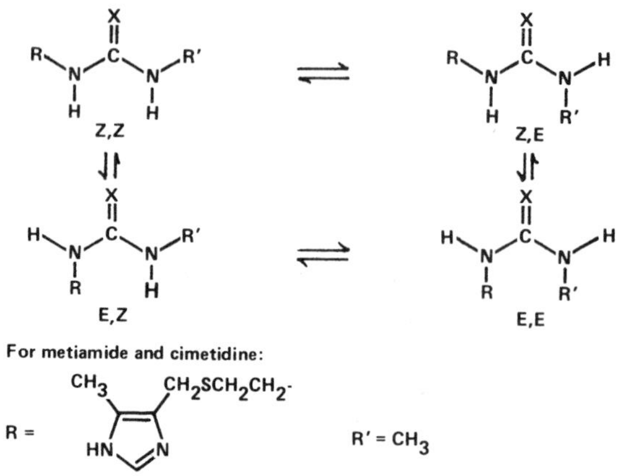

Figure 10. Possible planar conformations of N,N'-disubstituted thioureas (X = S), cyanoguanidines (X = NCN), and ureas (X = O), in equilibrium in solution.

that the two conformations (Z,E and E,Z) analogous to the cyanoguanidine are more active pharmacologically, but are energetically unfavorable for the urea.[53]

A laboratory synthesis of cimetidine is outlined in Figure 11. 4-Carboethoxy-5-methylimidazole, made from ethyl α-chloroacetoacetate by condensation with formamide in the Bredereck procedure, is reduced by lithium aluminum hydride to give 4-hydroxymethyl-5-methylimidazole.[30] This carbinol is then condensed with cysteamine in the presence of HCl or HBr and the resulting amine salt is collected and neutralized with aqueous potassium carbonate. The liberated amine is treated with dimethylcyanodithioimidocarbonate and then with methylamine.[64] Many variations of this synthesis have been developed. Cimetidine forms colorless crystals from water or methyl cyanide, m.p 141-142 °C.

The specificity of cimetidine as a histamine H_2-receptor antagonist is indicated by the results obtained *in vitro* (Table 9).[65] Cimetidine acts as a competitive antagonist of histamine on the guinea pig atrium and rat uterus; the apparent dissociation constants (K_B) were not significantly different, and the slope of the regression of log (DR - 1) on log (B) on each tissue was not significantly different from unity. At high concentrations cimetidine antagonized the action of isoprenaline on the atrium and uterus, and the actions of histamine and carbachol on the isolated guinea pig ileum, but the antagonism

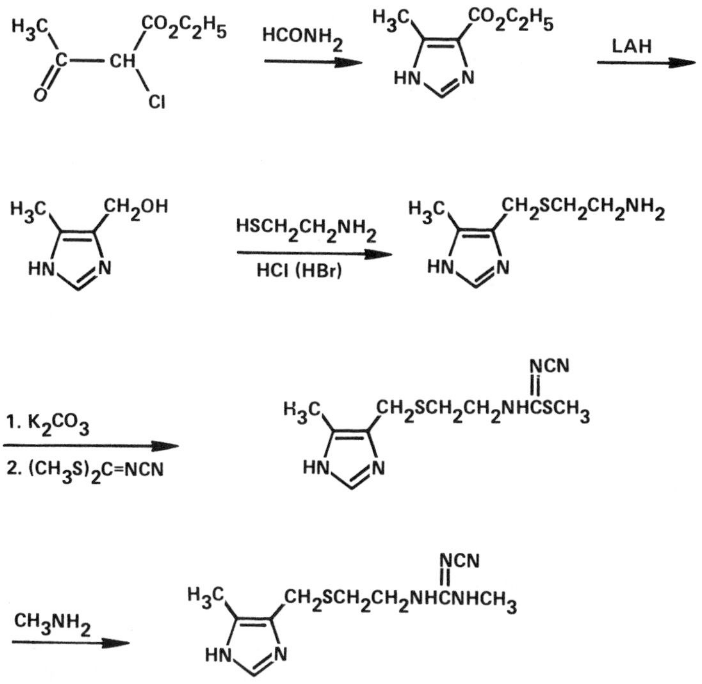

Figure 11.   Laboratory synthesis of cimetidine.

Table 9

The Antagonist Activity of Cimetidine on Isolated Tissues [65]

Tissue	Agonist	Cimetidine $(K_B \times 10^{-7}\ M)^a$	Slope of log (DR - 1) on log (B)^a
Atrium	Histamine	7.9 (6.8 – 9.2)	0.81 (0.62 – 1.00)
	Isoprenaline	1330 (410 – 6200)	1.44 (1.17 – 1.71)
Uterus	Histamine	8.1 (5.4 – 12.1)	0.96 (0.82 – 1.10)
	Isoprenaline	2620 (121 – 31,110)	0.61 (0.39 – 0.82)
Ileum	Histamine	4460 (2020 – 10,700)	1.47 (1.34 – 1.60)
	Carbachol	360 (208 – 658)	0.79 (0.72 – 0.86)

^{a}With 95% confidence limits.

Table 10

Inhibition of Gastric Acid Secretion *in vivo* **by Cimetidine**[65,89]

Animal	Preparation	Stimulant	Intravenous (ID$_{50}$ μmol/kg)
Rat[a]	Lumen-perfused stomach	Histamine	1.37
		Pentagastrin	1.40
Cat[a]	Lumen-perfused stomach	Histamine	0.85
		Pentagastrin	1.45
Dog[b]	Heidenhain pouch	Histamine	1.70
		Pentagastrin	2.00

[a]Anesthetized.

[b]Conscious.

was apparently noncompetitive. *In vivo,* cimetidine is effective at inhibiting histamine-stimulated gastric acid secretion in the rat, cat, and dog[65,89] (Table 10). Figure 12 shows the inhibition by a single intravenous injection of cimetidine on the near-maximal acid secretory response to an intravenous infusion of histamine, using the lumen-perfused stomach of the anesthetized rat.[89] The ID$_{50}$ values determined in the rat, cat, and dog were not significantly different from each other. Cimetidine was also shown to be active when administered orally, and a dose of 20 μmol/kg (approximately 5 mg/kg) produced a mean inhibition of 90% of maximal histamine-stimulated secretion in the dog.[65,89]

Cimetidine is also an effective inhibitor of pentagastrin-stimulated secretion. The ID$_{50}$ values shown in Table 10 indicate that the potency of cimetidine against pentagastrin-stimulated secretion is very similar to its potency against histamine-stimulated secretion. Cimetidine is less active against cholinergically stimulated secretion. Although the ability of cimetidine to inhibit gastric acid secretion evoked by a variety of stimulants could be interpreted as showing that it is a nonspecific antisecretory agent, the evidence from the *in vitro* studies on nongastric tissues, which clearly establish it as a specific competitive H$_2$-receptor histamine antagonist, argues against such a hypothesis.[89] The finding that H$_2$-receptor antagonists such as cimetidine inhibit pentagastrin-stimulated secretion clearly indicates that gastrin and histamine are somehow linked in the gastric secretory process. The results with these antagonists firmly establish that histamine has a physiological role in gastric acid secretion.

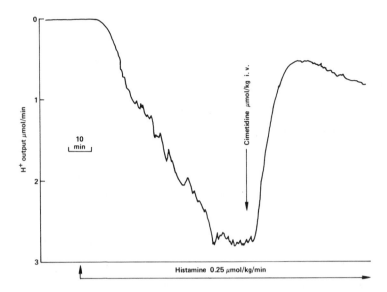

Figure 12. The inhibitory effect of a single intravenous injection of cimetidine on the near-maximal acid secretory response to an intravenous infusion of histamine, using the lumen-perfused stomach of the anesthetized rat. Reproduced with permission from Parsons.[89]

Cimetidine has been shown to be a specific competitive histamine H_2-receptor antagonist and an effective orally active inhibitor of stimulated gastric acid secretion in animals and in man, and to be as active as metiamide. Cimetidine has been extensively studied in man and its safety and efficacy have been established in the acute treatment of peptic ulcer. Cimetidine given orally as 1-1.2 g/day has been shown to relieve symptoms and promote healing of lesions in a majority of patients with peptic ulcer disease. Much of the seminal work with the new drug is published in the proceedings of an international symposium held in London in October 1976.[90] Cimetidine was marketed first in the United Kingdom in November 1976* and in the United States in August 1977, and by 1979 was sold in over 100 countries under the trademark Tagamet.

*This represents just over 4 years from the initial laboratory synthesis of cimetidine (in 1972). The progress was greatly assisted by the initial studies carried out with metiamide and is a testimony to the considerable ethusiasm and effort of all those involved in the development work and especially to the direction of Dr. W. A. M. Duncan.

3. POSTSCRIPTUM

It is self evident that any account of drug discovery must be incomplete and certainly only a small proportion of the total studies made have been described in this chapter. The large number of researchers involved in this project and the time span of 12 years from the start of the research work to the initial clinical studies ensures that it is impossible to be comprehensive. It would take an entire book to describe all the ideas investigated during the exploration of structural features in the attempts to improve upon activity throughout the course of this research. Many avenues examined turned out to be ineffective and since, in the main, these are not mentioned here, the net effect may be to make the work appear to be more rational and more perceptive than is warranted. Other studies sowed the seeds for further developments and led to the discovery of other

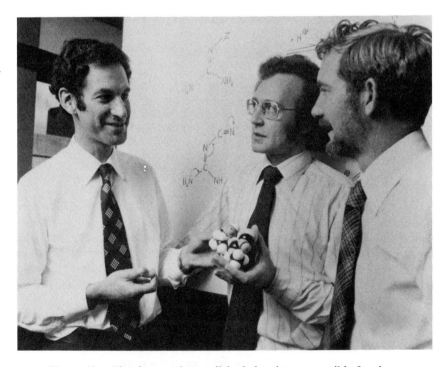

Figure 13.   The three senior medicinal chemists responsible for the design of the H_2-receptor histamine antagonists at the Research Institute, Smith Kline and French Research Limited, Welwyn Garden City, England. Left to right: Dr. C. Robin Ganellin, Dr. John C. Emmett, and Dr. Graham J. Durant, discussing the chemistry of cimetidine.

novel active structures as antagonists, for example, 1,1-diamino-2-nitro-ethylenes[91] and 2-aminopyrimid-4-ones (isocytosines).[92] The work also led to the characterization of selective agonists as pharmacological tools for exploring the pharmacology of histamine receptors, notably 2- and 4-methylhistamines,[31] 2-pyridylethylamine and 2-thiazolylethylamine,[93] and dimaprit,[94] and impromidine.[95]

This account has also concentrated on medicinal chemistry; it has touched on pharmacology and ignored the contributions from biochemistry and the numerous laboratory studies needed to develop cimetidine as a useful drug, namely, chemical production, chemical analysis, pharmaceutical formulation, long term safety assessment in animals, and human pharmacology. One area of glaring omission is that of chemical synthesis. For medicinal chemists most of their intellectual activity and working time is directed toward synthesis of the compounds to be tested. Deciding what to make is usually only a small part of the work. The medicinal chemist has to reconcile what structure he or she would ideally like to synthesize for testing with what is stable chemically and what is attainable by chemical synthesis. This means that one has to compromise and settle for what is feasible. Like politics, it is the art of the possible. Such debate is continuous and most certainly was a key factor in the discovery of cimetidine, as it must be in drug discovery in general. However, since the work outlined here did involve a very large medicinal chemical content the author has mainly addressed this aspect of the research. There is no shortage of published examples of the problems of chemical synthesis, whereas authors seem generally more reluctant to reveal medicinal chemical reasoning. The author sincerely hopes that readers will be tolerant of the lack of balance in this chapter. For an account identifying many of the ticklish decisions that had to be made during the development of cimetidine the reader should consult reference 96.

ACKNOWLEDGMENT

The work described here was a collaborative effort among Dr. J. W. Black, F. R. S. (now Sir James Black), Dr. G. J. Durant, Dr. J. C. Emmett, Dr. C. R. Ganellin, Dr. M. E. Parsons, and Dr. G. R. White. Major contributions were also made by R. C. Blakemore and A. C. Rasmussen (pharmacology), M. J. Graham, Dr. R. C. Mitchell and Dr. E. S. Pepper (physicochemical studies), and Dr. R. C. Young (correlation studies). Some 700 compounds were synthesized on the road to the discovery of cimetidine. Most of the compounds were novel; new syntheses had to be developed and methods established. More than 50 chemists contributed to the work of actually making the compounds over the years. The success of the project attests to their skill. Substantial technical contributions were made by Dr. M. E. Footit, A. J. Hayter, D. W. Hills, D. R. Hollyman, R. J. King, J. M. Loynes, P. D. Miles, H. D. Prain, W. Tertiuk, and C. S. Whyatt.

REFERENCES

1. H. H. Dale and P. P. Laidlaw, *J. Physiol. Lond.,* **41,** 318 (1910).
2. D. Bovet and A. M. Staub, *C.R. Soc. Biol. (Paris),* **124,** 547 (1937).
3. E. R. Loew, *Physiol. Rev.,* **27,** 542 (1947).
4. J. A. Wells, H. C. Morris, H. B. Bull, and C. A. Dragstedt, *J. Pharmacol. Exp. Ther.,* **85,** 122 (1945).
5. B. N. Halpern and G. Mauric, *C.R. Soc. Biol.,* **140,** 440 (1946).
6. H. O. Schild, *Br. J. Pharmacol.,* **2,** 189 (1947).
7. B. Folkow, K. Haeger, and G. Kahlson, *Acta Physiol. Scand.,* **15,** 264 (1948).
8. D. F. Hawkins and H. O. Schild, *Br. J. Pharmacol.,* **6,** 682 (1951).
9. O. Arunlakshana and H. O. Schild, *Br. J. Pharmacol.,* **14,** 48 (1959).
10. C. Robertson and M. I. Grossman, *Arch. Int. Pharmacodyn.,* **90,** 223 (1952).
11. U. Trendelenburg, *J. Pharm. Exp. Ther.,* **130,** 450 (1960).
12. P. B. Dews and J. D. P. Graham, *Br. J. Pharmacol. Chemother.,* **1,** 278 (1946).
13. M. I. Grossman, C. Robertson, and C. E. Rosiere, *J. Pharmacol. Exp. Ther.,* **104,** 277 (1952).
14. R. G. Jones, "Chemistry of Histamine and Analogs. Relationship between Structure and Pharmacological Activity," in *Handbook of Experimental Pharmacology XVIII/I. Histamine and Anti-Histaminics,* M. Rocha e Silva, Ed., Springer-Verlag, Berlin, 1966, p. 1.
15. A. S. F. Ash and H. O. Schild, *Br. J. Pharmacol. Chemother.,* **27,** 427 (1966).
16. C. Robertson and M. I. Grossman, *Arch. Int. Pharmacodyn.,* **91,** 1 (1952).
17. T. M. Lin, R. S. Alphin, F. G. Henderson, D. N. Benslay, and K. K. Chen, *Ann. N.Y. Acad. Sci.,* **99,** 30 (1962).
18. F. G. van den Brink, *"Histamine and Antihistamines; Molecular Pharmacology, Structure-Activity Relations, Gastric Acid Secretion,"* Drukkerij Gebr. Janssen N.V., Nijmegen, 1969, p. 179.
19. M. E. Parsons, "Quantitative Studies of Drug-Induced Acid Gastric Secretion," Ph.D. Thesis, University of London, 1969.
20. M. N. Ghosh and H. O. Schild, *Br. J. Pharmacol. Chemother.,* **13,** 54 (1958).
21. R. A. Gregory and H. J. Tracy, *Gut,* **5,** 103 (1964).
22. H. Gregory, P. M. Hardy, D. S. Jones, G. W. Kenner, and R. C. Sheppard, *Nature (Lond.),* **204,** 931 (1964).
23. M. I. Grossman, *Gastroenterology,* **52,** 882 (1967).
24. L. R. Johnson, *Gastroenterology,* **61,** 106 (1971).
25. C. F. Code, *Fed. Proc.,* **24,** 1311 (1965).
26. C. R. Ganellin, G. J. Durant, and J. C. Emmett, *Fed. Proc.,* **35,** 1924 (1976).
27. G. J. Durant, J. M. Loynes, and S. H. B. Wright, *J. Med. Chem.,* **16,** 1272 (1973).
28. E. J. Ariens and A. M. Simonis, *Arch. Int. Pharmacodyn.,* **127,** 479 (1960).
29. B. R. Baker, *J. Chem. Educ.,* **44,** 610 (1967).
30. G. J. Durant, J. C. Emmett, C. R. Ganellin, A. M. Roe, and R. A. Slater, *J. Med. Chem.,* **19,** 923 (1976).
31. J. W. Black, W. A. M. Duncan, G. J. Durant, C. R. Ganellin, and M. E. Parsons, *Nature (Lond.),* **236,** 385 (1972).
32. G. J. Durant, M. E. Parsons, and J. W. Black, *J. Med. Chem.,* **18,** 830 (1975).
33. P. van der Merwe, *Hoppe-Seyler's Z. Physiol. Chem.,* **177,** 301 (1928).
34. M. E. Parsons, R. C. Blakemore, G. J. Durant, C. R. Ganellin, and A. C. Rasmussen, *Agents Actions,* **5,** 464 (1975).
35. C. R. Ganellin, *J. Appl. Chem. Biotechnol.,* **28,** 183 (1978).

36. J. W. Black, G. J. Durant, J. C. Emmett, and C. R. Ganellin, British Patents 1,296,544 (1972); 1,305,546 (1973); 1,305,547 (1973); 1,305,549 (1973).
37. J. H. Wyllie, T. Hesselbo, and J. W. Black, *Lancet, 2,* 1117 (1972).
38. J. W. Black, G. J. Durant, J. C. Emmett, and C. R. Ganellin, *Nature (Lond.), 248,* 65 (1974).
39. M. Charton, *J. Org. Chem., 30,* 3346 (1965).
40. C. R. Ganellin, *J. Pharm. Pharmacol., 25,* 787 (1973).
41. Personal communication from M. J. Graham, The Research Institute, Smith Kline and French Research Limited, Welwyn Garden City, Hertfordshire, England.
42. L. Pauling, *The Nature of the Chemical Bond,* Cornell University, New York, 1960.
43. A. Bondi, *J. Phys. Chem., 68,* 441 (1964).
44. O. Exner, *Collect. Czech. Chem. Commun., 32,* 1 (1967).
45. A. Leo, P. Y. C. Jow, C. Silipo, and C. Hansch, *J. Med. Chem., 18,* 865 (1975).
46. C. Hansch and S. M. Anderson, *J. Org. Chem., 32,* 2583 (1967).
47. S. Anderson and C. Hansch, result quoted in A. Leo, C. Hansch, and D. Elkins, *Chem. Rev., 71,* 525 (1971).
48. G. G. Nys and R. F. Rekker, *Eur. J. Med. Chem., 9,* 361 (1974).
49. E. M. Arnett and G. Scorrano, in *Advances in Physical Organic Chemistry, Vol. 13,* V. Gold, Ed., Academic Press, London, 1976, p. 130.
50. C. Hansch, J. E. Quinlan, and G. L. Lawrence, *J. Org. Chem., 33,* 347 (1968).
51. G. J. Durant, J. C. Emmett and C. R. Ganellin, in *International Symposium on Histamine H_2-Receptor Antagonists,* C. J. Wood and M. A. Simkins, Eds., Smith Kline and French Laboratories Ltd., Welwyn Garden City, England, 1973, p. 13.
52. Personal communication from Dr. M. E. Parsons, The Research Institute, Smith Kline and French Research Limited, Welwyn Garden City, Hertfordshire, England.
53. G. J. Durant in *Proceedings of the 6th International Symposium on Medicinal Chemistry, Brighton, U.K., 1978,* A. Simkin, Ed., Cotswold, Oxford, 1979, p. 189.
54. G. J. Durant, J. C. Emmett, and C. R. Ganellin, (a) British Patent 1,338,169 (1973), (b) British Patent 1,397,436 (1975).
55. J. Bradshaw, R. T. Brittain, J. W. Clitherow, M. J. Daly, D. Jack, B. J. Price, and R. Stables, *Br. J. Pharmacol., 66,* P 464 (1979).
56. T. O. Yellin, S. H. Buck, D. J. Gilman, D. F. Jones, and J. M. Wardleworth, *Life Sci., 25,* 2001 (1979).
57. J. W. Black, W. A. M. Duncan, J. C. Emmett, C. R. Ganellin, T. Hesselbo, M. E. Parsons, and J. H. Wyllie, *Agents Actions, 3,* 133 (1973).
58. S. J. Haggie, C. G. Clark, J. W. Black, and J. H. Wyllie, *Fed. Proc., 35,* 1948 (1976).
59. R. E. Pounder, J. G. Williams, G. J. Milton-Thompson, and J. J. Misiewicz, *Br. Med. J.,* 307 (1975).
60. L. R. Celestin et al., *Lancet, 2,* 779 (1975).
61. J. A. H. Forrest, D. J. C. Shearman, R. Spence, and L. R. Celestin, *Lancet, 1,* 392 (1975).
62. M. Charton, *J. Org. Chem., 30,* 969 (1965).
63. G. J. Durant, J. C. Emmett, and C. R. Ganellin, see reference 90, p. 1.
64. G. J. Durant, J. C. Emmett, C. R. Ganellin, P. D. Miles, H. D. Prain, M. E. Parsons, and G. R. White, *J. Med. Chem., 20,* 901 (1977).
65. R. W. Brimblecombe, W. A. M. Duncan, G. J. Durant, J. C. Emmett, C. R. Ganellin, and M. E. Parsons, *J. Int. Med. Res., 3,* 86 (1975).
66. C. R. Ganellin, *Farm. Tijd. Belg., 55,* 4 (1978).
67. M. Truter, *Acta Crystallogr., 22,* 556 (1967).
68. J. E. Worsham, H. A. Levy, and S. W. Peterson, *Acta Crystallogr., 10,* 319 (1957).
69. P. Vaughan and J. Donohue, *Acta Crystallogr., 5,* 530 (1952).

70. E. W. Hughes, *J. Am. Chem. Soc.,* **62**, 1258 (1940).
71. N. V. Rannev, R. P. Ozerov, I. D. Datt, and A. N. Kshnyskina, *Kristallografiya,* **11**, 175 (1966).
72. J. M. Bryden, L. A. Burkardt, E. W. Hughes, and J. Donohue, *Acta Crystallogr.,* **9**, 573 (1956).
73. M. J. Janssen, *Rec. Trav. Chim. Pays-Bas,* **81**, 650 (1962).
74. D. W. Farlow and R. B. Moodie, *J. Chem. Soc. (B),* **1971**, 407.
75. R. C. Hirt, R. G. Schmitt, H. L. Strauss and J. G. Koren, *J. Chem. Eng. Data,* **6**, 610 (1961).
76. J. G. Bonner and J. C. Lockhardt, *J. Chem. Soc.,* **1958**, 3858.
77. M. Herlem, *Bull. Soc. Chim. Fr.,* **1965**, 3329.
78. G. Charlot and B. Tremillon, in *Les Réactions Chimiques dans les Solvents et les Sels Fondus,* Gauthier-Villars, Paris 1963, p. 90.
79. N. Kameyama, *J. Chem. Ind. (Jap.),* **24**, 1263 (1921); *Chem. Abstr.,* **16**, 2247 (1922).
80. J. E. DeVries and E. St. Clair Gantz, *J. Am. Chem. Soc.,* **76**, 1008 (1954).
81. Personal communication from Dr. R. C. Mitchell, The Research Institute, Smith Kline and French Research Limited, Welwyn Garden City, Hertfordshire, England.
82. W. D. Kumler and G. M. Fohlen, *J. Am. Chem. Soc.,* **64**, 1944 (1942).
83. W. C. Schneider, *J. Am. Chem. Soc.,* **72**, 761 (1950).
84. W. D. Kumler and P. T. Sah, *J. Org. Chem.,* **18**, 669 (1953).
85. M. L. Filleux-Blanchard and A. Durand, *Org. Magn. Reson.,* **3**, 187 (1971).
86. C. G. McCarty and D. M. Wieland, *Tetrahedron Lett.,* **1969**, 1787.
87. Personal communication from Dr. E. S. Pepper, The Research Institute, Smith Kline and French Research Limited, Welwyn Garden City, Hertfordshire, England.
88. C. R. Ganellin, "Chemistry and Structure-Activity Relationships of H_2-Receptor Antagonists," in *Handbook of Experimental Pharmacology XVIII/2, Histamine and Anti-Histaminics,* M. Rcha e Silva, Ed., Springer-Verlag, Berlin, 1977, p. 251.
89. M. E. Parsons, see reference 90, p. 13.
90. W. L. Burland and M. A. Simkins, Eds., *Cimetidine — Proceedings of the 2nd International Symposium on Histamine H_2-Receptor Antagonists,* Excerpta Medica, Amsterdam-Oxford, 1977.
91. G. J. Durant, J. C. Emmett, C. R. Ganellin, and H. D. Prain, British Patent 1,421,792 (1976).
92. G. J. Durant, J. C. Emmett, and C. R. Ganellin, British Patent 1,419,994 (1976).
93. G. J. Durant, C. R. Ganellin, and M. E. Parsons, *J. Med. Chem.,* **18**, 905 (1975).
94. M. E. Parsons, D. A. A. Owen, C. R. Ganellin, and G. J. Durant, *Agents Actions,* **7**, 31 (1977).
95. G. J. Durant, W. A. M. Duncan, C. R. Ganellin, M. E. Parsons, R. C. Blakemore and A. C. Rasmussen, *Nature (Lond.),* **276**, 403 (1978).
96. W. A. M. Duncan and M. E. Parsons, *Gastroenterology,* **78**, 620 (1980).

Clozapine

2

J. Schmutz and E. Eichenberger

1. DISCOVERY

In a recent clinical comparison of clozapine and chlorpromazine, Shopsin and his associates[1] wrote: "according to existing animal screening procedures, clozapine could hardly have been classified by pharmacologists as a potential neuroleptic agent. How it came to be used as a potential antipsychotic remains a mystery." We propose to lift the veil of mystery by outlining the investigations that led to the recognition of clozapine as a novel type of antischizophrenic agent.

In 1958 our group embarked on a program of synthesis of tricyclic compounds to be tested for pharmacological properties, including potential psychotropic actions. To date this program has yielded more than 1900 compounds exhibiting a large variety of pharmacological effects. Several of these, including clozapine itself, have found clinical application.

Our chemical program was based on the dibenzo-epine system 4 (Figure 1) containing a seven-membered central ring, which had previously received little attention. The N-5-aminoalkylated dibenzo[b,e][1,4]diazepines 1 and 2, which were the early targets of this program,[2] were considered of interest because of their structural similarity to the iminodibenzyl structure of imipramine. Indeed, compounds with pharmacological properties resembling those of imipramine were found among types 1 and 2 and also among the 11-aminoalkylated derivatives of types 3 and 5,[3,4] but none appeared of sufficient interest to warrant further development. However, we did obtain the very effective antidepressant dibenzepin (8) and the antihistamine clobenzepam (9) from the 10-aminoalkyl-lactam 6 (Z = 0). Meanwhile, our study of amidines of type 7

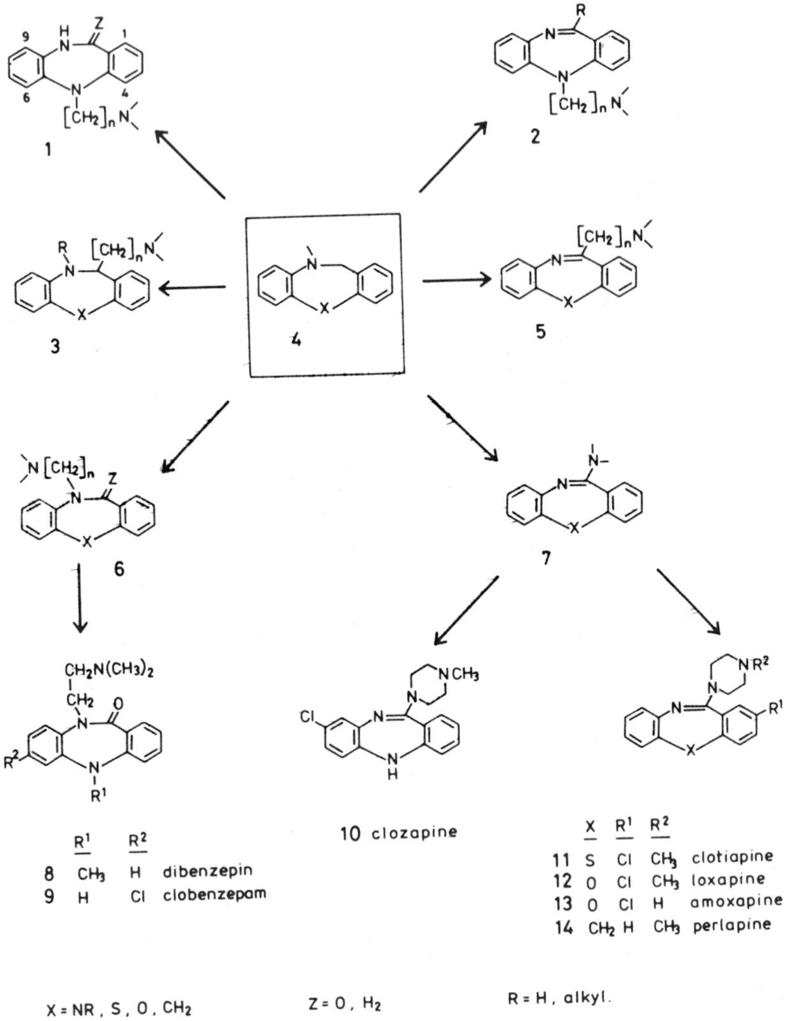
1
2
3
4
5
6
7
8 CH3 H dibenzepin
9 H Cl clobenzepam
10 clozapine
11 S Cl CH3 clotiapine
12 O Cl CH3 loxapine
13 O Cl H amoxapine
14 CH2 H CH3 perlapine
X = NR, S, O, CH2
Z = O, H2
R = H, alkyl.

Figure 1.

led, rather unexpectedly, to the discovery of a new class of tricyclic neuroleptic agents.[5,6] These included the classical neuroleptics clotiapine (11) and loxapine (12), the neuroleptic antidepressant amoxapine (13), and perlapine (14), which has been used as a hypnotic. Clozapine (10), the nitrogen member of this series (7, X = NH), differs markedly in its pharmacological profile from the classical neuroleptics and is an effective antipsychotic agent virtually devoid of extrapyramidal reactions. The essential elements in the action of clozapine, namely, psychomotor inhibition resembling that of the neuroleptics, but without catalepsy, and marked neurovegetative effects that might be expected as possible side effects in man, were clearly recognized in the early pharmacological testing.* In the first full pharmacological report, which appeared in January 1961, clozapine was characterized as follows:

> Compound HF-1854,† like chlorpromazine, has a central sedative action and strong antagonistic effects against adrenaline, noradrenaline, acetylcholine and histamine. Like chlorpromazine, it inhibits the effects of sympathetic stimulation without, however, producing ganglioplegic effects. HF-1854 differs from chlorpromazine in particular on account of its very strong inhibition of the pain reaction in the mouse and rabbit. Moreover, no real catalepsy such as that produced by chlorpromazine was seen with HF-1854. The substance may be classified as a neuroleptic agent with strong analgesic, parasympatholytic and sympatholytic actions. In man, the central neuroleptic effects may be expected to appear with lower doses than those affecting autonomic functions, but autonomic effects should be borne in mind as possible side effects. In the normal cat, only the higher dose levels produced autonomic effects alongside the tranquillizing action. We propose that the compound be tested in man.

The pharmacological data on which this early appraisal was based are shown in Table 1. The apomorphine gnawing test,[8] which later came to be widely used as a screening procedure for neuroleptics, was not available at that time. This was perhaps fortunate, since the lack of activity of clozapine in that test might have stopped its further development.

At the end of 1961, a more comprehensive report containing expanded pharmacological and toxicological data was prepared to serve as a basis for the first clinical trials. Table 2, comparing the pharmacological effects of clozapine with those of chlorpromazine, haloperidol, chlordiazepoxide, and barbiturates has been taken from that report. It is seen from this table that the pharmacological profile of clozapine closely resembles that of chlorpromazine, but clearly differs from those of the other drugs, including haloperidol. Again, the strong antinociceptive action of clozapine, which subsequently turned out to

*Clozapine was submitted for pharmacological testing in May 1960, and the first patent was applied for in August 1960.[7]
†Laboratory code number of clozapine.

Table 1

First Characterization of Clozapine in Comparison with Chlorpromazine (CPZ). Summary of Early Pharmacological Data (January 1961)

Test		Clozapine (mg/kg)	CPZ (mg/kg)
Inhibition of locomotion and behavior			
Mouse, jiggle cage	ID_{50} p.o.	2.5	3.5
Cat, indifference, passivity	ED_{min} p.o.	2	2
Somnolence, mydriasis, salivation, prolapse of nictitating membrane	ED_{min} p.o.	>4	4
Antinociceptive effects			
Mouse, phenylbenzoquinone syndrome	ID_{50} p.o.	3	5
Rabbit, tooth pulp stimulation threshold	$ED_{200\%}$ i.v.	~0.25	~1.5
Cardiovascular and autonomic effects			
Anaesthetized cat:			
Decrease in blood pressure	ED_{min} i.v.	0.1	0.2
Decrease in heart rate	ED_{min} i.v.	0.5	0

NA-induced increase in blood pressure	ID_{min} i.v.	0.2	>2
Nictitating membrane contraction after sympathetic stimulation	ID_{min} i.v.	0.1	0.5
Blood press. decrease after vagus stimulation	ID_{min} i.v.	0.1	0.2
Guinea pig, isolated ileum			
Acetylcholine-induced contraction	$IC_{>90\%}$	0.16[a]	0.25[a]
Histamine-induced contraction	$IC_{>90\%}$	0.01[a]	0.02[a]
Guinea pig, histamine-induced bronchospasm	ID_{50} p.o.	3.6	>5
Effects on rabbit EEG			
Slow waves, high voltage, synchron.	ED_{min} i.v.	0.02	0.2
Electrically stimulated arousal	ID_{block} s.c.	0.63	1.4
Anticonvulsive effects			
Mouse, pentetrazol (120 mg/kg s.c.)		No protection	
Mouse, strychnine nitrate (1.3 mg/kg s.c.)		with 50 mg/kg p.o.	

[a] μg/ml.

Table 2

Comparison of the Pharmacological Effects of Clozapine, Chlorpromazine (CPZ), Haloperidol, Chlordiazepoxide (CDP), and Barbiturates (December 1961)

Pharmacological effects	Clozapine	CPZ	Haloperidol	CDP	Barbiturates
Adrenolytic effects	+++	+++	0	0	0
Noradrenolytic effects	++	+	0	0	0
Sympatholytic effects (peripheral)	+++	+++	(+)	0	0
Parasympatholytic effects (peripheral)	++	+	+	0	0
Antihistaminic/antianaphylactic action	++	+		0	0
Antiserotonin effects (peripheral)	++	+++			0
Antinociceptive effects	+++	+	+	0	0
Decrease in spontaneous motility	Wide dose range	Wide dose range	Wide dose range	Wide dose range	Narrow dose range
Cataleptic effects	0	+	+++	0	0
Inhibition of decerebration rigidity	+++	+++	+	+ (incompl.)	+
Anticonvulsive action	0	0		+++	++
Pentobarbital potentiation	+++	+++	+++	+	Additive
EEG arousal inhibition	+++	++	0	0	++
Inhibition of conditioned suppression	0	0		+++	+

be, in part at least, an artifact,* and the absence of cataleptic effects were emphasized. However, the latter feature was not thought to be particularly important for the therapeutic action since some effective neuroleptic agents, such as thioridazine, were known to be only feebly cataleptic. Also, it was already suspected that there was no relation between the cataleptic action of a drug in animals and its therapeutic, antischizophrenic action, and it was suggested that the cataleptic action was more likely to be connected with the Parkinson-like and psychomotor side effects of neuroleptic drugs.[9,10] In 1971 full reports containing the pharmacological, toxicological, and metabolic data then available were published.[11-13] A comprehensive review of the pharmacological and biochemical properties followed in 1975.[14]

Let us now turn to the early clinical trials of clozapine for which doses similar to those of chlorpromazine were suggested. The first two open clinical studies, both of which were completed in 1962, did not agree in their conclusions. In one of these, involving 19 patients, 12 of whom were chronic schizophrenics, previously prescribed treatment was gradually replaced by clozapine, starting with 3 x 20 mg and increasing to 3 x 160 mg daily. In this trial the drug was judged not to be an effective antipsychotic, producing considerable untoward, mainly neurovegetative, effects but not extrapyramidal syndrome (EPS), except hypersalivation, which was considered as a possible sign of EPS. The other trial, conducted by Gross and Langner in Vienna, involved 28 schizophrenic patients on a dose schedule similar to that outlined above. Here the antipsychotic effect was judged as very good or good in 21 and questionable in 2 patients. In the remaining 5 patients clozapine was discontinued either because of lack of therapeutic effect or because of side effects. The findings from this trial were subsequently included in publications by Gross and Langner.[15-18]

The conclusions reached by Gross and Langner were confirmed in 1966 by Hippius in Berlin, who in an internal report classified clozapine as a rapid-acting neuroleptic with antipsychotic and sedative effects. Another internal report by Engelmeier from Essen gave further support to these conclusions, so that by the end of 1966, on the basis of the experience gained from these three clinical trials involving some 100 schizophrenic patients, there was a wide consensus on the antipsychotic effectiveness of clozapine, and it was decided to extend the clinical examination of the drug. This was done as soon as the necessary additional toxicological data became available in the summer of 1967.

On completion of these trials, conducted at numerous psychiatric centers in

*In the dental pulp stimulation test in the rabbit, the salivation induced by clozapine caused short-circuiting of the electrodes, leading to an exaggerated rise in the stimulation threshold.

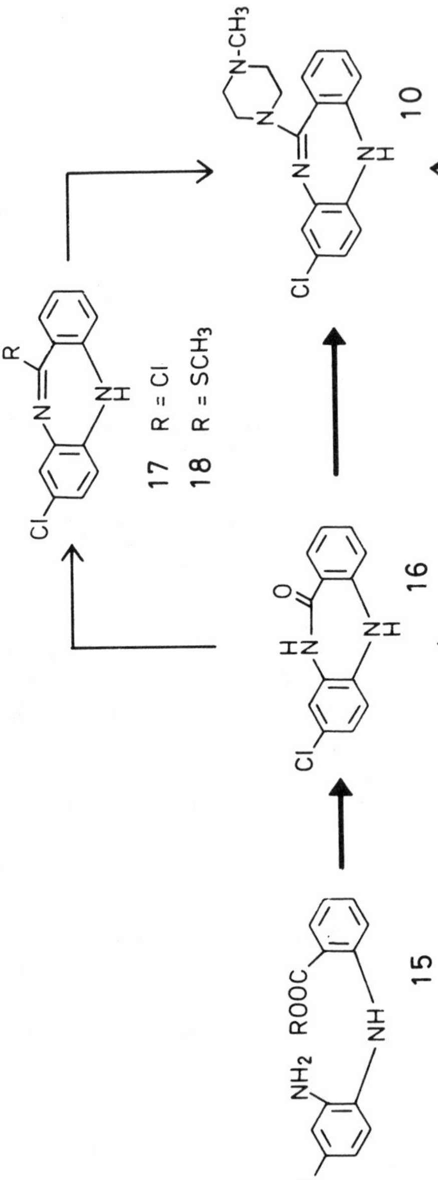

Figure 2.

17 R = Cl
18 R = SCH₃

15

16

19

10

46

Austria, Germany, Italy, and Switzerland[17-24] and involving more than 2200 patients, registration of clozapine was begun in 1971. In 1972 the drug was launched under the brand name Leponex, initially in Switzerland and Austria.

The clinical results have to a large extent confirmed our pharmacological predictions concerning the actions and side effects of clozapine. The drug proved to be antipsychotic and practically free of extrapyramidal side effects, but gave rise to neurovegetative side effects, such as hypotension, tachycardia, and salivation, which caused a few difficulties, especially at the onset of treatment. In spite of this, however, acceptance was excellent. Clozapine has been called a unique neuroleptic because it exerts a strong antipsychotic effect without inducing EPS.[20,21,25]

In 1975 the successful progress of clozapine was checked by an unforeseen event that remains unexplained to this day, despite the many efforts made.[26,27] Soon after the introduction of clozapine in Finland a high incidence of agranulocytosis was reported in patients treated with clozapine in hospitals and clinics situated in the southwestern part of that country. Numerous drugs, including the tricyclic psychotropic agents, were known to cause this unpredictable, rare, but life-endangering side effect and clozapine was no exception in this respect. However, the incidence of agranulocytosis associated with clozapine had been within the known range for other tricyclic neuroleptics, for example, chlorpromazine (up to 0.1%), until the Finnish cases were reported.

Despite the restrictions that now limit its use, clozapine continues to be prescribed relatively frequently, mainly, it appears, because of its low propensity for producing EPS and tardive dyskinesias.[25]

2. SYNTHESIS

Clozapine is 8-chlor-11-(4-methyl-1-piperazinyl)-5H-dibenzo[b,e][1,4]diazepine (10). The key intermediate for its synthesis[28] is the lactam 16 (Figure 2), which is obtained in good yield either by thermal cyclization of the aminocarboxylic acid 15 (R = H) in boiling xylene or by base-catalyzed cyclization of its ester (15; R = Me) in dioxane.[29] The aminocarboxylic acid 15 is readily obtained from 2-bromo-5-chloronitrobenzene by condensation with anthranilic acid in the presence of potassium carbonate and powdered copper according to Ullmann's method, followed by reduction of the nitro group, preferably with sodium dithionite in aqueous alkali. Catalytic hydrogenation is not suited because of the tendency of the chlorine substituent to undergo hydrogenolysis.

The lactam 16 is readily converted to clozapine in a one-stage reaction with a complex of N-methylpiperazine and titanium tetrachloride,[30] in a modification of the amidine synthesis first described by Fryer et al.[31] The preparation of clozapine by way of the imido chloride 17 is less convenient, since the latter, with a free NH group in position 5, is not very stable. Aminolysis of the thioether 18 proceeds very slowly, but the thiolactam 19 reacts readily with

N-methylpiperazine. However, the best and simplest method is the direct reaction between lactam **16** and the TiCl₄ complex of N-methylpiperazine.

3. MOLECULAR PROPERTIES

As is evident from an inspection of its structure (**10**), the clozapine molecule incorporates the partial structures of both a 1,4- and a 1,5-benzodiazepine. The amidine moiety has a pK_a of 3.70 and, unlike the distal nitrogen of the piperazine ring, is not protonated at physiological pH. Compound **20** which

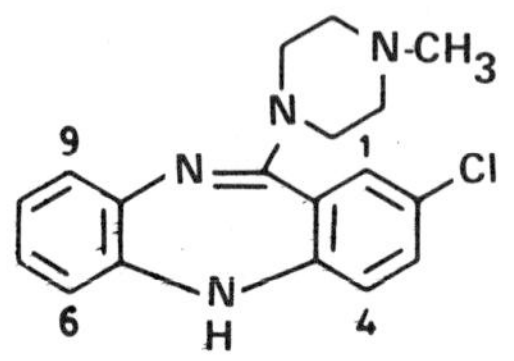

20 (HF-2046)

is isomeric with clozapine, has practically the same pK_a value as the latter. Moreover, there is no difference in the partition coefficients of the two isomers[32] or in their conformational properties as determined by X-ray analysis[33] (see Figure 3). In both compounds the tricyclic system is folded along a line running approximately through the nitrogen atom in position 5 and the center of the C-N double bond. The dihedral angle between the planes of the two aromatic rings was found to be 115° in clozapine (**10**) and 117.5° in the isomer **20**. The central seven-membered heterocyclic ring occurs in the boat conformation. The C-N bond connecting the ring to the piperazine ring has considerable double bond character as evidenced by its shorter-than-normal bond length. These molecular properties confer upon the ring system of clozapine a certain degree of rigidity that is further increased by the close contact that exists between the piperazine ring and the unsubstituted benzene ring. This is clearly demonstrated in Figure 3. As a result of this increase, the piperazine ring, which occurs in a chair conformation, lies in a plane roughly parallel to that of the other, 8-substituted, benzene ring. Quantum-chemical calculations also indicate an appreciable barrier for the rotation of the piperazine ring relative to the tricyclic nucleus.[34]

The methyl group attached to the distal nitrogen of the piperazine ring is in an equatorial position, whereas the lone pair of electrons that is important for binding to receptors extends in an axial direction. The distances between that distal nitrogen atom and the centers of the two aromatic rings are 6.03 and 7.71 Å, respectively.

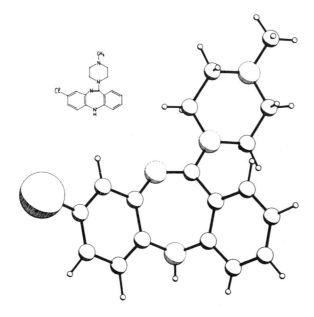

Figure 3. Computer-drawn perspective view of clozapine showing the molecular conformation as determined by X-ray analysis of the crystalline base.[33]

4.   STRUCTURE-ACTIVITY RELATIONSHIPS

4.1   Clozapine versus Classical Neuroleptics

Clozapine differs structurally from the classical tricyclic neuroleptics such as clotiapine (11) and loxapine (12) by having its chloro substituent not in position 2, but in position 8 of the tricyclic system. This positional isomerism has a decisive influence on the pharmacological properties. This is illustrated in Table 3, which compares clozapine with its positional isomer **20**, loxapine (**12**), and chlorpromazine in a number of pharmacological and biochemical test models.

The most striking distinguishing feature of clozapine is that it is practically devoid of cataleptic action and does not inhibit apomorphine-induced gnawing in the rat. Classical neuroleptics, such as **12**, **20**, and chlorpromazine, are very active in both these tests. On the other hand, clozapine is very effective in antagonizing the hypermotility induced in mice by 4,α-dimethyl-*m*-tyramine (H 77/77), its potency being of the same order of magnitude as that of the classical neuroleptics.[35] This test, which probably also involves DA-antagonism, is suitable for screening both cataleptogenic and noncataleptogenic neuroleptics.

Table 3
Comparison of Some Pharmacological and Biochemical Properties of Clozapine and Classical Neuroleptics[a]

		Clozapine (10)	Isomer (20)	Loxapine (12)	CPZ	Ref.
Locomotion, M	ID_{50} mg/kg p.o.	2.5	6.0	0.05	4.0	37
Catalepsy, R	ED_{30}'' mg/kg p.o.	0	3.5	0.35	3.8	37
Apomorphine-gnawing, R	ID_{50} mg/kg s.c.	0	1.7	0.07	2.6	37
H77/77-Hypermotility, M	ID_{50} mg/kg i.p.	0.08	—	0.02	0.22	35
DA adenylate cyclase inhibition, striatum R	K_i (nM)	170	18	45	48	38
³H-Haloperidol binding, striatum R	IC_{50} (nM)	231	29[b]	16	24	39
³H-Clozapine binding, whole brain R	IC_{50} (nM)	5	7.5[b]	98	28	40
³H-QNB binding, whole brain R	IC_{50} (μM)	0.3	0.2	3	3	37

[a] 0 = inactive at 20 mg/kg, M = mouse, R = rat.
[b] Unpublished results.

The difference between clozapine and the classical neuroleptics can also be demonstrated biochemically. Thus the inhibitory activity of clozapine on DA-stimulated adenylate cyclase is much weaker than that of its 2-chloro isomer **20**. Similarly, the affinity of clozapine for the binding site in the [³H]haloperidol assay *in vitro* is very weak compared with the affinities of the isomer **20** and loxapine (**12**), which are, respectively, 8 and 15 times as great in this test. Clozapine has, however, been shown to bind specifically and with high affinity to rat brain membranes,[36] but the binding sites are heterogenous, with about two-thirds being muscarinic cholinergic receptors.

The affinity of clozapine for muscarinic cholinergic receptors, as measured *in vitro* by the [³H]quinuclidinyl benzilate ([³H]QNB) assay, is of the same order as that of the isomer **20**. Loxapine and CPZ, on the other hand, are only roughly one-tenth as potent. There appears to be some correlation between the affinities for the clozapine and QNB binding sites.

In general, it must be recognized that it is difficult to make firm assertions concerning structure-activity relationships in this group of noncataleptogenic, "atypical" neuroleptics in the absence of a specific screening test that is relevant to and correlates with their clinical activity. However, some conclusions may be drawn from the central depressant effects of these agents as measured by their action on the locomotor activity of mice and their central anticholinergic activity determined by the [³H]QNB assay *in vitro*.

4.2 Influence of the Bridging Moiety X

Clozapine, as well as the analogously substituted morphanthridine, dibenz[*b,f*][1,4]oxazepine and dibenz[*b,f*][1,4]thiazepine derivatives **21**, **22**, and **23**, all exhibit varying degrees of CNS-depressing activities (Table 4). The most potent of these analogues are clozapine and the dibenzoxazepine **22**. All, except the oxazepine **22**, show fairly strong anticholinergic effects, the thiazepine **23** being the most active. *N*-Alkylation of clozapine in position 5 (compounds **24**, **25**, **26**) results in some reduction of the locomotor-inhibitory effects. The anticholinergic action, on the other hand, is retained or even enhanced by 5-*N*-alkylation.

4.3 Substitution in Position 8

Of the 8-substituted dibenzodiazepines studied the chloro and fluoro derivatives **10** and **32** exhibit maximal CNS-depressant effects as evidenced by inhibition of locomotor activity in mice (Table 4). The influence of substituents in position 8 on the central inhibitory activity decreases in the following order:

$$\geqslant Cl > F > Br = CH_3 > H > CF_3 \sim SCH_3 > OCH_3 > NO_2 \gg OH$$

Only the methyl and methoxy derivatives (**28**, **29**) exhibit weak cataleptic effects, and the methoxy compound and the fluoro analogue **32** of clozapine are

Table 4

Influence of the Bridging Moiety and Aromatic Substituents on Biological Activity[a]

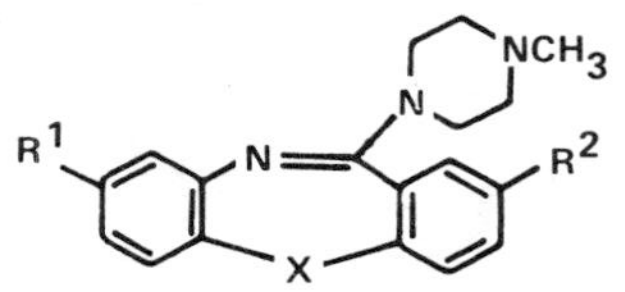

Compd.	X	R[1]	R[2]	Motor activity M, ID_{50} (mg/kg p.o.)	Catalepsy R, $ED_{30''}$ (mg/kg s.c.)	Apo-gnawing R, IC_{50} (mg/kg s.c.)	^{3}H-QNB IC_{50} (μM)	Ref.
10	NH	Cl	H	2.5	0	0	0.3	37
21	CH$_2$	Cl	H	8.1	0	0	0.3	37
22	O	Cl	H	2.5	0	0	1.0	37
23	S	Cl	H	23	0	0	0.07	37
24	NMe	Cl	H	9.0	0	0	0.1 [b]	41
25	NEt	Cl	H	6.0[b]	0[b]	0[b]	0.4 [b]	
26	NPr	Cl	H	3.2[b]	0[b]	0[b]	—	
27	NH	H	H	10	0	0	1.0	37

28	NH	Me	H	7.5	34	0^b	—	41
29	NH	OMe	H	28	45	20^b	0.82^b	41
30	NH	OH	H	$\gg100$ ^{b}	—	—	—	
31	NH	SMe	H	25	0	0^b	0.32^b	41
32	NH	F	H	3.2^b	—	31^b	0.14^b	
33	NH	Br	H	6.0^b	0^b	0^b	0.29^b	
34	NH	NO$_2$	H	>10 ^{b}	—	0^b	0.10^b	
35	NH	CF$_3$	H	24	0	0^b	0.55^b	41
36	NH	Cl	F	2.2	0	9.0	0.5	37
37	NH	Cl	Cl	2.0	8.0	16	0.3	37

^{a}0 = inactive at 20 mg/kg, M = mouse, R = rat.
^{b}Unpublished results.

the only members of the series to display some antiapomorphine activity. The unsubstituted dibenzodiazepine **27** still retains CNS-depressant and anticholinergic properties, but both activities are reduced to about one-quarter of those of clozapine.

It is noted that in this series there appears to be no relation between the electronic effects or the lipophilicity of the aromatic substituents and the pharmacological activities. Similar findings have been reported for analogously substituted dibenzo[*b,f*]thiepins of the type illustrated by structure **48**, using the rotating rod test on mice as a measure of neuroleptic activity.[42-44]

In contrast to these findings for 8-substituted dibenzoepines, we have found that in a series of dibenzothiazepines and dibenzoxazepines substituted in position 2 of the ring system, the most strongly electron-withdrawing substituents conferred the highest neuroleptic activity as measured by the apomorphine test in the rat.[6] When such a "neuroleptic" substituent is introduced in position 2 of clozapine, the 2,8-substituted derivatives obtained (e.g., **36** and **37**) again display properties characteristic of the classical neuroleptics, coupled with strong anticholinergic activities.

It may be deduced from these results that the two aromatic rings of the dibenzoepine system relate to different pharmacological properties of these compounds. It is postulated that the 2-substituted benzene ring of the cataleptogenic neuroleptics is concerned in the interaction of the molecule with dopaminergic receptors. The unsubstituted dibenzodiazepines, dibenzothiazepines, and dibenzoxazepines show only weak or no activity in the catalepsy or apomorphine tests.[6,37] The substituents in position 2 thus determine the affinity and quantitatively affect the biological activity. The other benzene ring is thought to be involved in the interaction at the muscarinic-cholinergic site. The 8-substituted dibenzoepines **10**, **21**, **22**, and **23** (Table 4) all are roughly three times as potent in the [³H]QNB test as the corresponding unsubstituted compounds.[37] The nature of the substituent in position 8 in the dibenzodiazepine series has little influence on the anticholinergic activity, as is seen from the activities of compounds **28-35**, all of which are of the same order of magnitude. The effect of introducing a chloro substituent in position 2 of the unsubstituted dibenzoepines is not consistent: clotiapine (**11**) is only about one-tenth as potent as the unsubstituted thiazepine in the [³H]QNB assay, whereas loxapine (**12**) is approximately equipotent with its unsubstituted analogue[37] and, in the diazepine series, the 2-chloro derivative **20** is five times as active as the unsubstituted compound **27**. The introduction of a further halogen atom in position 2 of the clozapine molecule has no appreciable effect on its anticholinergic activity (see compounds **10**, **36** and **37**).

Table 5

Influence of Basic Substituent in Position 11 of the Clozapine Molecule on Biological Activity

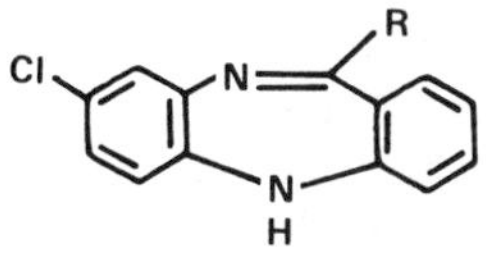

Compd.	R	Motor activity M, ID_{50} (mg/kg p.o.)	^{3}H-QNB assay IC_{50} (μM)	Ref.
38	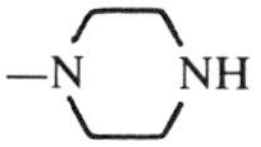 —N͡NH	40	1.4[a]	41
10	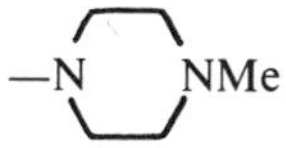 —N͡NMe	2.5	0.3	37
39	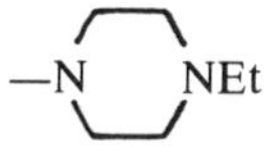 —N͡NEt	7.0	—	41
40	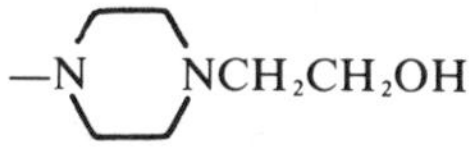 —N͡NCH$_2$CH$_2$OH	14	9.0	37
41	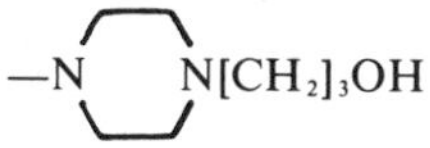 —N͡N[CH$_2$]$_3$OH	19	20	37
42	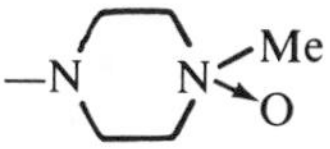 —N͡N⟨Me, O	40	$\gg$10	45
43	—N⌐NMe$_2$	>32	1.6	45
44	—NHCH$_2$CH$_2$NMe$_2$	14	4.4[a]	41
45	—NCH$_2$CH$_2$NMe$_2$ | Me	40	—	41

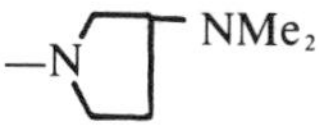

[a]Unpublished results.

4.4   Nature of the Basic Group

A 4-substituted piperazinyl group in the dibenzodiazepines is essential for strong CNS-depressant activity (Table 5). The open-chain ethylenediamine derivatives **44** and **45**, the dimethylaminopyrrolidine **43**, and the unsubstituted piperazinyl derivative **38** (i.e., desmethylclozapine) all are very weak CNS depressants. The tricyclic system of the pyrrolidine derivative **43** has been shown by X-ray crystal structure analysis to have the same conformation as clozapine iteself, but the distances between the exocyclic nitrogen atom and the two benzene rings of **43** are different from those of clozapine.[45] Thus the exocyclic nitrogen of compound **43** is unable to occupy the same relative position as the distal piperazinyl nitrogen in clozapine, and receptor interaction is impeded.

Hydroxyalkylation of the distal piperazine nitrogen leads to compounds **40** and **41**, which are much weaker than clozapine in regard to both CNS-depressant and anticholinergic effects; and clozapine-N-oxide (**42**) is weaker still. In the formation of the N-oxide the axial lone pair of electrons on the distal piperazine nitrogen of clozapine is occupied by an oxygen atom; this probably renders any contact with receptors impossible.

4.5   Other Modifications of the Tricyclic System

The influence of changes in the bridging group X is discussed earlier. Let us now briefly consider the effect of some other modifications involving the central heterocyclic ring or one of the aromatic nuclei.

The thieno[3,4-*b*][1,5]benzodiazepine **46**, which is an isostere of clozapine, was found, rather surprisingly, to be cataleptogenic;[46] it is therefore likely to be a classical neuroleptic. However, the thieno[3,2-*c*][1]benzazepine **47**[39,47] is noncataleptogenic, but shows a distinct apomorphine-antagonistic action, in constrast to the isosteric morphanthridine derivative **21**, which is devoid of such activity (Table 4). The thieno derivative **47** was found to have antipsychotic activity in man without any appreciable extrapyramidal side effects.[50]

Finally, some noncataleptogenic agents that appear to resemble clozapine in their pharmacological properties have been reported among a series of piperazinyldibenzo[*b,f*]thiepins.[42-44] Thus compounds **48** and **49** likewise lack apomorphine-antagonistic action and are even more strongly centrally depressant than clozapine in the rotating rod test on the mouse.

In general, it may be said that a complete tricyclic 6-7-6 or 6-7-5 system seems to be necessary for clozapine-like pharmacological properties. So far at least, efforts to find clozapine-like agents among bicyclic epines have failed.[48,49] Thus, for example, the benzodiazepine **50** proved to have no neuroleptic properties.

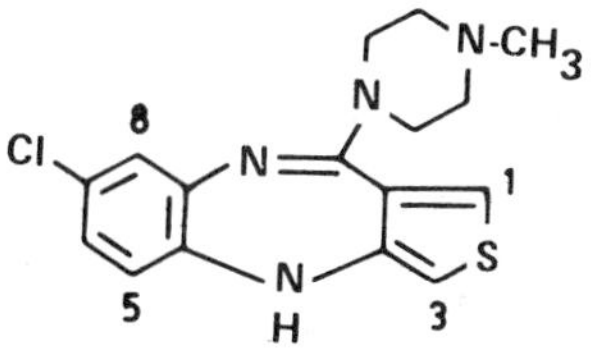

46

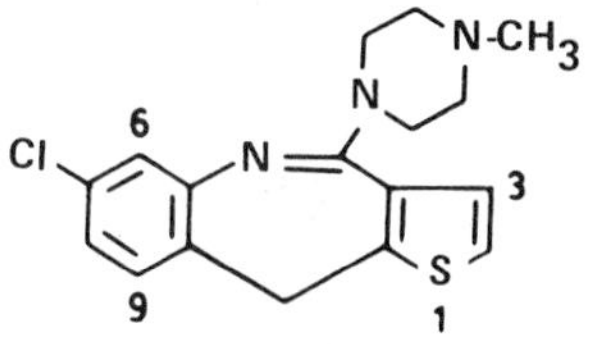

47 (NT 104-252)

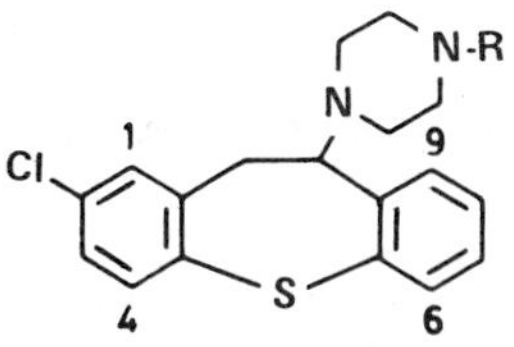

48 R = CH$_3$

49 R = CH$_2$CH$_2$OH

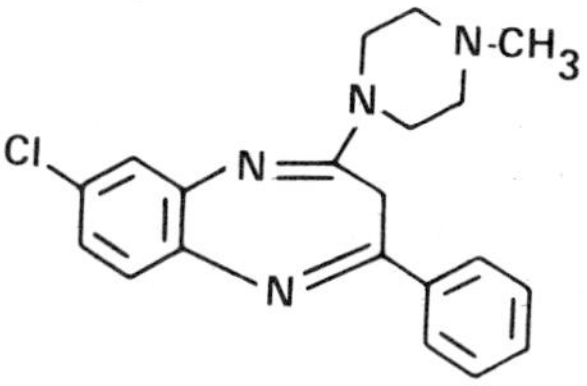

50

5. CONCLUSIONS

Clozapine has generated widespread scientific interest mainly because, on the basis of its pharmacological and biochemical actions, it cannot be classed among the classical neuroleptics. However, the actual mechanism of the antipsychotic action of clozapine is not yet understood. The situation as it is today presents us with three major challenges: first, for the medicinal chemist, the clozapine structure is an interesting model for molecular modification with the aim of achieving greater specificity of action with fewer neurovegetative side effects; second, for the biologist, it remains to establish which of the different pharmacological components of clozapine contribute to or are responsible for its unique antipsychotic action; and third, the high incidence of agranulocytosis in southern Finland has led to an intensification of efforts to find methods for recognizing, at the laboratory level, the risk of a toxic action on leucopoiesis.

ACKNOWLEDGMENT

The story we present here is the result of over 20 years' research effort involving so many colleagues in different fields that it is quite impossible to name them here. Our thanks are due to all of them. However, we do wish to record our special indebtedness to the following colleagues from preclinical research, who have been particularly closely associated with this work for much of those 20 years and who have contributed greatly to its successful outcome: Drs. H. R. Bürki, R. Fischer, and F. Hunziker, Mr. F. Künzle, Drs. H. Lauener, A. C. Sayers, and G. Stille, and Mr. T. G. White. We wish also to thank Dr. C. W. Picard for critical discussions and help in the preparation of this manuscript.

REFERENCES

1. B. Shopsin, H. Klein, M. Aaronsom, and M. Collora, *Arch. Gen. Psychiat.* **36**, 657 (1979).
2. F. Hunziker, F. Künzle, and J. Schmutz, *Helv. Chim. Acta,* **46**, 2337 (1963).
3. F. Hunziker, F. Künzle, O. Schindler, and J. Schmutz, *Helv. Chim. Acta,* **47**, 1163 (1964).
4. F. Hunziker, F. Künzle, and J. Schmutz, *Helv. Chim. Acta,* **49**, 244 (1966).
5. G. Stille, H. Lauener, E. Eichenberger, F. Hunziker, and J. Schmutz, *Arzneim.-Forsch. (Drug Res.),* **15**, 841 (1965).
6. J. Schmutz, *Arzneim.-Forsch. (Drug Res.),* **25**, 712 (1975).
7. J. Schmutz and F. Hunziker, *Swiss Patent* 398 620 to Wander Ltd. (1965); see also *U.S. Patent* 3 539 573; see *Chem. Abstr.,* **64**, 8219 (1966).
8. P. A. J. Janssen, C. J. E. Niemeegers, and A. H. M. Jageneau, *Arzneim.-Forsch. (Drug Res.),* **10**, 1003 (1960).
9. S. Courvoisier, R. Ducrot, J. Fournel, L. Julou, and D. Leau, *C. R. Soc. Biol.,* **152**, 1371 (1958).
10. J. R. Boissier, *Therapie,* **15**, 73 (1960).
11. G. Stille, H. Lauener, and E. Eichenberger, *Farmaco (Pavia), Ed. Prat.,* **26**, 603 (1971).
12. S. Lindt, H. Lauener, and E. Eichenberger, *Farmaco (Pavia), Ed. Prat.,* **26**, 585 (1971).
13. R. Gauch and W. Michaelis, *Farmaco (Pavia), Ed. Prat.,* **26**, 667 (1971).
14. A. C. Sayers and H. A. Amsler, in *Pharmacological and Biochemical Properties of Drug Substances,* Vol. 1, M. E. Goldberg, Ed., American Pharmaceutical Association and Academy of Pharmaceutical Sciences, Washington, 1977, p. 1.
15. H. Gross and E. Langner, *Wien. Med. Wochenschr.,* **40**, 814 (1966).
16. H. Gross and E. Langner, *Excerpta Med. Int. Congr. Ser.,* **180**, 477 (1969).
17. H. Gross and E. Langner, *Arzneim.-Forsch. (Drug Res.),* **19**, 496 (1969).
18. H. Gross and E. Langner, *Int. Pharmacopsychiat.,* **4**, 220 (1970).
19. D. Bente, M. P. Engelmeier, R. Heinrich, H. Hippius, and W. Schmitt, *Excerpta Med. Int. Congr. Ser.,* **129**, 977 (1967).
20. J. Angst, D. Bente, P. Berner, H. Heimann, H. Helmchen, and H. Hippius, *Pharmakopsychiatry,* **4**, 201 (1971).
21. J. Angst, W. Jaenicke, A. Padrutt, and C. Scharfetter, *Pharmakopsychiatry,* **4**, 192 (1971).
22. H. Berzewski, H. Helmchen, H. Hippius, H. Hoffmann, and S. Kanowski, *Arzneim.-Forsch. (Drug Res.),* **19**, 495 (1969).
23. M. Balassa, E. Deisenhammer, and H. Scherrer, *Wien. Med. Wochenschr.,* **121**, 90 (1971).
24. D. de Maio, *Arzneim.-Forsch. (Drug Res.),* **22**, 919 (1972).
25. F. J. Ayd, *Int. Drug Ther. Newslett.,* **9**, 5 (1974).

26. H. A. Amsler, L. Teerenhovi, K. Barth, K. Harjula, and P. Vuopio, *Acta Psychiat. Scand.,* **56,** 241 (1977).
27. S. Knuutila, E. Helminen, L. Knuutila, S. Leisti, M. Siimes, P. Tammisto, and T. Westermarck, *Hum. Genet.,* **38,** 77 (1977).
28. F. Hunziker, E. Fischer, and J. Schmutz, *Helv. Chim. Acta,* **50,** 1588 (1967).
29. F. Hunziker, H. Lauener, and J. Schmutz, *Arzneim.-Forsch. (Drug Res.),* **13,** 324 (1963).
30. J. Schneider, *German Patent* 2,316,438 to Wander Ltd.; *Chem. Abstr.,* **80** 14969 (1974).
31. R. I. Fryer, J. V. Earley, G. F. Field, W. Zally, and L. H. Sternbach, *J. Org. Chem.,* **34,** 1143 (1969).
32. J. Schmutz, *Pharm. Acta Helv.,* **48,** 117 (1973).
33. T. J. Petcher and H. P. Weber, *J. Chem. Soc., Perkin Trans.* **II,** 1415 (1976).
34. J. P. Tollenaere, H. Moereels, and M. H. J. Koch, *Eur. J. Med. Chem.,* **12,** 199 (1977).
35. C. Rüdeberg, *Psychopharmacol.,* **59,** 247 (1978); C. Rudeberg, in *Biological Psychiatry Today,* J. Obiols, C. Ballus, E. Gonzales Monclus, and J. Pujol, Eds., Elsevier North Holland Biomedical Press, 1979, p. 119.
36. D. Hauser and A. Closse, *Life Sci.,* **23,** 557 (1978).
37. H. R. Bürki, A. C. Sayers, W. Ruch and H. Asper, *Arzneim.-Forsch. (Drug Res.),* **27 (II),** 1561 (1977).
38. R. J. Miller, A. S. Horn, and L. L. Iversen, *Mol. Pharmacol.,* **10,** 759 (1974); R. J. Miller and C. R. Hiley, *Naunyn-Schmiedeberg's Arch. Pharmacol.,* **292,** 289 (1976).
39. H. R. Bürki, *Life Sci.,* **23,** 437 (1978).
40. H. R. Bürki, *Life Sci.,* **26,** 2187 (1980).
41. J. Schmutz, F. Hunziker, G. Stille, and H. Lauener, *Chim. Ther.,* 424 (1967).
42. K. Šindelář, A. Dlabač, J. Metyšová, B. Kakáč, J. Holubek, E. Svátek, Z. Šedivý, and M. Protiva, *Collect. Czech. Chem. Commun.,* **40,** 1940 (1975).
43. K. Šindelář, A. Dlabač, B. Kakáč, E. Svátek, J. Holubek, Z. Šedivý, E. Princová, and M. Protiva, *Collect. Czech. Chem. Commun.,* **40,** 2649 (1975).
44. J. O. Jílek, K. Šindelář, M. Rajšner, A. Dlabač, J. Metyšová, Z. Votava, J. Pomykáček, and M. Protiva, *Collect. Czech. Chem. Commun.,* **40,** 2887 (1975).
45. H. R. Bürki, R. Fischer, F. Hunziker, F. Künzle, T. J. Petcher, J. Schmutz, H. P. Weber, and T. G. White, *Eur. J. Med. Chem.,* **13,** 479 (1978).
46. J. B. Press, C.M. Hofmann, N. H. Eudy, W. J. Fanshawe, I. P. Day, E. N. Greenblatt, and S. R. Safir, *J. Med. Chem.,* **22,** 725 (1979).
47. F. Hunziker, *Swiss Patent* 560 220 to Wander Ltd. (1975); *Chem. Abstr.,* **83,** 58881t (1975).
48. C. R. Ellefson, C. M. Woo, A. Miller, and J. R. Kehr, *J. Med. Chem.,* **21,** 952 (1978).
49. M. J. Kukla, *J. Heterocycl. Chem.,* **14,** 933 (1977).
50. F. Hunziker, R. Fischer, P. Kipfer, J. Schmutz, H. R. Bürki, E. Eichenberger, and T. G. White, *Eur. J. Med. Chem.,* (1981) in press.

Butaclamol

L.G. Humber

3

An account of the development of the antipsychotic agent butaclamol (**1**) must begin with the discovery of chlorpromazine, the prototype antipsychotic drug. Chlorpromazine (**2**) descendant of the sedative-antihistamine promethazine, was synthesized by Charpentier in 1950.[1] Within a period of only 4 years Delay et al. in France[2] and Lehmann and Hanrahan in Montreal[3] had determined chlorpromazine to be the first effective drug in the treatment of psychotic disorders.

Almost simultaneously, in 1951, imipramine (**3**) was synthesized by Haflinger and Schindler.[4] In view of the common structural features evident in

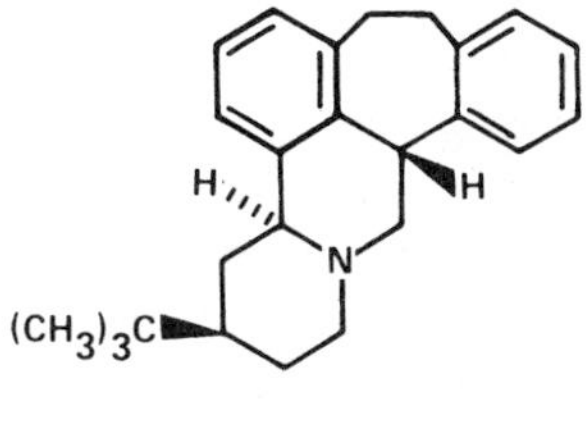

1

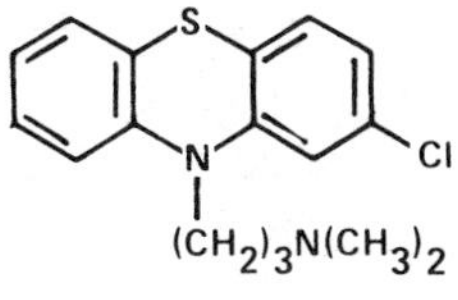

2

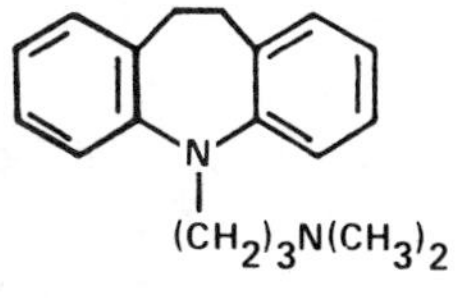

3

chlorpromazine and imipramine, the latter was investigated in man by Kuhn[5] in 1957 for antipsychotic properties. Imipramine was devoid of such activity but was identified as the first effective non-monoamine oxidase inhibitor for the treatment of depressive states.[5]

A third significant event transpired in 1958 with the disclosure[6] that the thioxanthene chlorprothixene (**4**) had a pharmacological profile suggestive of clinical antipsychotic activity. The thioxanthenes represent today another class of widely used antipsychotic agents.

$CH(CH_2)_2N(CH_3)_2$

4

$CH(CH_2)_2N(CH_3)_2$

5

It is evident from a cursory inspection of the structures of imipramine and chlorprothixene, both inspired by the phenothiazines, that the stage was set for the synthesis of amitryptiline (**5**). In fact, no less than 15 independent groups in Europe and North America were involved in the study of amitriptyline and related dibenzo[a,d]cycloheptenes.[7] The competition to synthesize amitriptyline was so fierce that five applicants were involved in a patent interference declared in the United States Patent office.[8]

Among those who had developed amitriptyline were Winthrop et al.[9] and Herr et al[10] at the Ayerst Laboratories in Montreal, so that when the present author had the opportunity, in the mid-1960s, to initiate a project aimed at the development of novel types of psychotropic agents, there existed in our laboratories a veritable store of chemical intermediates, as well as chemical and pharmacological expertise concerning dibenzo[a,d]cycloheptenes.

The strategy selected was to utilize the readily available precursor of amitriptyline, 10,11-dihydro-5H-dibenzo[a,d]cyclohepten-5-one[6], as the starting material for the synthesis of novel carbocyclic and heterocyclic ring systems. It was hoped that suitable derivatives of these ring systems would retain features that might permit recognition by the then putative "receptors" that mediated the actions of the "tricyclic" drugs discussed above and that better therapeutic agents might be obtained. Targets were selected with sufficient chemical novelty so that they would not likely be the goal of other research groups.

Our first tactic was to transform the tricyclic ketone **6** into 1,6,7,11b-tetra-hydro-2H-dibenz(c,d)azulen-2-one (**9**). It was envisaged that this tetracyclic ketone would serve as the precursor to a series of potentially interesting bridged

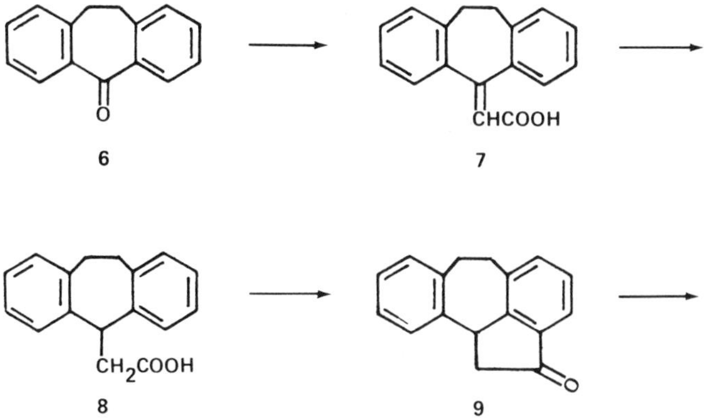

Figure 1.

analogues of amitriptyline. The sequence of reactions by which the synthesis of
9 was achieved[11] is summarized in Figure 1.

A full characterization of the dibenz[c,d]azulenone **9** had hardly been completed when a paper by Van der Stelt et al.[12] appeared describing a synthesis of
9 and its utilization for the preparation of a series of 2-amino derivatives of
type **10**. Within a matter of months Galantay et al., at a regional American
Chemical Society meeting[13], also described the synthesis of the
dibenz[c,d]azulenone **9**, as well as the 1,11b-dehydro and the 1,6,7,11-dehydro
derivative. A later publication by the Galantay group[14] described the preparation of a series of bridged amitriptyline analogues of type **11**.

Our desire for exclusivity in the field of dibenz[c,d]azulenes was thus shat-
tered at a very early stage in the project. We nevertheless elected to take a
calculated risk and to explore further the chemistry of the dibenz[c,d]azulenone
(**9**). Among the reactions studied was the Beckmann rearrangement of the oxime of **9**. Under numerous sets of conditions no rearrangement product could
be obtained. In contrast, the treatment of **9** with sodium azide in molten

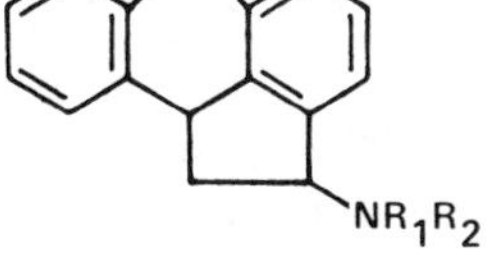

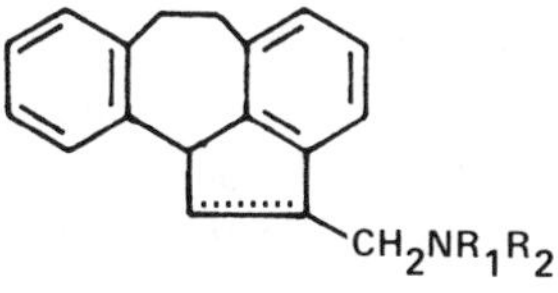

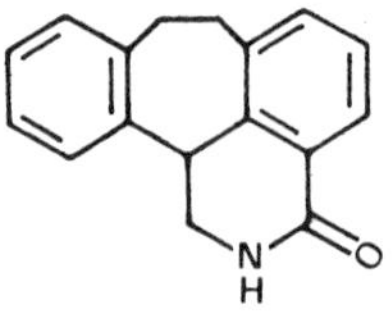

12

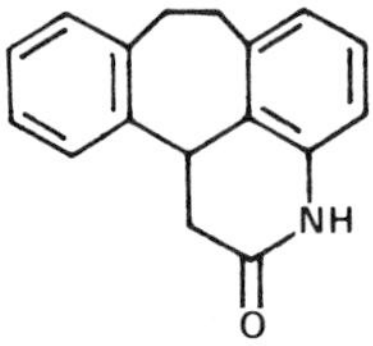

13

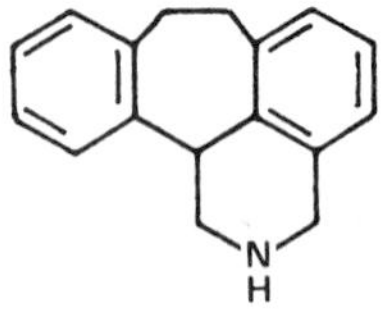

14

trichloroacetic acid at 70 °C afforded a single lactam, **12,** ν_{max} (CHCl$_3$), 1672 cm^{-1}, in 80% yield.[11] Initially we assumed that the dihydrocarbostyril **13** had been formed, in view of the expected behavior of cyclic aralkyl ketones in the Schmidt rearrangement,[15] where aryl migration is generally observed. However, examination of the ultraviolet spectrum of **14,** the lithium aluminum hydride reduction product from lactam **12,** showed that it was unchanged when taken as the free base or as the hydrochloride salt. This indicated that the precursor lactam at hand was the dihydroisocarbostyril **12,** a structural assignment that was fully confirmed by subsequent studies.

The unexpected formation of the isocarbostyril **12** was ascribed[11] to the rigidity of the dibenz[c,d]azulene system **9** which imposes a configurational preference on an assumed iminodiazonium ion intermediate wherein aryl migration would impose a high degree of strain in the transition state.

Compounds **12** and **14** were the first representatives of the hitherto unknown benzo[1,2]cyclohepta[3,4,5-de]isoquinoline ring system and, inasmuch as no reports on the synthesis of this ring system appeared in the then current literature by competing groups, we elected to use this tetracyclic system as the template for the design of a series of derivatives for pharmacological evaluation. It transpired that our exclusivity in the domain of the benzo[1,2]cyclohepta [3,4,5-de]isoquinolines was never challenged. The possibility of such a challenge had not, however, been very remote, as evidenced by a 1967 report by Galantay[16] that the Schmidt rearrangement of **15a** (Figure 2), the 1,11b-dehydro analogue of **9,** proceeded normally to afford the carbostyril derivative **15b.** The same reaction, though, apparently had not been tried by them on **9** itself.

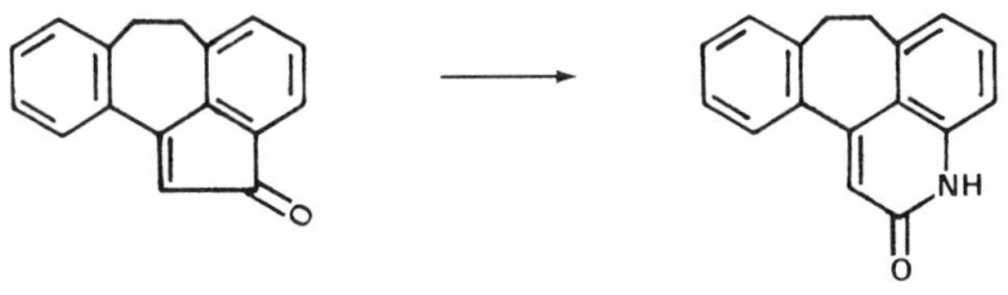

15a   15b

Figure 2.

The most pressing need at this stage was for a convenient method for the synthesis of **12** or **14** that did not involve the use of the hazardous sodium azide-molten trichloroacetic process. In view of the isoquinolinic nature of the target compounds, we readily developed alternative routes to various oxidation levels of the benzo[1,2]cyclohepta[3,4,5-*de*]isoquinoline ring system, and these are summarized in Figure 3.

The aminomethyl compound **18** was a key intermediate and was obtained from the nitrile **19** as described previously[11] or by hydrolysis of the isocyanate **20**, derived from the acetic acid **8**.[17] Alternatively, **18** was obtained by reduction of the oxime **17**, which was prepared from ketone **6** by way of carbinol **16a** and aldehyde **16b**.[17] The aminomethyl compound **18** was converted to the carbamate **23**, the carbamoyl chloride **22**, or the formamide **21**. The last intermediate was also obtained by a facile one-step reduction of the isocyanate **20**.[18] The carbamic acid derivatives **22** and **23** were cyclized to the isocarbostyril **12**, previously obtained from the dibenz[*c,d*]azulenone **9**, and the formamide **21** was cyclized under Bischler-Napieralski conditions to afford the Schiff's base **24**, which was readily reduced to the tetrahydroisoquinoline derivative **14**. The tetracyclic Schiff's base **24**, as we see below, proved to be a very accessible and a most versatile intermediate.

The chemistry of the Schiff's base **24** was extensively explored and various types of benzo[1,2]cyclohepta[3,4,5-*de*]isoquinoline derivatives were evaluated pharmacologically.[19] No outstanding psychotropic properties were found. The prospects of obtaining useful psychotropic agents from this project appeared extremely remote until it was observed[20] that 2-ethyl-1,2,3,7,8,12b-hexahydro-benzo(1,2]cyclohepta[3,4,5-*de*]isoquinoline **25**,[21] as well as various 2,3-dialkyl derivatives **26**,[17] exhibited pronounced taming effects in animals. Optimal activity was observed with taclamine (**27**), the benzo[6,7]cyclohepta [1,2,3-*de*]pyrido[2,1-*a*]isoquinoline analogue obtained by formally joining together the alkyl groups at the positions 2 and 3 in **26**.

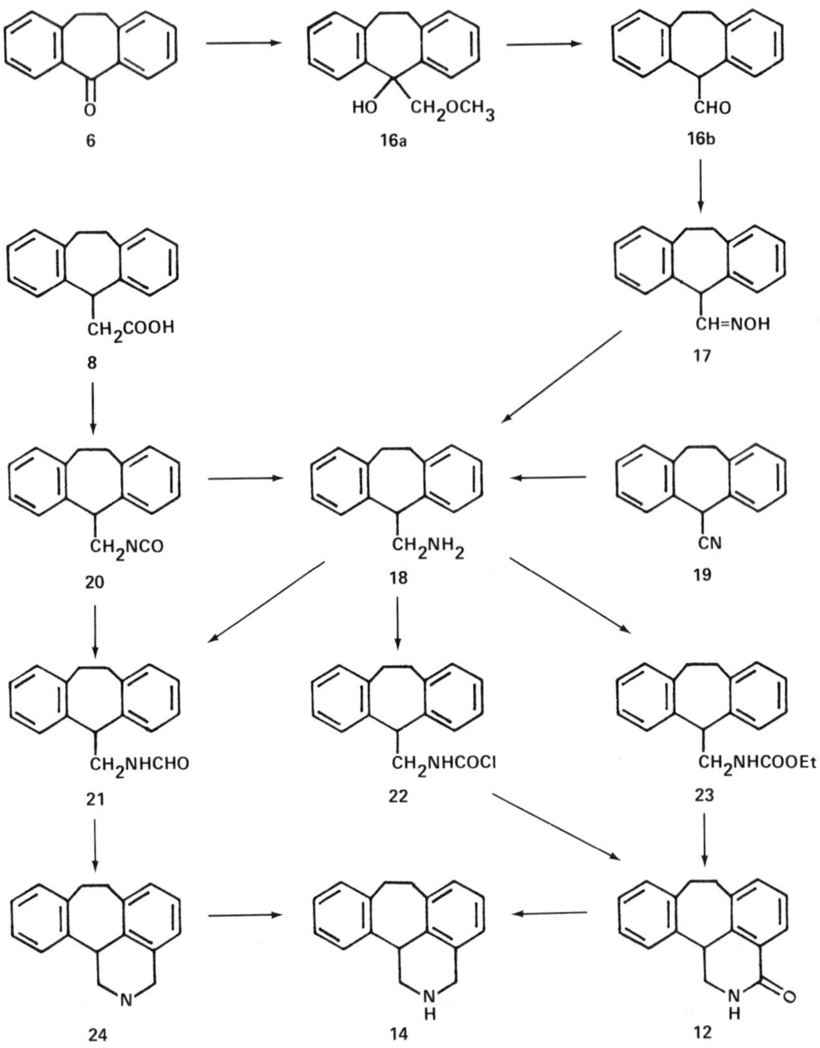

Figure 3.

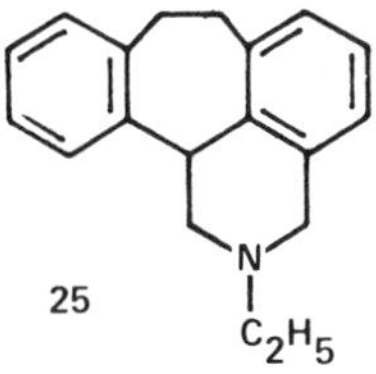

Voith and Herr found[22] that taclamine exerted a taming effect in septal-lesioned rats and in isolation-induced, aggressive mice. Low doses attenuated conflict behavior and there was a wide separation between doses causing behavioral and ataxic effects. Taclamine showed only weak anticonvulsant activity.

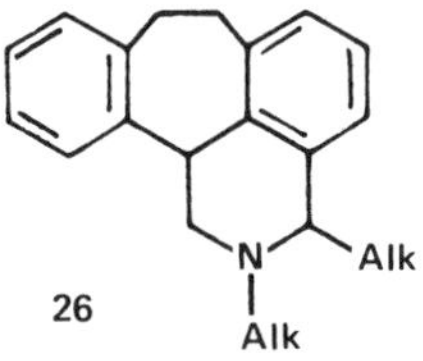

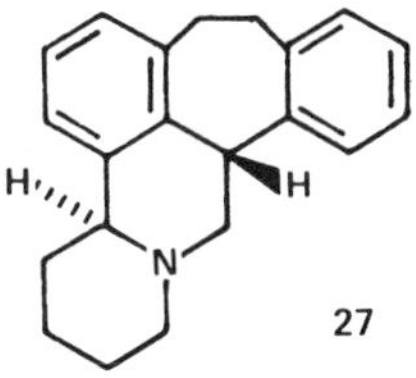

Taclamine was not commercially developed; however, studies on its synthesis and stereochemistry were instrumental in the subsequent development of butaclamol. In our early studies with the Schiff's base 24,[19] we reacted it with methyl vinyl ketone to afford a mixture of the *cis* and *trans* pentacyclic aminoketones 28 and 29 (Figure 4), which were not separated. Several years later when the reaction was repeated, the isomeric aminoketones, formed in a 1:5 ratio, were separated chromatographically and each was deoxygenated by desulfurization of its ethylene thioketal derivative. The product from the more abundant aminoketone afforded taclamine, while the less abundant isomer afforded a product, 30, devoid of taming effects.

At that time the 4a,13b-configurations in the pentacyclic derivatives 27-30 were unknown. An examination of the NMR spectra of taclamine 27 and its isomer 30 revealed that the benzhydrilic C13b proton in taclamine appeared as a triplet centered at 4.9δ, while the similar proton in 30 appeared as a doublet centered at 4.5δ. Inspection of Dreiding models of the most stable conformations of the *cis* and *trans* isomers revealed that the dihedral angles between the C13b proton and those at C_{14} were markedly different in the isomer pair. The Newman projection, shown in Figure 5, revealed angles of 20 and 90° for 30, and 35 and 146° for 27. On this basis taclamine (27) was assigned a 4a,13b-*trans* configuration.

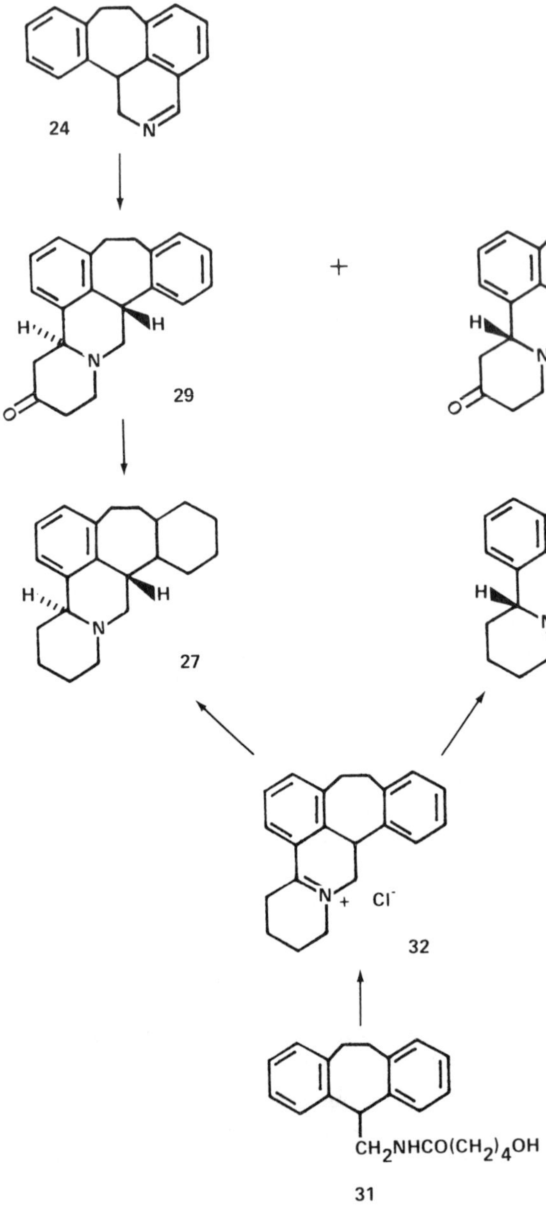

Figure 4.

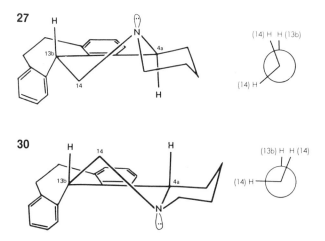

Figure 5.

We subsequently developed a simpler and more direct synthesis for taclamine, a stereomechanistic consideration of which serves to support the configurational assignments made above. Thus **31**, the adduct formed from the aminomethyl compound **18** and valerolactone (Figure 4), was subjected to a double cyclization with phosphorous oxychloride to afford the pentacyclic quinolizinium salt **32**. Catalytic reduction of this salt would be expected to proceed by way of adsorbtion of the planar rings' CDE region to the catalyst from the less-hindered β-face whence hydrogen would be delivered to generate a 4a,13b-*cis* relative configuration. Indeed, catalytic hydrogenation afforded the isomer **30**, which had been assigned a 4a,13b-*cis* configuration on the basis of NMR considerations. In contrast, reduction with zinc and hydrochloric acid afforded taclamine **27**, which had been assigned a *trans* configuration.

In this way the elucidation of the stereochemistry of taclamine also clarified the stereochemistry of the aminoketone **29**, the major product of the addition of methyl vinyl ketone to the Schiff's base. The ready availability of this *trans*-aminoketone, now no longer required for the synthesis of taclamine, prompted a study of its chemistry. Reaction of **29** with ethyl magnesium bromide afforded the tertiary ethyl carbinol **33**, which was found to antagonize amphetamine stereotyped behavior, suggestive of neuroleptic activity. The ethyl carbinol was about as active as chlorpromazine.

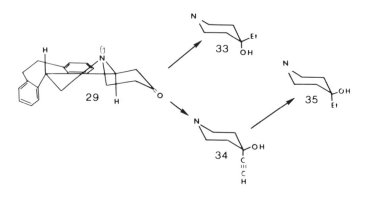

Figure 6.

The synthesis of the tertiary ethyl carbinol introduced a new stereochemical element in that the configuration at position 3 was unknown. This problem was resolved to our satisfaction by the observation that the reaction of the *trans*-aminoketone **29** with sodium acetylide (Figure 6) afforded the acetylenic carbinol **34**, which on catalytic reduction, afforded **35**, an isomer of ethyl carbinol **33**. We concluded that the small linear acetylide anion reacted with the carbonyl group by an axial attack to generate, after reduction, the isomer **35** with an equatorial hydroxyl group, while the bulkier ethyl anion was restricted to attack from the least hindered equatorial direction to give **33** with an axial hydroxyl group, that is, a 3(OH),13b(H)-*trans* relative configuration.

A variety of tertiary carbinols (see Table 1) were synthesized from the appropriate Grignard reagent or aryllithium.[24,25] On the basis of the above considerations, they were assigned 3(OH),13b(H)-*trans* relative configurations whenever the 3-substituent was bulkier than an ethyl group. These stereochemical assignments, as well as the 4a,13b-*trans* relative configurations deduced earlier on the basis of mechanistic and spectral considerations, were fully confirmed for the (+)-3-isopropyl and the (±)3-*tert*-butyl analogues dexclamol and butaclamol by x-ray crystallographic studies.[26]

The tertiary carbinols in Table 1 were evaluated for neuroleptic activity. The primary screen was the antagonism of amphetamine-induced stereotypy in rats,[27] one of the most selective and sensitive tests for typical neuroleptics[28] since amphetamine-induced stereotypy can be regarded as an animal model of human psychosis.[29] Neuroleptic drugs antagonize amphetamine-induced

Table 1

Effects on (+)-Amphetamine-induced Stereotype of 3-Substituted Benzo[6,7]-cyclohepta[1,2,3-de]pyrido[2,1-a]isoquinolin-3-ols[24,25]

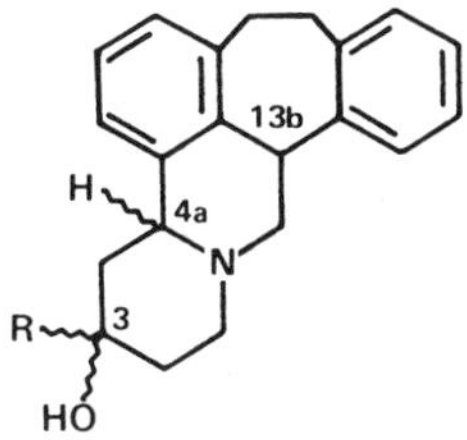

Compound No.	R =	Relative Configuration		Antagonism of ASB MED (mg/kg, i.p.)[a]
		4a,13b	3(OH),13b(H)	
1	tert-C₄H₉	trans	trans	0.62
33	C₂H₅	trans	trans	10.0
34	C≡CH	trans	cis	Inactive
35	C₂H₄	trans	cis	Inactive
36	CH₃	trans	Unknown	>20.0
37	C₂H₅	cis	cis	Inactive
38	C≡CH	cis	cis	Inactive
39	n-C₃H₇	trans	trans	15.0
40	cyclo-C₃H₅	trans	trans	1.25
41	iso-C₃H₇	trans	trans	1.25
42	CH₂CH=CH₂	trans	Unknown	>20.0
43	n-C₄H₉	trans	trans	10.0
44	tert-C₄H₉	cis	trans	Inactive
45	n-C₆H₁₃	trans	trans	5.0
46	cyclo-C₆H₁₁	trans	trans	1.25
47	C₆H₅	trans	trans	2.5
48	2-CH₃-C₆H₄	trans	trans	1.25
49	C₆H₅CH₂	trans	trans	>20.0
50	2(OCH₃)C₆H₄	trans	trans	0.63
51	3(OCH₃)C₆H₄	trans	trans	1.25
52	4(OCH₃)C₆H₄	trans	trans	2.5
53	3,4(OCH₃)₂-C₆H₃	trans	trans	5.0
54	2,4(OCH₃)₂-C₆H₃	trans	trans	10.0

Table 1 (contd.)

Compound No.	R =	Relative Configuration 4a,13b	3(OH),13b(H)	Antagonism of ASB MED (mg/kg, i.p.)[a]
55	2-ClC$_6$H$_4$	trans	trans	2.5
56	3-F-C$_6$H$_4$	trans	trans	5.0
57	4-Br-C$_6$H$_4$	trans	trans	20.0
58	2-CF$_3$-C$_6$H$_4$	trans	trans	10.0
59	2-Thienyl	trans	trans	2.5
60	3-Thienyl	trans	trans	5.0
61	2-Furyl	trans	trans	5.0
62	3-Pyridyl	trans	trans	5.0
63	Chlorpromazine			7.5
64	Fluphenazine			0.5

[a]MED = minimal effective dose, defined as the dose that antagonized all the behavioral effects of amphetamine (10 mg/kg, i.p.) during the entire 4-hour experimental period.

stereotyped behavior through blockade of postsynaptic dopamine receptors. The antipsychotic activity in schizophrenic patients is probably also mediated by this mechanism, since a positive correlation exists between antiamphetamine activity and therapeutic effect.[30,31]

The antiamphetamine effects of the tertiary carbinols are shown in Table 1 and the results are expressed as the minimal effective dose (MED), arbitrarily defined as the lowest dose that antagonized *all* the behavioral effects of amphetamine. Chlorpromazine and fluphenazine were used as reference standards.

The *tert*-butyl derivative, butaclamol, was about equipotent to fluphenazine, having a MED of 0.62 mg/kg, i.p., and was selected for detailed evaluation.

It was demonstrated that butaclamol antagonized amphetamine toxicity in aggregated mice and apomorphine-induced emesis in dogs. It depressed both discriminated avoidance and continuous lever pressing behavior in rats and inhibited ambulation and rearing in the open field. At higher doses, butaclamol induced catalepsy. Adrenergic blocking activity, measured by the antagonism of epinephrine-induced mortality, was weak.[27]

Butaclamol was also shown to induce an increase in rat striatal homovanillic acid concentration *in vivo* and to block the dopamine-induced increase in adenylate cyclase activity of homogenates of the olfactory tubercule.[32] In addition, butaclamol was shown to directly increase brain dopamine turnover.[33]

On the basis of this pharmacological and biochemical profile, it was predicted that butaclamol would be a potent antipsychotic drug, with a potency comparable to that of fluphenazine. These predictions were fully substantiated in open and double-blind clinical studies.[34-40]

The development of a novel molecular entity that possesses the predicted clinical activity and is a useful agent in man is usually regarded as an end point of pharmaceutical research and a source of satisfaction to those involved. In the case of butaclamol, useful benefits extended beyond the not unsubstantial development of a clinically active drug to include the development of a dopamine receptor binding assay and the description of topographical features of the dopamine receptor macromolecule.

The pharmacological, biochemical, and clinical studies referred to above were all performed with racemic (±)-butaclamol. When (±)-butaclamol was resolved it was shown that all the activity, both *in vivo*[41,42] and *in vitro*,[43] resided exclusively in the (+)-enantiomer (see Table 2), which had been shown through crystallographic studies to have 3S,4aS, and 13bS absolute configurations.[26] At the time, (±)-butaclamol was the only neuroleptic that exhibited absolute enantiospecificity at the dopamine receptor. Since then several such neuroleptic enantiomer pairs have been uncovered.[44]

The *in vivo* findings with the butaclamol enantiomers were first disclosed in abstract form[45] in early 1974, just after the first demonstration of high-affinity, specific binding of [³H]naloxone to the opiate receptor by Pert and Snyder[46] using the enantiomer pair (-)-levorphanol and (+)-dextrorphan to distinguish between specific and nonspecific binding, and just after the confirmation of these findings had been published by Terenius[47] and by Simon et al.[48] It was apparent that the enantiospecificity displayed by the dopamine receptor toward the butaclamol enantiomers could lead to a dopamine receptor binding assay, and within a short time after the publication of our abstracts, requests for samples were received from Prof. Seeman at the University of Toronto and from Prof. Snyder at Johns Hopkins University. Both groups were successful in developing independently, an assay for the dopamine receptor and their results were published, coincidentally, in the same issue of the *Proceedings of the National Academy of Science* in late 1975.[49,50]

This binding assay has contributed substantially to knowledge of dopamine receptors in normal, as well as diseased, states. It has been shown, for example,

Table 2
Dopamine Receptor Antagonist Properties of Butaclamol and Analogues

Compound	Antagonism of ASB MED[a] (mg/kg, i.p.)	Inhibition of [³H]haloperidol binding IC_{50} $(nM)^{b}$
(±)-Butaclamol·HCl	0.62	3.5
(+)-Butaclamol·HBr	0.31	1.4
(−)-Butaclamol·HBr	>50 [c]	>1000[d]
(±)-Isobutaclamol·HCl	0.62	1.7
(+)-Isobutaclamol·HBr	0.31	0.8
(+)-Isobutaclamol·HBr	>25 [c]	>1000[d]
(±)-Anhydrobutaclamol·HCl	0.62	9.5
(±)-Deoxybutaclamol·HCl	0.62	6.3

[a]Minimal effective dose antagonizing amphetamine stereotypy. For methodology see reference 27.
[b]For methodology see reference 43.
[c]Highest dose tested.
[d]Highest concentration tested.

that in postmortem brains of parkinsonian[51] and schizophrenic patients[52,53] the number of dopamine receptors was increased. Furthermore, chronic treatment of rats with neuroleptic drugs resulted in an enhanced behavioral sensitivity to dopamine receptor stimulants such as apomorphine. Several investigators[54-56] have demonstrated, using the binding assay, that in such chronically treated animals, the total number of dopamine receptors in the basal ganglia was increased. Supersensitivity following chronic neuroleptic treatment is regarded as a model of tardive dyskinesia, which is a late clinical complication of prolonged neuroleptic therapy.

In our own laboratories, we studied the molecular structure of butaclamol and its congeners in an attempt to define its mode of interaction with the dopamine receptor and to identify topographical features of the dopamine receptor.

It was recognized early[42] that there existed common structural features in (+)-butaclamol and (-)-apomorphine (65), a widely studied dopamine receptor agonist, the (+)-enantiomer of which is devoid of dopaminergic activity.[57] Thus, in common with (-)-apomorphine, (+)-butaclamol contains within its molecular framework, two phenethylamine moieties, one of which is con-

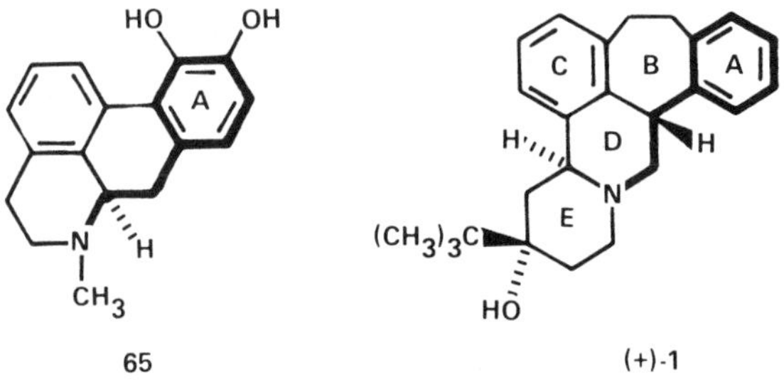

Figure 7.

strained within an isoquinolinic system while the other is in an extended form. Studies on the dopaminergic activity of (-)-apomorphine, and various analogues and fragments thereof, have established that this activity is associated with its dihydroxylated extended phenethylamine moiety (see Figure 7).[58] The topography of this unit, which likely represents also the receptor-site conformation of the endogenous neurotransmitter dopamine, was quantitatively defined in terms of parameters derived from crystallographic data.[59] The parameters, namely, the values of key torsion angles τ, the radial distance from the nitrogen to the center of ring A, and the out-of-plant displacement of the nitrogen with respect to ring A are shown in Table 3. A positive value for the last parameter implies that the nitrogen atom lies above the plane of ring A with the molecules oriented as in Figure 7. Values for parameters defining the topography of (+)-butaclamol's extended phenethylamine moiety are also shown in Table 3, for the conformer A extant in the crystal structure and for the conformer B obtained by rotation about the CH_2-CH_2 bond of the cycloheptane ring (see Figure 8).

The data in Table 3 permitted a comparison of the topographies of the extended phenethylamine moieties of (-)-apomorphine with those of conformers A and B of (+)-butaclamol. It was shown[26,42] that the phenethylamine groupings of (-)-apomorphine and conformer B of (+)-butaclamol can be aligned with the phenyl rings A coplanar and concentric and with the nitrogen atoms coincident. On the basis of the common topographical features in these two molecules, conformer B of (+)-butaclamol was designated as its receptor-site conformation.

These observations led to the definition of the *neuroleptic pharmacophore* as a phenyl ring and a nitrogen atom, oriented such that the values for the distance of the nitrogen from the plane of the phenyl ring and the radial distance from the nitrogen to the center of the phenyl ring are similar to those for

Table 3

Parameters Associated with the Conformations of the Phenethylamine Moieties in (+)-Butaclamol and (−)-Apomorphine[26]

Parameter	(+)-Butaclamol		(−)-Apomorphine[a]
	Conformer A[a]	Conformer B[b]	
$\tau(C_{13a}C_{13b}\text{-}C_{14}\text{-}N)$	-169°	-155°	—
$\tau(C_{13}\text{-}C_{13a}\text{-}C_{13b}\text{-}C_{14})$	17°	5°	—
$\tau(C_{7a}\text{-}C_7\text{-}C_{6a}\text{-}N)$	—	—	178, 178°
$\tau(C_8\text{-}C_{7a}\text{-}C_7\text{-}C_{6a})$	—	—	-146, -135°
Distance of N from Ring A plane	0.19A	-0.9A	-0.9, -1.23A
Distance of N from center of ring A	5.1 A	5.1A	5.12, 5.09A

[a]Derived from crystallographic data.
[b]Derived from measurements on Dreiding models.

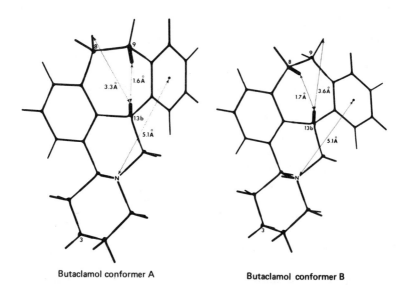

Butaclamol conformer A   Butaclamol conformer B

Figure 8. Shadowgraphs of Dreiding models of the nuclei of (+)-butaclamol conformers (the distances shown are from measurements on Dreiding models).

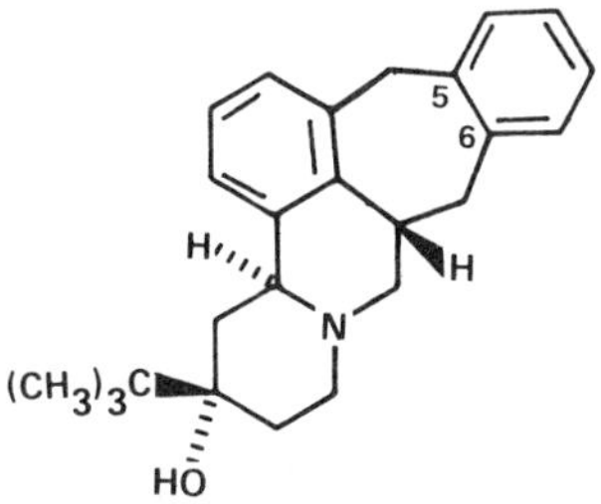

66

(-)-apomorphine and (+)-butaclamol, conformer B, as shown in Table 3. This pharmacophore has since been found to be present, or potentially present, in a wide range of dopamine receptor agonists, as well as antagonists.[60] Based on this pharmacophore and complementary binding sites on the dopamine receptor, we have proposed a model of the dopamine receptor in which the elements of the pharmacophore are uniquely oriented in a cartesian coordinate system.[61]

An additional feature of the model derived from a study of isobutaclamol (**66**), a benzo[5,6]cyclohepta analogue of butaclamol, whose synthesis, resolution, absolute configuration, and crystal structure have recently been reported.[62-64] (+)-Isobutaclamol was found to be equipotent to (+)-butaclamol both *in vivo* and *in vitro* (see Table 2), while (-)-isobutaclamol was devoid of dopamine antagonist properties. (+)-Butaclamol and (+)-isobutaclamol interact with the same receptor and both ligands should adopt similar conformations to facilitate these interactions. The conformer B of (+)-isobutaclamol (Figure 9) was designated as its receptor-site conformation. It differs from the conformation seen in the crystal structure (Figure 10),[64] in that ring E, which exists in the crystal with a cisoid rings DE fusion, is assumed to undergo nitrogen inversion by way of the deprotonated species to afford a conformation with a transoid DE fusion, as was observed in the crystal structure of butaclamol (Figure 11). In contrast, unlike butaclamol, (+)-isobutaclamol exists in the crystal with its cycloheptane ring in conformation B, which is similar to the deduced receptor-site conformation of (+)-butaclamol.

An analysis of the molecular structure of (+)-isobutaclamol, conformer B, revealed that while the out-of-plane displacement of the nitrogen with respect to phenyl ring A is the same as in (+)-butaclamol conformer B (0.9 Å), the radial distance from the center of ring A to the nitrogen (6.4 Å) is markedly different from that in (+)-butaclamol, conformer B (5.1 Å), suggesting that these

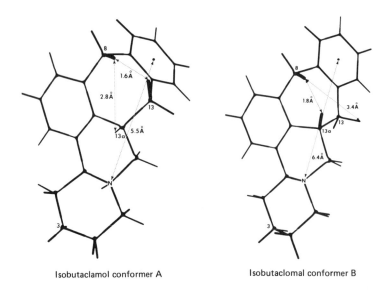

Isobutaclamol conformer A   Isobutaclomal conformer B

Figure 9.   Shadowgraphs of Dreiding models of the nuclei of (+)-iso-butaclamol conformers (the distances shown are from measurements on Dreiding models).

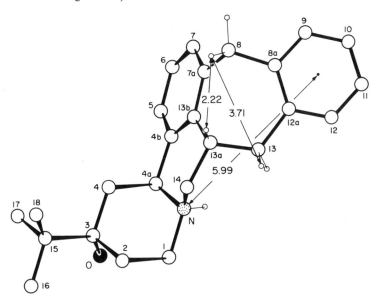

Figure 10.   Crystal structure of (+)-isobutaclamol hydrobromide (the distances indicated in Å are calculated from the crystallographic data).

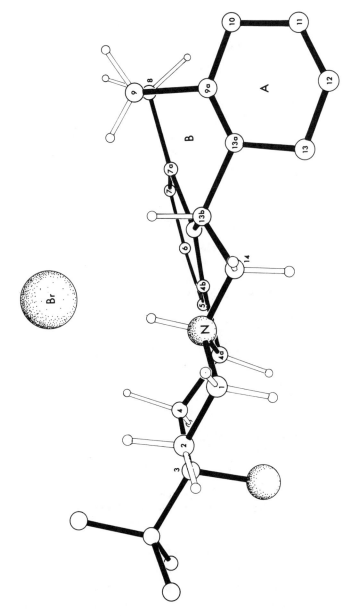

Figure 11. Crystal structure of (±)-butaclamol hydrobromide.

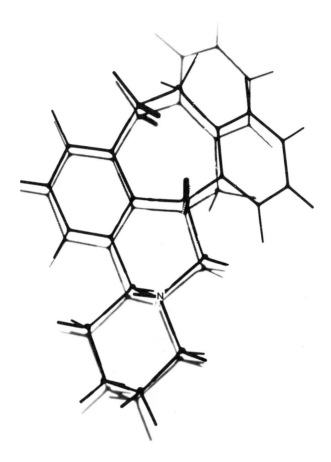

Figure 12. Superimposed shadowgraphs of Dreiding models of the nuclei of B conformers of (+)-butaclamol and (+)-isobutaclamol.

two ligands would be incapable of presenting the same pharmacophore. When, however, Dreiding models of the two ligands are superimposed (Figure 12), corresponding atoms of each of the pair are found to be coincident, with the exception of three-carbon atom segments of the rings A of each (Figure 12). Further, the phenyl rings A of both ligands were found to lie in the same plane and to be immediately adjacent to each other. It was concluded that the dopamine receptor macromolecule contains a planar phenyl ring binding site that has the dimensions of at least two adjacent benzene rings.

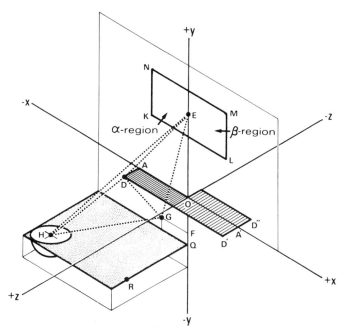

Figure 13. Representation of the lipophilic binding site and the primary binding sites on the dopamine receptor (see text). The figure is drawn to a scale of 1 cm = 1Å. Key distances are: $Q\text{-}E = 4.7$; $A\text{-}D = 0.9$; $D\text{-}E = 5.7$; $A\text{-}Q = 3.2$; $D\text{-}G = 2.6$; $H\text{-}E = 9.6$; $D\text{-}H = 4.5$; $O\text{-}F = 1.8$; $O\text{-}Q = 2.5$; $H\text{-}G = 6.5$; $Q\text{-}R = 5.0$; $H\text{-}R = 4.0$; $F\text{-}Q = 0.7$; $N\text{-}K = M\text{-}L = 2.4$; $K\text{-}L = M\text{-}N = 4.8$.

This conclusion was incorporated into our model of the dopamine receptor (Figure 13) in terms of a planar aromatic binding site composed of α- and β-regions that are occupied by the phenyl rings A of (+)-butaclamol and (+)-isobutaclamol, respectively, when they interact with the receptor.

The distances in Figure 13 were obtained from models of the conformers B of (+)-butaclamol and (+)-isobutaclamol, oriented in a cartesian coordinate system calibrated in angstroms, such that rings A were located in the xy plane with their centers positioned at the centers of the α- and β-regions, respectively, at a distance above the x-axis proportional to 4.7 Å and with the nitrogen atom located at point D in the $-x + z$ plane.

The model also shows the coordinates of point G, the location of an electronegative atom that was proposed to participate in hydrogen bond formation with the nitrogen atom. Arguments based on this model have been used[62] to rationalize the observed enantiospecificity of the dopamine receptor toward the butaclamol enantiomers.

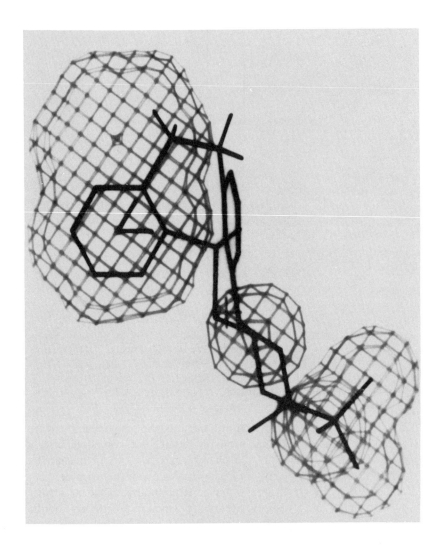

Figure 14. Model of the dopamine receptor, with the (+)-isobutaclamol molecule superimposed, generated by the MMS-X computer-based molecular modeling and graphic display system. (Courtesy of Dr. G. Marshall, Washington University, St. Louis.)

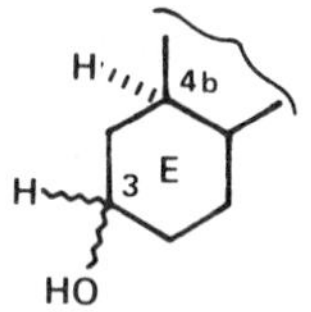

67 (3H,4b-H-*Trans*)
68 (3H,4b-H-*Cis*)

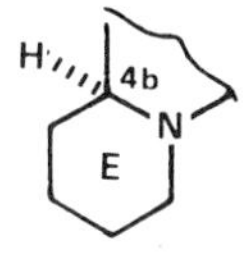

69

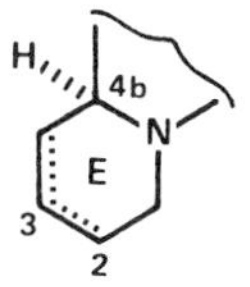

70

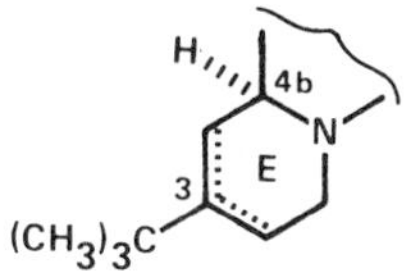

71

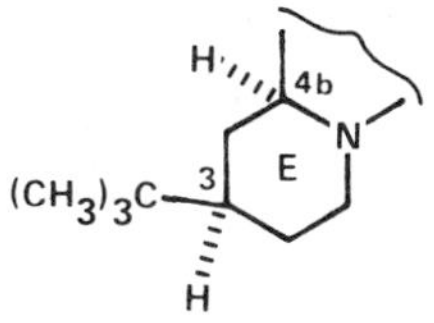

72

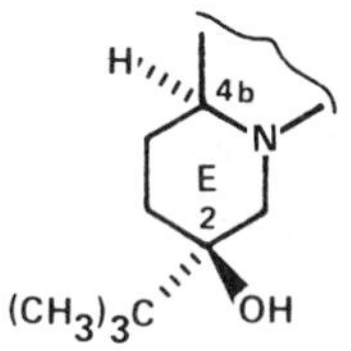

73

Another important feature of the model derived from a study of congeners of butaclamol involving modifications in ring E.[61] Of the analogues studied (67-73), only (±)-anhydrobutaclamol (71) and (±)-deoxybutaclamol (72) retained dopamine receptor blocking properties, being about equipotent to (±)-butaclamol both *in vivo* and *in vitro* (Table 2). Clearly, all the analogues that lacked a *tert*-butyl group at position 3 were inactive, while all active analogues retained this feature. It was apparent that dopamine receptor blocking activity in the benzocycloheptapyridoisoquinoline series is critically dependent on the presence of a *tert*-butyl or similar bulky group attached equatorially to the 3-position of the nucleus.

This conclusion led to the incorporation into the model of the dopamine receptor of an accessory lipophilic binding site on the receptor macromolecule, centered at position H, that binds strongly to the *tert*-butyl group of butaclamol and accounts for a major portion of its observed affinity for the dopamine receptor. The coordinates and volume of this lipophilic binding site were derived from crystallographic data.

Figure 14 is another representation of the receptor model, generated with the MMS-X computer-based molecular modeling and graphic display system.[65] Input data comprised the $x\,y\,z$ coordinates of those atoms of (+)-butaclamol and (+)-isobutaclamol, in their receptor-site conformations, that served to define the α- and β-regions of the aromatic binding site, the nitrogen atom location site, and the lipophilic accessory binding site. The coordinates were obtained either from crystallographic results, or from a program that generates coordinate data from bond lengths and angles.[66] The display, Figure 14, is in the form of an electron density map of the atoms referred to above, contoured to their van der Waals radii (light lines). The display also shows the molecule of (+)-butaclamol (heavy lines) superimposed on the receptor model.

This form of the receptor model has proved to be of great value for conveniently examining known and candidate dopamine receptor ligands for the presence of a pharmacophore compatible with the requirements of the dopamine receptor.

In conclusion, this account of the development of butaclamol constitutes another example from the annals of medicinal chemistry, where a speculative, but goal-oriented chemistry program, combined with unexpected pharmacological findings, has led to drugs with high potency and great specificity. In addition, the unique properties of butaclamol and its congeners have allowed some insights to be gained into the nature of various aspects of the dopamine receptor.

ACKNOWLEDGMENTS
I acknowledge the efforts of Drs. Francois Bruderlein and Adolf Philipp, my principal chemical collaborators during the course of work described, and Dr. Katherine Voith, who was responsible for uncovering the psychopharmacological profile of butaclamol.

REFERENCES

1. T. Charpentier, U.S. Patents 2,519,886 and 2,530,451 (1950).

2. J. Delay, T. Deniker, and J. M. Harl, *Ann. Med. Psychol. Fr.* **110**, 112 (1952).

3. H. E. Lehmann and G. E. Hanrahan, *A.M.A. Arch. Neurol. Psychiat.*, **71**, 227 (1954).

4. F. Haflinger and W. Schindler, U.S. Patent 2,554,736 (1951).

5. R. Kuhn, *Schweiz. Med. Wochenschr.*, **87**, 1135 (1957).

6. P. V. Petersen, N. Lassen, T. Holm, R. Kopf, and I. Moller-Nielsen, *Arzneim.-Forsch.*, **8**, 395 (1958).

7. For a review see M. Protiva, *Farmaco, Ed. Sci.,* **21**, 76 (1966).

8. File wrapper of U.S. patent application, S.N. 802, 298, filed March 27, 1959, now U.S. Patent 3,384,663, issued to G. Rey-Bellet and H. Spiegelberg and assigned to Hoffmann-LaRoche. Other applications cited in the file wrapper are: (a) S.N. 855,981, E. L. Engelhard (Merck), filed Nov. 30, 1959; (b) S.N. 828,722, F. J. Villani (Schering), filed July 22, 1959; (c) S.N. 27,267, S. O. Winthrop (Ayerst), filed May 6, 1960; (d) J. Mills (Lilly), filing date and serial number not disclosed.

9. S. O. Winthrop, M. A. Davis, G. S. Myers, J. G. Gavin, R. Thomas, and R. Barber, *J. Org. Chem.*, **27**, 230 (1962).

10. F. Herr, J. Stewart, and M. P. Charest, *Arch. Int. Pharmacodyn.,* **134**, 328 (1961).

11. L. G. Humber, M. A. Davis, R. A. Thomas, R. Otson, and J. R. Watson, *J. Heterocycl. Chem.*, **3**, 247 (1966).

12. C. Van Der Stelt, A. Haasjes, H. M. Tersteege, and W. Th. Nauta, *Rec. Trav. Chim.*, **84**, 1466 (1965).

13. E. Galantay, H. Agahigian, and N. Paolella, Abstracts, American Chemical Society, Middle Atlantic Meeting, Philadelphia, PA, Feb. 3-4, 1966, subsequently published in *J. Am. Chem. Soc.,* **88,** 3875 (1966).
14. E. Galantay, C. Hoffman, N. Paolella, J. Gogerty, L. Iorio, G. Leslie, and J. H. Trapold, *J. Med. Chem.,* **12,** 444 (1969).
15. P. A. S. Smith, *Molecular Rearrangements,* Part I, P. de Mayo, Ed., John Wiley, New York, 1963, p. 522.
16. E. Galantay, U.S. Patent 3,310,565 (March 21, 1967).
17. L. G. Humber, C. H. Chou, M. A. Davis, M. Georgiades, and F. T. Bruderlein, Canadian Patent 1,000,071 (Nov. 30, 1976).
18. C. H. Chou, A. Asselin, K. Pelz, and L. G. Humber, Canadian Patent 1,047,031 (Jan. 23, 1979).
19. L. G. Humber, M. A. Davis, G. Beaulieu, and M. -P. Charest, *Can. J. Chem.,* **46,** 2981 (1968).
20. K. Voith, personal communication.
21. L. G. Humber and M. A. Davis, U.S. Patent 3,403,157 (Sept. 24, 1968).
22. K. Voith and F. Herr; Abstracts of papers, 5th International Congress of Pharmacology, San Francisco, 1972, Abstract No. 1457.
23. F.T. Bruderlein, L. G. Humber, and K. Pelz, *Can. J. Chem.,* **52,** 2119 (1974).
24. F. T. Bruderlein, L. G. Humber, and K. Voith, *J. Med. Chem.,* **18,** 185 (1975).
25. K. Voith, F. T. Bruderlein, and L. G. Humber, *J. Med. Chem.,* **21,** 694 (1978).
26. P. Bird, F. T. Bruderlein, and L. G. Humber, *Can. J. Chem.,* **54,** 2715 (1976).
27. K. Voith and F. Herr, *Psychopharmacologia (Berl.),* **42,** 11 (1975).
28. P. A. J. Janssen, C. J. E. Niemegeers, and K. H. L. Schellekens, *Arzneim.-Forsch.,* **15,** 104 (1965).
29. A. Randrup and I. Munkvad, *Proc. Int. Symp. Amphetamines Relat. Compd.,* **1969,** 695-713 (1970).
30. H. M. van Praag, *Br. J. Psychiat.,* **130,** 463 (1977).
31. I. Creese, D. R. Burt, and S. H. Snyder, *Science,* **192,** 481 (1976).
32. W. Lippmann, T. A. Pugsley, and J. Merker, *Life Sci.,* **16,** 213 (1975).
33. W. Lippmann and T. A. Pugsley, *Pharmacol. Res. Commun.,* **7,** 371 (1975).
34. D. H. Mielke, D. M. Gallant, T. Oelsner, C. M. Kessler, W. K. Tomlinson, and G. H. Cohen, *Dis. Nerv. Syst.,* **36,** 7 (1975).
35. L. E. Hollister, K. L. Davis, and P. A. Berger, *Psychopharmacol. Commun.,* **1,** 493 (1975).
36. J. M. Gallart-Capdevila, *Arch. Neurobiol.,* **38,** 545 (1975).
37. F. Imaz, T. A. Ban, and H. E. Lehmann, *Psychopharmacol. Bull.,* **12,** 31 (1976).
38. M. L. Clark, A. Paredes, J. P. Costiloe, and F. Wood, *J. Clin. Pharmacol.,* **17,** 529 (1977).
39. M. L. Clark, J. P. Costiloe, F. Wood, A. Paredes, and G. Fulkerson, *Dis. Nerv. System.,* **38,** 943 (1977).
40. J. H. Nesteros, H. E. Lehmann, and T. A. Ban, *Int. Pharmacopsychiat.,* **13,** 138 (1977).
41. K. Voith and J. R. Cummings, *Can. J. Physiol. Pharmacol.,* **54,** 551 (1976).
42. L. G. Humber, F. T. Bruderlein, and K. Voith, *Mol. Pharmacol.,* **11,** 833 (1975).
43. T. A. Pugsley and W. Lippman, *J. Pharm. Pharmacol.,* **31,** 47 (1979).
44. P. Seeman, K. Westman, M. Protiva, J. Jilek, A. Saxena, N. Anand, L. Humber, and A. Philipp, *Eur. J. Pharmacol.,* **57,** 247 (1979).
45. L. G. Humber and F. T. Bruderlein, Abstracts of Papers, National Meeting of the American Chemical Society, Los Angeles, Medi-5, 174; K. Voith, *ibid.,* Medi-6.
46. C. B. Pert and S. H. Snyder, *Science,* **179,** 1011 (1973).
47. L. Terenius, *Acta Pharmacol. Toxicol.,* **32,** 317 (1973).

48. E. J. Simon, J. M. Hiller, and I. Edelman, *Proc. Natl. Acad. Sci. U.S.,* **70,** 1947 (1973).
49. P. Seeman, M. Chau-Wong, J. Tedesco, and K. Wong, *Proc. Natl. Acad. Sci., U.S.,* **72,** 4376 (1975).
50. D. S. Burt, S. J. Enna, I. Creese, and S. H. Snyder, *Proc. Natl. Acad. Sci.,* **72,** 4655 (1975).
51. T. Lee, P. Seeman, A. Rajpup, I. Farley, and O. Hornykiewicz, *Nature,* **273,** 59 (1978).
52. T. Lee, P. Seeman, W. W. Tourtellotte, I. J. Farley and O. Hornykiewicz, *Nature,* **274,** 897 (1978).
53. F. Owen, T. Crow, M. Poulter, A. Cross, A. Longden, and G. Riley, *Lancet,* **2,** 223 (1978).
54. D. R. Burt, I. Creese, and S. H. Snyder, *Science,* **196,** 326 (1977).
55. P. Muller and P. Seeman, *Life Sci.,* **21,** 1751 (1977).
56. A. Hitri, W. Weiner, R. Borison, B. Diamond, P. Nausieda, and H. Klawans, *Ann. Neurol.,* **3,** 134 (1978).
57. W. S. Saari, S. W. King, V. J. Lotti, and A. Scriabine, *J. Med. Chem.,* **17,** 1086 (1974).
58. For a review see P. C. Jain and N. Kumar, *Progress in Drug Research,* Vol. 21, E. Jucker, Ed., Birkhauser Verlag, Basel, 1977, p. 409.
59. J. Giesecke, *Acta Crystallogr.,* **B29,** 1785 (1973); **B33,** 302 (1977).
60. G. R. Marshall, D. A. Dunn, C. D. Barry, and L. G. Humber, unpublished.
61. L. G. Humber, F. T. Bruderlein, A. H. Philipp, M. Gotz, and K. Voith, *J. Med. Chem.,* **22,** 761 (1979).
62. A. H. Philipp, L. G. Humber, and K. Voith, *J. Med. Chem.,* **22,** 768 (1979).
63. L. G. Humber, A. H. Philipp, K. Voith, T. Pugsley, W. Lippmann, F. R. Ahmed, and M. Przybylska, *J. Med. Chem.,* **22,** 899 (1979).
64. F. R. Ahmed and M. Przybylska, *Acta Crystallogr.,* **B35** 2169 (1979).
65. C. D. Barry, H. E. Bosshard, R. A. Ellis, and G. R. Marshall, *Fed. Proc.,* **33,** 2368 (1974).
66. G. R. Marshall, personal communication.

Clonidine

4

Helmut Stähle

Discovery needs luck, invention, intellect; neither can do without the other.

J.W.v. GOETHE

And in due respect to Goethe's genius I might add: But patience, hope, and expectation also play an important part.

1. INTRODUCTION

It is in the imagination of the synthetic organic chemist that new molecules are conceived. Unfortunately, attempts to realize such structural ideas are often hindered by unexpected pitfalls and a successful reduction to practice is not guaranteed. Seldom can a chemist work on his own free-wheeling ideas and conceptions, undisturbed by extraneous regulations and obligations.

A synthetic chemist may choose from among a multitude of approaches for the design of his targets. Among the more reliable of such approaches is that which patterns synthetic goals on structures with established efficacy, and the chemist tries to improve the therapeutic effect of these structures by molecular modifications. This is very likely the approach chosen by a young chemist starting his career among a team of experienced research experts in the pharmaceutical industry. In my case this happened in 1960. I was not in fact a pure-bred chemist but a pharmacist with medicinal chemical ambitions.

2. THE SYNTHETIC TASK

In the beginning of the sixties I was asked to synthesize a peripherally active α-adrenergic compound that would be useful for nasal decongestion as simple

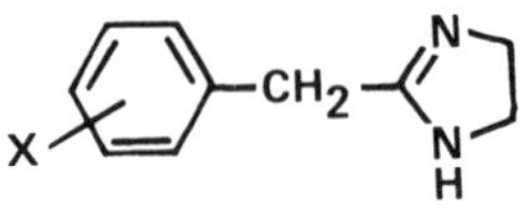

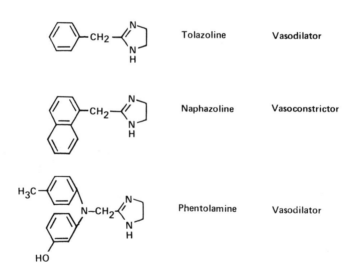

Figure 1. General structure of the classical imidazolines with α-adrenergic activity.[2]

nose drops. Swelling of blood vessels of the mucous membranes of the nasal passage, nasal discharge, and obstruction are some of the most distressing symptoms of the common cold. A locally acting α-adrenergic vasoconstrictor agent was expected to provide relief by shrinking the swollen nasal membranes and producing an unobstructed air passage. I quickly found out that most of the newer decongestive agents were derived from the imidazoline structure (Figure 1).[1] The task of designing a new analogue was not particularly challenging, but nevertheless there was some hope that it might result in an unexpected activity, as I noticed that some related imidazolines (Figure 2) did have other pharmacological actions. Tolazoline and phentolamine, for example, had α-blocking activity and were highly effective vasodilators, although, unfortunately, they were useful only in a limited range in therapeutics because of their side effects.[2]

Tolazoline	Vasodilator
Naphazoline	Vasoconstrictor
Phentolamine	Vasodilator

Figure 2. Imidazolines as therapeutics.

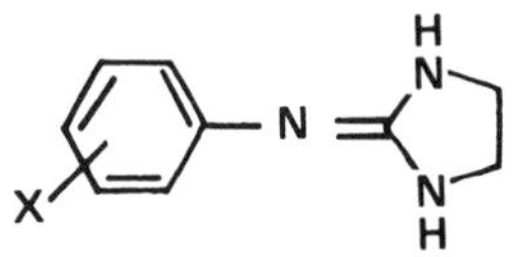

Figure 3. General structure of 2-(arylimino)imidazolidines.

The decongestive imidazolines are substituted amidines in which the amidine function is incorporated into an imidazoline ring. Additionally, this portion is connected with an aromatic nucleus by way of a methylene (—CH$_2$—) bridge. The first fundamental alteration of this basic structure was reported by several research teams,[3] who replaced the —CH$_2$— bridge by an —NH— group. This resulted in a new general structure shown in Figure 3, which in effect builds a guanidine-like function into the molecule. However, at that time a replacement of the —CH$_2$— bridge by an —NH— group had not been achieved chemically in compounds substituted at both the 2- and 6-positions of the phenyl ring. Clearly, steric hindrance by the two *ortho* substituents was an obstacle to the successful synthesis of such compounds by conventional methods,[3] and 2,6-di-substituted 2-(arylimino)imidazolidines (Figure 4) were to remain unknown in the literature until the completion of our work.

When planning my synthetic targets I was fascinated by the idea of achieving a synthesis of the 2,6-disubstituted 2-(arylimino)imidazolidines which had been attempted so often, but without success. My analysis of structure and activity of the 2-(arylmethyl)imidazolines had indicated that compounds with this substitution pattern would represent the most effective substances.[4] Thus I explicitly expected good vasoconstrictive and decongestive activity from the 2,6-disubstituted 2-(arylimino)imidazolidines.

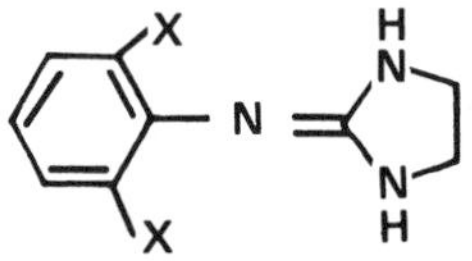

Figure 4. General structure of 2,6-disubstituted 2-(arylimino)imidazolidines.

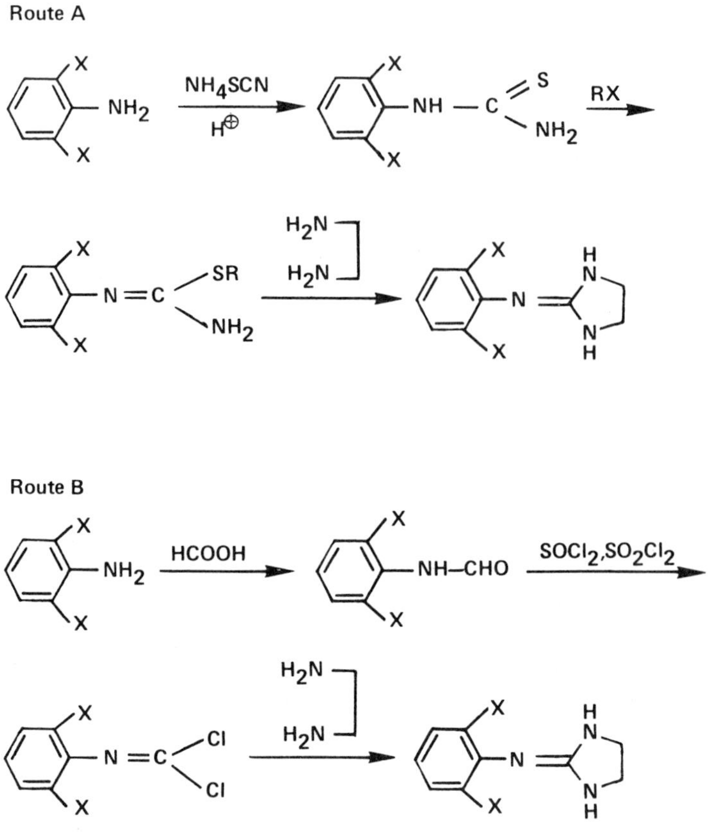

Route A

Route B

Figure 5. Synthetic routes for the synthesis of 2,6-disubstituted 2-(arylimino)imidazolidines.

3. CHEMICAL DISCOVERY

At first, the realization of the synthesis encountered problems. The usual methods for preparation of iminoimidazolidines were useful only for obtaining a limited number of molecules and were not applicable to the preparation of the 2,6-disubstituted analogues. Two approaches finally provided access to the desired 2,6-disubstituted 2-(arylimino)imidazolidines. The first of these was a modification of the synthesis carried out by Bloom (Figure 5, route A).[5] The other approach, which we developed at C. H. Boehringer Sohn, involved the

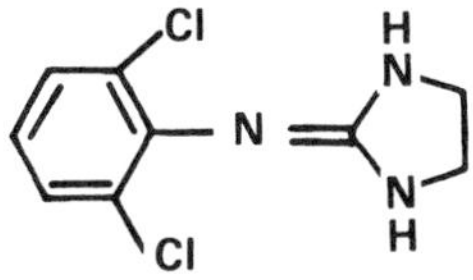

Figure 6. Structure of clonidine.

reaction of 2,6-disubstituted *N*-(dichloromethylene)anilines with ethylene-diamine (Figure 5, route B).[6,7] In retrospect, I believe that probably my most important contribution to the discovery of clonidine (Figure 6) was the idea of introducing chlorine atoms as substituents in the 2- and 6-position of the phenyl ring. At that time, a double halogen substitution was still unusual for pharmaceuticals and the prevailing opinion — based on what was then known from the literature[8,9] — was that compounds with several halogen atoms would be useful at most as pesticides. When in spite of these prejudices I proceeded to synthesize the 2,6-dichloro-substituted compound and submitted it under the code number St 155 for pharmacological screening, it turned out that this drug had indeed a remarkably high vasoconstrictive and decongestive effect at unusually low dosage levels.[10]

The decongestive effect was determined by Dr. Hoefke according to the method described by Binet and Araudinet.[11] In anaesthetized dogs the connection between nose and pharynx was blocked by paraffin soaked cotton wool. Additionally, the nostrils were closed by a special balloon catheter. By these means the changes in volume within the nose could be plethysmographically determined by use of a Marey capsule. The changes in volume within the nasal cavity could be recorded on a smoked drum.

4. DISCOVERY OF THE BLOOD-PRESSURE LOWERING ACTIVITY

On the basis of the early pharmacological findings a small sample of St 155 was supplied to the medical department of C. H. Boehringer Sohn to be used to test its nasal decongestive properties in man. Dr. Wolf, a physician and a member of the trial group, allowed his secretary Mrs. Schwandt — at that time still Miss Nickel — to administer to herself a few drops of a 0.3% solution in her nostrils, since she had a cold. However, there was some surprise and embarrassment when the lady fell asleep for 24 hours. She also developed a rather low blood pressure, a marked bradycardia and dryness of the mouth. The dose amounted — as determined later — to the equivalent of approximately 20 tablets of Catapres.*[12-14]

*Tradename of clonidine.

Table 1

Effects of Clonidine in Animal Experiments[17]

Effect	Threshold dose (μg/kg)	Experimental animal
Sedation	10	Dogs, cats
Secretory inhibition	50	Rats
Contraction of nictitating membrane	10	Dogs, cats
Blood sugar increase	10	Rats
Analgesia (several tests)	20-400	Mice
Adrenolysis	100	Rabbits, cats
Increase in blood pressure (initial)	1	Dogs, cats, rabbits
Decrease in blood pressure	1	Dogs, cats, rabbits
Local anesthesia	0.1%	Guinea pigs
Bradycardia	1	Dogs, cats, rabbits

After this first trial in a human it became clear to Dr. Wolf that the drug's decongestant properties were far less interesting than its potent antihypertensive activity. The compound was thereupon developed for this new indication and was introduced into therapy in 1966. Since then clonidine has been quite a useful antihypertensive drug.

The spectrum of activity of clonidine is shown in Table 1. When administered intravenously, clonidine causes a transient rise in arterial blood pressure that is followed by a prolonged hypotensive action. While the initial hypertensive effect is the expression of peripheral α-adrenoreceptor stimulating properties of the drug, the subsequent and more important decrease in blood pressure is due primarily to a stimulation of central α-adrenoreceptors that causes a reduced activity of the peripheral sympathetic nervous system. Clonidine was the first antihypertensive agent with a clearcut central site of action. Besides its therapeutic value, clonidine has proved to be an important pharmacological tool and has provided valuable insight into the importance of central α-adrenoreceptors and the physiology of central blood pressure regulation. The pharmacology of clonidine has been reviewed in detail by Kobinger[15] and Walland.[16]

Introduction of the two *ortho* chlorine atoms in the 2-(arylimino)imidazolidine molecule indeed proved crucial for the activity of clonidine. First, the two *ortho* substituents forced the molecule into a nonplanar conformation such that it met the steric requirements to fit into the α-adrenoreceptor (Section 5). Second, the two chlorine atoms also made the molecule sufficiently lipophilic to penetrate the blood-brain barrier.

There is considerable evidence that the central α-adrenoreceptor responsible for the hypotensive action of clonidine and the peripheral receptor are quite similar. Clearly, therefore, the activity of clonidine would be determined not only by its ability to activate the central receptors, but also by its ability to reach the site of action — distribution of the α-adrenoreceptor-stimulating agent between the brain and blood would determine whether peripheral vasoconstriction or centrally mediated depression of the cardiovascular system predominates. In the case of clonidine, the balance of hydrophilic and hydrophobic properties (as gauged by the partition coefficient between octanol and buffer) is such that the molecule readily penetrates the CNS. From among the hundreds of imidazolidines synthesized, clonidine appears to be optimal with respect to both distribution and its ability to stimulate the central receptors (Section 6).

5. MOLECULAR AND CONFORMATIONAL STRUCTURE

It could be shown by means of spectroscopic investigation[18,19] that the tautomeric equilibrium in the clonidine molecule lies quantitatively on the side of the iminoimidazolidine form (Figure 7). Although the highest negative charge is found on the imidazolidine ring nitrogen atoms,[20] the protonation of clonidine base takes place at the bridge nitrogen atom, since only then can stabilization of the molecule occur through delocalization of the positive charge in the guanidine portion. This leads to the structure depicted in Figure 8. In the protonated form of clonidine the π electrons of the double bond are delocalized and the positive charge is dispersed over the three nitrogen atoms.

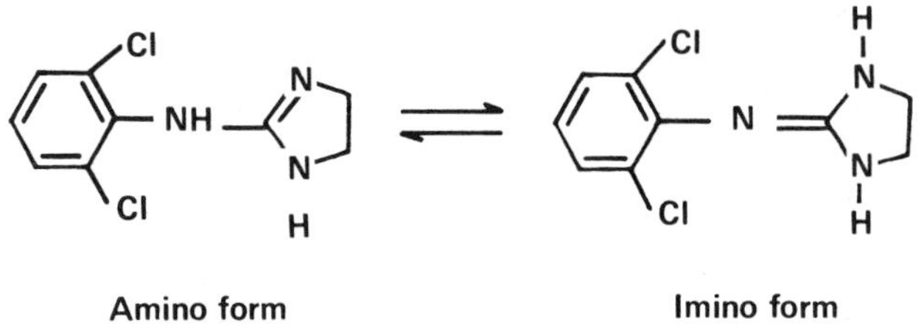

Amino form   Imino form

Figure 7. Tautomeric equilibrium between imino and amino forms in clonidine free base.

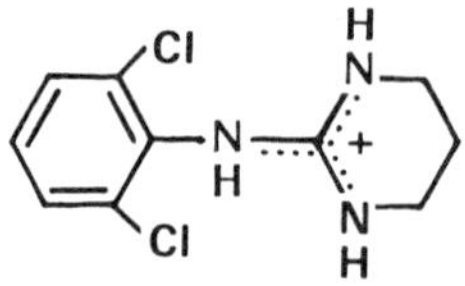

Figure 8.   Structure of protonated clonidine.

Stereo models show that clonidine is hindered in its rotation around the C-N-axis because of the two chlorine atoms in the *ortho* position (Figure 9). It can only exist in a conformation with nonplanar arrangement with the two rings approximately perpendicular to each other. This is supported by X-ray structure analysis,[22] which shows that the torsion angle between the two ring planes amounts to 75° in the crystal (Figure 10).

The α-adrenergic effects of clonidine and other imidazolidine compounds may be explained on the basis of a structural overlap between clonidine and noradrenaline. The latter may be taken as an example of a substance acting on the α-receptor. According to Pullman and Coubeils, the distance between the cationic center N^+ and the center of the aromatic ring of noradrenaline is between 5.1 and 5.2 Å, while the nitrogen is situated between 1.2 and 1.4 Å above the plane of the aromatic nucleus.[23,24] In clonidine the corresponding intramolecular distances in the nonplanar conformation have been calculated to be approximately 5.0-5.1 Å and 1.28-1.36 Å.[25] This fits rather well with the model of the α-adrenoreceptor derived from measurements of interatomic distances calculated for noradrenaline[23,24] (Figure 11).

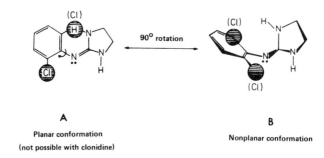

90° rotation

A

Planar conformation
(not possible with clonidine)

B

Nonplanar conformation

Figure 9.   Conformation (B) of clonidine according to Jen et al.[21]

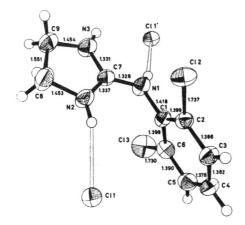

Figure 10. Perspective view of the crystal structure of clonidine hydrochloride. Reproduced with permission from Byre et al.[22]

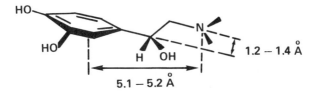

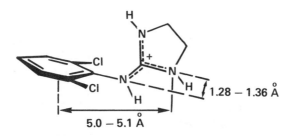

Figure 11. Appropriate structures of noradrenaline and clonidine for interaction with the postulated α-adrenergic receptors. According to Pullman et al.[23], Coubeils et al.,[24] and Wermuth et al.[25]

Furthermore, in contrast to noradrenaline, which can assume several conformations in its interaction with the α-adrenergic receptor, clonidine can alter its conformation much less readily because of the presence of the *ortho,ortho'*-dichloro substitution preventing free rotation of the two rings. This, perhaps, contributes to the better complementary picture presented at the α-adrenergic receptor by clonidine than noradrenaline.

6. STRUCTURE-ACTIVITY RELATIONSHIPS

Since the discovery of clonidine, structural modifications have been made in this molecule primarily to obtain information about the molecular features underlying the hypotensive property.

In the molecule of clonidine, at least three possibilities for a structural modification are present: the aromatic portion (a), the bridge (b) and the imidazolidine moiety (c) (Figure 12).

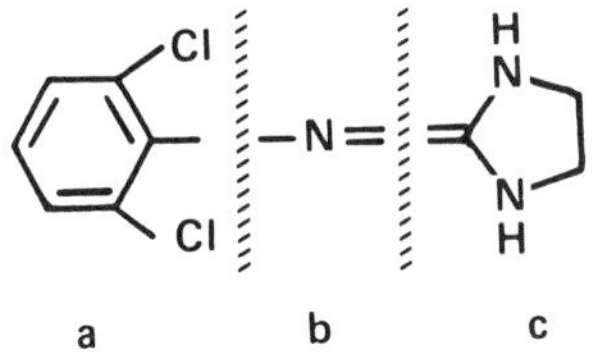

a   b   c

Figure 12.   Subdivision of clonidine into three fundamental structural parts.

6.1   Structural Changes in the Aromatic Part

As a first step, we chemically modified the aromatic part (a) of clonidine and correlated the new derivatives with their blood-pressure-lowering activity. It became clear that the non-planar conformation of clonidine has a decisive effect on the drug-receptor interaction. Compounds with a planar conformation, as, for example, the 3,4-dichloro isomer, show practically no blood-pressure-decreasing activity though they are able to penetrate the blood-brain barrier and thus reach the central site of action (Table 2).[26] An adjustment to the planar conformation is possible with such molecules that do not carry any bulky substituents in the *ortho* position of the aromatic ring and are therefore able to freely rotate around the C-N-axis.

Of all phenyl-substituted clonidine-like imidazolidines the 2,6-dihalogenated derivatives are the most potent.[26-28] If the phenyl ring contains no substituent or is substituted with more than three groups, it results in compounds with significantly lower hypotensive properties. Monosubstitution is only beneficial at the *ortho* position and when it is performed with substituents favoring

Table 2

**Influence of the Molecular Conformation in
Dichlorophenyliminoimidazolidines on Hypotensive Activity
in Anesthetized Rabbits Following Intravenous Administration[a]**

Compound	Molecular conformation	log P^b	ED_{20} $(mg/kg)^c$
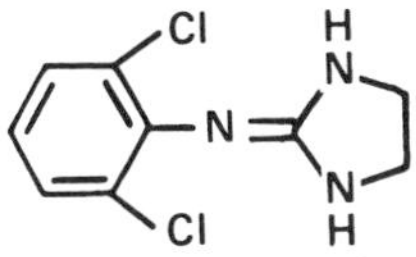 Clonidine	Nonplanar	0.47	0.01
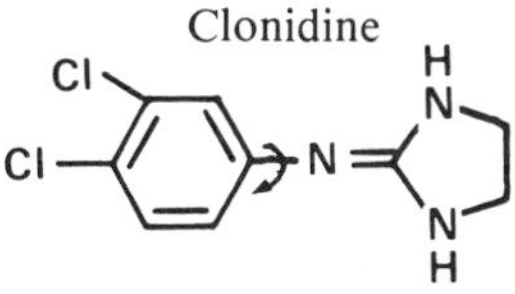	Planar	0.34	3.0

[a]By analogy with Stahle[26] and Hoefke.[27]

[b]P = partition coefficient in octanol/buffer (pH = 7.4).

[c]ED_{20} = effective dose (mg/kg), lowering arterial blood pressure by 20 mm Hg.

lipophilicity.[26-28] The influence of one, two, or three chlorine atoms in the phenyl ring is shown in Table 3. In general, disubstitution increases hypotensive activity over monosubstitution, provided that the substituents are attached to the correct positions of the phenyl ring and that the compounds are lipophilic enough (Table 4).[28] It is noteworthy that the 2,3-dihalogenated derivatives possess a relatively high effectiveness.

Replacement of chlorine by bromine and trifluoromethyl decreases the hypotensive activity. The difluoro analogue is much less active (Table 5).

Substitution of one or both chlorines by a different halogen or an alkyl group, or elimination of one or both chlorines also leads to a decrease of hypotensive activity (Table 6). The substitution of alkyl groups in the 2-, 4- and 6-positions shows no clearcut relationship in structure and activity. While monosubstitution with a methyl or an ethyl group in the *ortho* position shows a low activity, the 2,6-disubstituted methyl and ethyl compounds are totally inactive. The 2-methyl-6-ethyl compound, however, is capable of lowering the blood pressure. The 2,4,6-trisubstituted derivatives are highly active (Table 7).

Table 3

**Influence of One, Two, or Three Chlorine Atoms in
2-aryliminoimidazolidines on Hypotensive Activity in
Anesthetized Rabbits after i.v. Injection[a]**

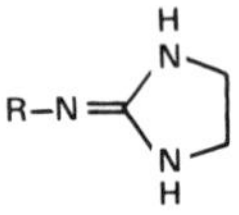

R	$\log 1/C$[b]	ED_{20} (mg/kg)
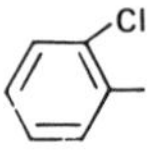	0.00	1.00
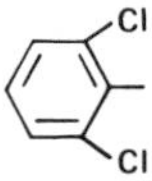	2.00	0.01
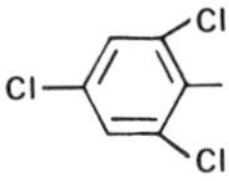	1.04	0.09

[a]By analogy with Stahle and Hoefke.[26-28]
[b]$C = ED_{20}$ = effective dose (mg/kg), lowering blood pressure by 20 mm Hg.

Table 4
Influence of the Substitution Pattern in Dichlorophenyliminoimidazolidines on Hypotensive Activity in Anesthetized Rabbits after i.v. Injection[a]

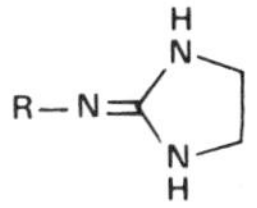

R	$\log 1/C^b$	ED_{20} (mg/kg)
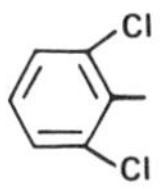	2.00	0.01
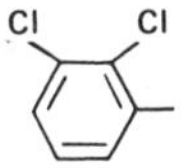	1.70	0.02
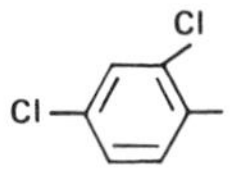	0.77	0.17
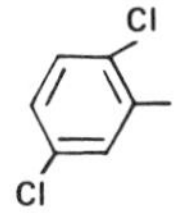	0.60	0.25
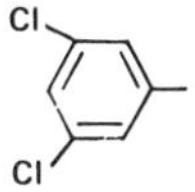	−0.48	3.00
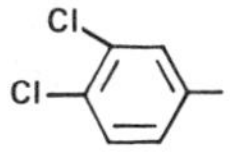	< −0.48	>3.00

[a]By analogy with Stahle and Hoefke.[26-28]
[b]$C = ED_{20}$ = effective dose (mg/kg), lowering blood pressure by 20 mm Hg.

Table 5
Influence of Replacement of Chlorine Atoms in the
2,6-Postion of the Phenyl Ring in
2-aryliminoimidazolidines by Bromine,
Trifluoromethyl, and Fluorine on Hypotensive Activity
in Anesthetized Rabbits after i.v. Injection[a]

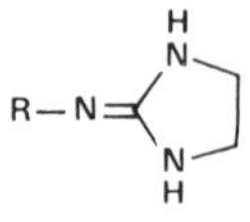

R	$\log 1/C^b$	ED_{20} (mg/kg)
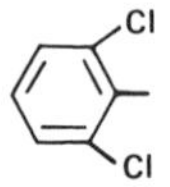	2.00	0.010
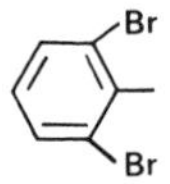	1.35	0.045
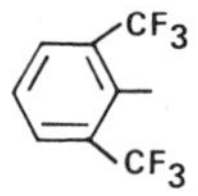	1.22	0.060
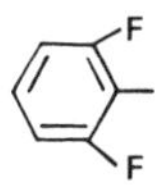	< -0.48	> 3.000

[a]By analogy with Stahle and Hoefke.[26-28].
^bC = ED_{20} = effective dose (mg/kg), lowering blood pressure by 20 mm Hg.

Table 6

**Influence of Alteration of the Substituents in the
2,6-Position of 2-aryliminoimidazolidines on the
Hypotensive Activity in Anesthetized Rabbits
following Intravenous Administration[a]**

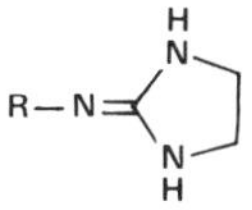

R	$\log 1/C$[b]	ED_{20} (mg/kg)
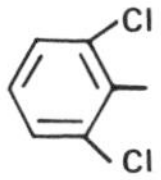	2.00	0.01
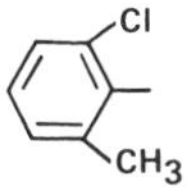	1.30	0.05
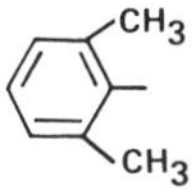	—	—
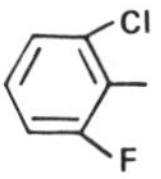	1.40	0.04
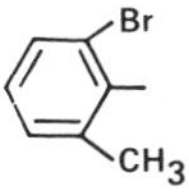	0.22	0.60
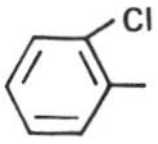	0.00	1.00
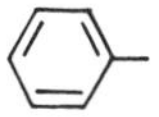	< -0.48	> 3.00

[a]By analogy with Stahle and Hoefke.[26-28]
[b]$C = ED_{20}$ = effective dose (mg/kg), lowering blood pressure by 20 mm Hg.

Table 7

Influence of Alkyl Groups in the Phenyl Ring of 2-aryliminoimidazolidines on Hypotensive Activity in Anesthetized Rabbits after i.v. Injection[a]

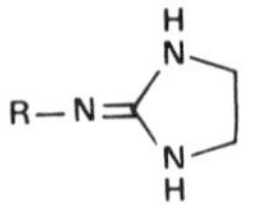

R	log $1/C$[b]	ED_{20} (mg/kg)
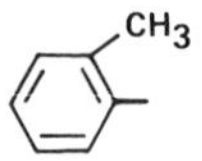 (o-CH$_3$)	− 0.08	1.20
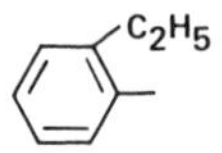 (o-C$_2$H$_5$)	0.40	0.40
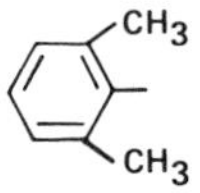 (2,3-diCH$_3$)	—	—
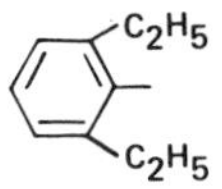 (2,3-diC$_2$H$_5$)	—	—
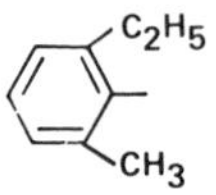 (C$_2$H$_5$, CH$_3$)	0.52	0.30
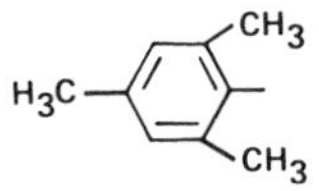 (CH$_3$, CH$_3$, CH$_3$)	1.52	0.03
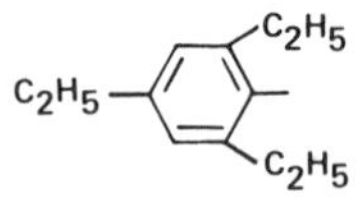 (C$_2$H$_5$, C$_2$H$_5$, C$_2$H$_5$)	1.52	0.03

[a]By analogy with Stahle and Hoefke.[26-28]

[b]C = ED_{20} = effective dose (mg/kg), lowering blood pressure by 20 mm Hg.

Table 8
Hypotensive Activity of Monoatomic Bridge Analogues
of Clonidine following Intravenous Administration
to Anesthetized, Normotensive Rats

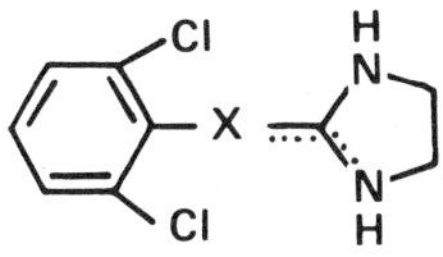

X	log 1/C	$ED_{30}{}^{a}$ (mg/kg)
—N=	2.00	2.7
—S—	0.73	50
—CH_2—	0.56	72
—O—	− 1.33	5750

$^{a}ED_{30}$ = dose causing a 30% decrease in mean arterial blood pressure.[28]

Here again, the partition coefficient is of importance. The monosubstituted and, to a larger extent, disubstituted compounds show low values for partition coefficients between octanol and phosphate buffer at pH 7.4, whereas the trisubstituted compounds show high values (see Section 7).

6.2 Structural Changes in the Bridge
Replacement of the bridge nitrogen atom of clonidine by a -CH_2- group, sulfur, or oxygen yields bridge analogues of clonidine with reduced hypotensive activity (Table 8).[28] Extension of the bridge between the phenyl ring and the imidazolidine ring is also accompanied by a loss of hypotensive activity (Table 9).[26-28]

6.3 Structural Changes in the Imidazolidine Ring
A decrease of hypotensive activity is also noted on enlargement of the five-membered imidazolidine ring of clonidine into a six-, seven-, or eight-membered nucleus (Table 10).[26-28]

Table 9
The Influence of Extension of the Nitrogen
Bridge in Clonidine on Hypotensive Activity after
i.v. Injection to Anesthetized Rabbits[a]

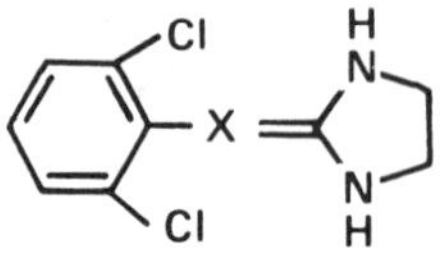

X	log $1/C$[b]	ED_{20} (mg/kg)
—N =	2.00	0.01
—CH_2—N =	0.07	0.85
—NH—N =	0.62	0.24
—CH = N—N =	0.62	0.24
—OCH_2CH_2—NH—N =	– 0.40	2.50

[a]By analogy with Stahle and Hoefke.[26-28]
[b]C = ED_{20} = effective dose (mg/kg), lowering blood pressure by 20 mm Hg.

Substitution of one of the imidazolidine nitrogen atoms by a CH_2— group, sulfur, or oxygen atom again leads to a diminution of hypotensive activity (Figure 13).[29] The imidazolidine ring has also been structurally altered by ring closure reactions into annellated bi- and tricyclic structures.[30] The hypotensive activity of these annellated clonidine molecules was distinctly less than that of clonidine, with the exception of some compounds in the imidazo[1,2-a]s-triazine series (Figure 14).[26,27]

As shown by these few examples, all significant departures from the structure of clonidine led to a considerable decrease of activity. The variation of the substituents in the aromatic ring led only to further substances with a blood-pressure-lowering activity comparable to that of clonidine.

Table 10

**The Influence of Expansion of the
Imidazolidine Ring of Clonidine (n = 2)
on the Hypotensive Activity in Anesthetized
Rabbits after i.v. Application**[a]

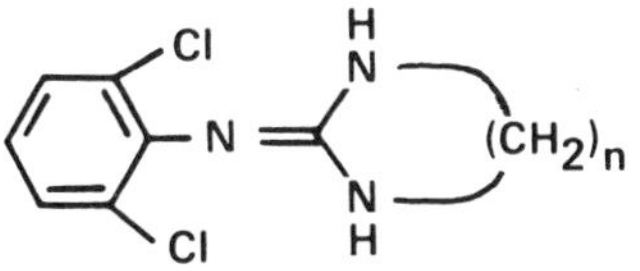

n	$\log 1/C$[b]	ED_{20} (mg/kg)
2	2.00	0.01
3	− 0.48	3.0
4	− 0.48	3.0
5	0.00	1.0

[a]By analogy with Stahle and Hoefke.[26-28]

[b]C = ED_{20} = effective dose (mg/kg), lowering blood pressure by 20 mm Hg.

7. QUANTITATIVE STRUCTURE-ACTIVITY RELATIONSHIPS

To determine quantitative structure-activity relationships within the series of 2-(arylimino)imidazolidines, regressions analyses according to Hansch were carried out by several teams.[31-35] Of the numerous quantitative correlations I give one example here: For 13 imidazolidines closely related to clonidine (Figure 15) a clear quantitative dependence of the blood-pressure-lowering activity on the partition coefficient could be demonstrated.[35] All imidazolidines included in Figure 15 are hindered from free rotation around the C-N axis. The lipophilicity of drugs, as expressed by their octanol-water partition coefficients, is the most widely and frequently used parameter for structure-activity studies in biological systems. It is suitable in many cases to describe drug transport processes. Also hydrophobic interactions between drug and receptor can often be explained by this molecular parameter (for review see Hansch,[36,37] and Lien[38]).

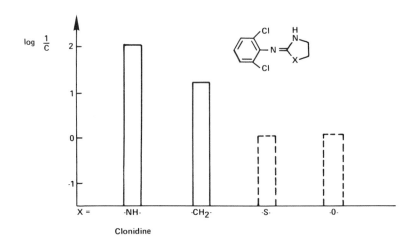

Figure 13. Influence of replacement of the imidazolidine part of clonidine by various hetero ring systems on the hypotensive activity in anesthetized rabbits after i.v. application. $C = ED_{20}$ = effective dose (mg/kg), lowering blood pressure by 20 mm Hg. Dotted bars indicate that the thiazolidine and oxazolidine derivative showed no activity up to 1 mg/kg. From Stahle and Hoefke.[29]

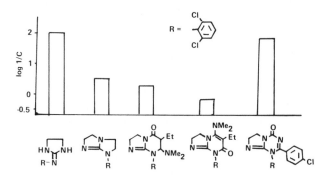

Figure 14. Hyptensive activity of some annellated structures of clonidine following intravenous administration to anesthetized rabbits. C = dose (mg/kg), decreasing mean arterial blood pressure by 20 mm Hg. From Stahle[26] and Hoefke.[27]

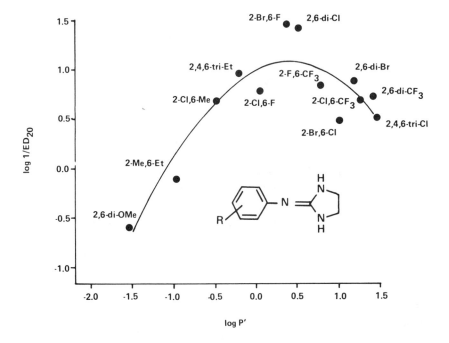

$$\log 1/ED_{20} = 0.372 \log P - 0.484 (\log P)^2 + 1.019$$

$$n = 13, r = 0.903, s = 0.260, F = 22.09 \ (P < 0.001)$$

Figure 15. 2-(Arylimino)imidazolidines that are closely related to clonidine. The relationship between hypotensive activity after intravenous administration to anesthetized rabbits and the partition coefficient is shown. ED_{20} = effective dose (mg/kg), lowering blood pressure by 20 mm Hg. P = partition coefficient in octanol/buffer (pH = 7.4). From Stahle and Hoefke.[28]

As can be seen from Figure 15, the relationship begins with an increasing hypotensive effect up to clonidine and then shows a decreasing hypotensive activity as the log P values increase. It seems that the blood-pressure-lowering effect is maximal when the log P value is about 0.4, quite close to the log P value found for clonidine (0.48). The equation shown in Figure 15 explains 82% of the variance in blood-pressure-lowering activity in the rabbit, which is very acceptable.

Among the hundreds of clonidine-like compounds that have been synthesized, only a few have been found to possess blood-pressure-lowering activity comparable with that of clonidine, indicating that clonidine represents an optimal chemical structure stimulating central α-receptors.

The results of the structure-activity correlations therefore disclose the following structural features for a drug lowering blood pressure by stimulating central α-adrenoreceptors:

1. A guanidine moiety fixed within the iminoimidazolidine system.
2. An aromatic N-substituent.
3. A conformationally nonplanar structure of the molecule obtained by the introduction of substituents in the *ortho* position of the phenyl ring.
4. A decrease in basicity of the guanidine grouping by means of the introduction of electronegative substituents, for example, chlorine atoms, in the aromatic ring.
5. A log P value of about 0.4.

8.   CONCLUSION

With the discovery of clonidine the central α-adrenergic receptors first became known to chemists, pharmacologists, and physicians. Clonidine poses a continuous and increasing challenge and promise for research on central neuronal transmitter substances having variable actions and expectations.

The relationship between structure and activity of clonidine-like central α-stimulants found in the series led to a completely new and nearly paradoxical conception concerning the adrenergic activity and modulation in the central nervous system.

Clonidine decreases intraocular pressure and has definitive advantages in treating glaucoma.[39] Also, some types of migraine can be treated successfully.[40] Moreover, it can improve the condition in children suffering from Tourette's syndrome. This syndrome, described by the French psychiatrist Gilles de la Tourette, is a rare and bizarre psychiatric disorder in children, characterized by incoordinated motor and multiple psychic disturbances, compulsive actions, and other behavioral symptoms. Prominent features are echolalia and coprolalia, meaning that these unfortunate children repeat strange words, and in particular obscene ones, continuously over and over again. Most of these children are socially intolerable. They cannot attend school and within the family they are unbearable. In more severe cases there is a marked tendency to self-destruction and even mutilation. Until now there has been no satisfactory therapy for these unfortunate children. High doses of the neuroleptic drug haloperidol achieve a slight improvement of this condition, but at the price of an excessive sedation and semicoma. Clonidine, however, in fairly low doses of 0.1-0.2 mg improves the mental and motor condition of these children extraordinarily so that they become almost completely adjusted to family, school, and social life.[41]

Another unexpected and extraordinary centrally induced action of clonidine is the stimulation of human growth hormone,[42] which has been found to occur less in endogenous than in exogenous depression.[43] Preliminary clinical trials with clonidine have been published,[43] but it has not yet been definitively determined whether these tests are reliable and predictive. If they are, the therapy of mental depression can be made more specific and effective.

Clonidine decreases, by a mechanism not yet fully elucidated, the output of nearly all secretory glands, for example, lacrimal, salivary, gastric secretory, and particularly the sweat glands. There is a rather rare condition, called "gastatory sweating," where sweating in the lower face and neck region is induced by eating particularly spicy food. This is socially and personally quite disturbing. Antisecretory drugs, such as anticholinergic compounds, are poorly effective in this condition. Low doses of clonidine, about 0.2 mg daily, inhibit this local sweating.[45]

The recent finding that clonidine can alleviate or even obviate the severe symptoms of opiate withdrawal indicates effects on central noradrenergic transmitter and modulator functions, which are not related to hypertension.[46-47] These new indications might be a clue and incentive for further pharmacological and clinical investigations using the manifold derivatives of clonidine already in existence or to be synthesized in the future.

If serendipity is defined as "something extraordinary" that has not been searched or looked for but has been detected by plain curiosity, meticulous observation, sagacity, and lateral thinking, then the clonidine story certainly is a significant and pertinent example. Conceived as a vasoconstrictor, clonidine was delivered in due time as a centrally acting blood-pressure-lowering drug and was finally developed into a cure for several other diseases and symptoms. Quite unexpectedly it also went on to become a useful tool for pharmacologists.

ACKNOWLEDGMENTS
I would like to thank, most sincerely, Prof. Dr. Zeile for entrusting me with the experimental work with the imidazolidines in 1960. My special thanks are due to my friend and coinventor Dr. Wolf for his great help and encouragement over many years. My thanks go also to Miss E. Janecek and to Mr. A. Reiner and Mr. G. Giesler for their conscientious technical assistance during very many experiments.

REFERENCES

1. F. Soldan, E. Druckrey, G. Hartfelder, I. Hoffmann, and B. Mencke, "Kreislaufmittel-Sympathomimetica und Sympatholytica (Adrenolytica)," in G. Ehrhart and H. Rusching, Ed., *Arzneimittel, Vol. 2, 2nd ed.,* Verlag Chemie, Weinheim/Bergstr., 1972, p. 131.
2. W. T. Comer and A. W. Gomoll, "Antihypertensive Agents," in *Medicinal Chemistry,,* A. Burger, Ed., 3rd ed., Wiley-Interscience, New York, 1970, p. 1050.
3. H. Najer, R. Giudicelli, and J. Sette, *Bull. Soc. Chim. Fr.,* **1961**, 2114.
4. H. Stahle, unpublished data, 1961.
5. Chas. Pfizer & Co., Inc., New York (inventor: B. M. Bloom): "Synthesis of 1,3-Diazacyclo-alkenes-2," U.S. Patent 2,899,426 (Augut 11, 1959); *Chem. Abstr.,* **54**, 588 (1960).
6. C. H. Boehringer Sohn, Ingelheim/Rhein (inventors: H. Stahle and K. Zeile): "Verfahren zur Herstellung von 2-substituierten Phenylamino-1,3-diazacycloalkenen-(2) und deren Saureaddi-tionssalze," German Patent 1,670,162 (June 29, 1978/October 31, 1966).
7. C. H. Boehringer Sohn, Ingelheim/Rhein (inventors: K. Zeile, H. Stahle, and K.-H. Haupt-man): "Disubstituierte 2-Phenylamino-1,3-diazacyclopentene-(2)," German Patent 1,303,141 (October 9, 1961/January 11, 1973).
8. W. Perkow, *Die Insektizide. Chemie, Wirkungsweise und Toxizitat,* 1st ed., Alfred Huthig Verlag, Heidelberg, 1956.
9. P. Muller, Ed., *DDT. Insecticides,* Vol. 1, Birkhauser Verlag, Basel, 1955.
10. W. Hoefke, personal communication, 1962.
11. L. Binet and L. Araudinet, *Presse Med.,* **1929**, 1637.
12. M. Wolf, personal communication, 1962.
13. W. Graubner and M. Wolf, *Arzneim.-Forsch. (Drug Res.),* **16**, 1055 (1966).
14. M. Wolf and H. Morr, "Imidazoline — New Facets of a Cinderella Molecule," in *Future Trends in Therapeutics. Principles and Techniques of Human Research and Therapeutics,* Vol. 15, F. G. McMahon, Ed., Futura Publishing, Mount Kisco, New York, 1978, p. 179.
15. W. Kobinger, *Rev. Physiol. Biochem. Pharmacol.,* **81**, 39 (1978).
16. A. Walland, "Clonidine," in *Pharmacological and Biochemical Properties of Drug Substances,* Vol. 1, M. E. Goldberg, Ed., American Pharmaceutical Association, Washington, 1977, p. 67.
17. W. Kobinger and W. Hoefke, "Pharmakologische Untersuchungen uber Angriffspunkt und Wirkungsmechanismus eines neuen Hochdruckmittels," in *Hochdruck-Therapie, Symposion uber 2-(2,6-Dichlorphenylamino)-2-imidazolinhydrochlorid am 20. und 21. Oktober 1967 in Ulm,* L. Heilmeyer, H.-J. Holtmeier, and E.F. Pfeiffer, Eds., Georg Thieme Verlag, Stutt-gart, 1968, p. 4.
18. B. Rouot, G. Leclerc, and C.G. Wermuth, *Chim. Ther.,* **1973**, 545.
19. K.-H. Pook, H. Stahle, and H. Daniel, *Chem. Ber.,* **107**, 2644 (1974).
20. H. Stahle, W. Heel, and J. Becker, unpublished data, 1971.
21. T. Jen, B. Dienel, H. Bowman, J. Petta, A. Helt, and B. Loev, *J. Med. Chem.,* **15**, 727 (1972).
22. G. Byre, A. Mostad, and C. Rømming, *Acta Chem. Scand.,* **B30**, 843 (1976).
23. B. Pullman, J. L. Coubeils, P. Courriere, and J. P. Gervois, *J. Med. Chem.,* **15**, 17 (1972).
24. J. L. Coubeils, P. Courriere, and B. Pullman, *J. Med. Chem.,* **15**, 453 (1972).
25. C. G. Wermuth, J. Schwartz, G. Leclerc, J. P. Garnier, and B. Rouot, *Chim. Ther.,* **1973**, 115.

26. H. Stahle, "Medicinal Chemistry Related to the Central Regulation of Blood Pressure. I. Chemical Part." in *Medicinal Chemistry IV. Proceedings of the 4th International Symposium on Medicinal Chemistry, Noordwijkerhout, The Netherlands, September 9-13, 1974,* J. Maas, Ed., Elsevier, Amsterdam, 1974, p. 75.

27. W. Hoefke, "Centrally Acting Antihypertensive Agents," in *Antihypertensive Agents,* E. L. Engelhardt, Ed., ACS Symposium Series, Vol. 27, R. F. Gould, Ed., American Chemical Society, Washington, DC, 1976, p. 27.

28. P. B. M. W. M. Timmermans, W. Hoefke, H. Stahle, and P. A. van Zwieten, "Structure-Activity Relationships in Clonidine-like Imidazolidines and Related Compounds," in *Progress in Pharmacology,* H. Grobecker, G. F. Kahl, W. Klaus and P. A. van Zwieten, Eds., Gustav Fischer Verlag, Stuttgart, in press, 1980.

29. H. Stahle and W. Hoefke, unpublished data.

30. H. Stahle and H. Koppe, Justis *Liebigs Ann. Chem.,* **1973,** 1275.

31. H. Struyker Boudier, J. de Boer, G. Smeets, E. J. Lien, and J. van Rossum, *Life Sci.,* **17,** 377 (1975).

32. W. Hoefke, W. Kobinger, and A. Walland, *Arzneim.-Forsch. (Drug Res.),* **25,** 786 (1975).

33. B. Rouot, G. Leclerc, and C. G. Wermuth, *J. Med. Chem.,* **19,** 1049 (1976).

34. P. B. M. W. M. Timmermans, and P. A. van Zwieten, *J. Med. Chem.,* **20,** 1636 (1977).

35. H. Stahle and W. Hoefke, unpublished data; submitted for publication in *Progress in Pharmacology.*

36. C. Hansch, "Quantitative Structure-Activity Relationships in Drug Design," in *Drug Design,* Vol. 1, E. J. Ariens, Ed., Academic Press, New York, 1971, p. 271.

37. C. Hansch, "Quantitative Approaches to Pharmacological Structure-Activity Relationships," in *Structure-Activity Relationships,* Vol. 1, C. J. Cavallito, Ed., Pergamon Press, London, 1973, p. 75.

38. E. J. Lien "The Relationship between Chemical Structure and Drug Absorption, Distribution and Excretion," in *Medicinal Chemistry IV. Proceedings of the 4th International Symposium on Medicinal Chemistry, Noordwijkerhout, The Netherlands, September 9-13, 1974,* J. Maas, Ed., Elsevier, Amsterdam, 1974, p. 319.

39. R. Harrison and C. S. Kaufmann, *Arch. Ophthalmol.,* **95,** 1368 (1977).

40. M. Wilkinson, *Res. Clin. Stud. Headache,* **3,** 315 (1972).

41. D. J. Cohen, J. G. Young, J. A. Nathanson, and B. A. Shaywitz, *Lancet,* **2,** 551 (1979).

42. I. Gil-Ad, E. Topper, and Z. Laron, *Lancet,* **2,** 278 (1979).

43. N. Matussek, M. Ackenheil, H. Hippius, H.-Th. Schroder, H. Schultes, and B. Wasilewski, "Effect of Clonidine on HGH Release in Psychiatric Patients and Controls," 6th World Congress of Psychiatry, Hawaii, 1977.

44. N. Matussek, *Nervenarzt,* **49,** 569 (1978).

45. H. U. Janka, E. Standl, and H. Mehnert, *Ann. Intern. Med.,* **91,** 130 (1979).

46. M. S. Gold, D. G. Redmond, and H. D. Kleber, *Lancet,* **1,** 929 (1978).

47. M. S. Gold, D. E. Redmond, Jr., and H. D. Kleber, *Am. J. Psychiatr.,* **136,** 100 (1979).

Atenolol   5

D.J. Le Count

The last two decades have witnessed a revolution in the treatment of ischemic heart disease and hypertension, a revolution that has come about by the discovery of a class of compounds known as the β-adrenoceptor blocking agents. Their use in the treatment of high blood pressure and in the prophylaxis of anginal attacks has provided a novel therapeutic advance and it may be justly claimed that their discovery has been the most significant single development in the treatment of cardiovascular disease. Since β-adrenoceptor blocking drugs combine low incidence of side effects with excellent efficacy, they are currently among the first choice in the treatment of hypertension, either alone or in combination with other antihypertensive agents. The importance these drugs have achieved in such a short time puts them into that group of drugs that includes such compounds as the benzodiazepines and the β-lactam antibiotics, classes whose names are synonymous with both a disease area and a chemical structure.

A discovery of this magnitude does not cease after the development of a single drug. Development of the initial concept is crucial. Few, if any, drugs are pure in their pharmacological profile, the β-adrenoceptor blocking agents being no exception. It was considered to be of prime importance to establish the contribution of each property within the pharmacological profile to the clinical action. It was in this atmosphere of scientific curiosity that atenolol was synthesized to give a β-adrenoceptor blocking agent with a pharmacological profile not possessed by any other member of this class. To appreciate the position of atenolol in the overall concept of β-adrenoceptor blockade a brief review of the historical developments is presented here.

1. THE HISTORICAL BACKGROUND OF ATENOLOL

The nervous system, which coordinates many functions of the body, is divided into two branches, the somatic system, which controls activity of the skeletal or voluntary muscles, and the autonomic system, which controls the internal development of the body. For example, by means of autonomic responses, cold causes reflex vasoconstriction of the blood vessels of the skin to conserve body heat, and increased CO_2 levels in the blood result in increased ventilation to reduce that CO_2 level. The autonomic nervous system is further divided into the parasympathetic and the sympathetic systems. The sympathetic system is unique in using noradrenaline (**1**) as its chemical transmitter. Noradrenaline is released from the fine nerve endings by the electrical impulses traveling down the nerve and then interacts with specific sites or receptors on the effector organs, thereby modulating their responses.

$$
\begin{array}{ll}
1 & R = R' = H \\
2 & R = CH_3, R' = H \\
3 & R = H, R' = CH_3 \\
4 & R = R' = CH_3 \\
5 & R = CH(CH_3)_2, R' = H
\end{array}
$$

This chronicle of division and subdivision within the peripheral nervous system does not end here. As early as 1906 a study by Dale[1] on the influence of ergot alkaloids on the effects of adrenaline (**2**) and sympathetic nerve stimulation provided experimental evidence for the existence of two distinct classes of sympathetic responses. He found that the excitatory responses of various organs to adrenaline and electrical sympathetic nerve stimulation were inhibited by the ergot alkaloids, whereas inhibitory responses were unaffected. Dale interpreted his results to mean that two "sympathetic myoneural junctions" were activated by adrenaline and sympathetic nerve (or adrenergic) stimulation and only the type responsible for excitatory responses was blocked by the ergot alkaloids. From another study[2] on the pharmacological effects of adrenaline and related phenethylamines Dale was able to conclude that the myoneural junctions or parts thereof concerned with inhibition were not identical in their affinities for chemical substances with those concerned with excitatory effects.

The original concepts of Dale were extended by the now classical studies of Ahlquist[3], who investigated the differentiation of the receptors on the basis of the order of potency of a series of sympathetic amines in producing responses in each of a variety of sympathetically innervated organs. Ahlquist used the endogenous catecholamines adrenaline and noradrenaline (by then recognized as the chemical transmitter of the sympathetic system), as well as the synthetic analogues α-methylnoradrenaline (3), α-methyladrenaline (4) and isoprenaline (5). The last substance had been synthesized by Konzett[4] in 1940 in the search for a bronchodilator and was the first synthetic catecholamine derivative to achieve clinical importance. It has played an important part in the development of the concept of β-adrenoceptor blockade. The amines chosen by Ahlquist were tested in intact dogs, cats, and rabbits and on isolated tissues from these and other animal species. He found the following relative potencies for producing excitation of the smooth muscles of the peripheral blood vessels (vasoconstriction), nictitating membrane, uterus, and ureter and inhibition of the smooth muscle of the intestine: adrenaline > noradrenaline > α-methylnoradrenaline > α-methyladrenaline > isoprenaline; however, the relative potencies for producing inhibition of the smooth vasculature (vasodilation) and the uterus and excitation of the heart he found to be: isoprenaline > adrenaline > α-methyladrenaline > α-methylnoradrenaline > noradrenaline. These two distinct rankings of potency prompted him to conclude also that there were two distinct adrenoceptor populations associated with the pharmacological responses he had measured. Those receptors associated with the first order of potency and which would be blocked by the adrenergic blocking agents then available he termed *alpha* adrenoceptors and those associated with the second order of potency he called *beta* adrenoceptors. From this work it became apparent that isoprenaline was a pure β-adrenoceptor stimulant devoid of α-adrenoceptor effects, that noradrenaline was acting mainly at the α-adrenoceptor with little β-action, and that adrenaline acted on both α- and β-adrenoceptors.

This proposal of Ahlquist's, now universally accepted, was initially not well received, partly because there was no compound then available that could block the responses at β-adrenoceptors. It was not until 1958 that the situation began to change, for in that year scientists of the Eli Lilly laboratories reported[5] on the competitive blockade of inhibitory adrenoceptors by the dichloro analogue of isoprenaline, DCI (6). It was found, for example, that the depressor effect produced by isoprenaline was much reduced in cats pretreated with DCI and that the isoprenaline-induced reversal of bronchoconstriction was also blocked by this substance, these effects being observed at doses that did not inhibit adrenergic smooth muscle stimulatory responses. Thus, DCI was the first

6

β-adrenoceptor blocking agent, representing the missing link in the Ahlquist classification, and as a consequence of its discovery the *alpha* and *beta* classification of adrenoceptors became more widely accepted. However, although DCI was shown to be capable of blocking some of the β-adrenergic responses to isoprenaline, it was itself a stimulant and it has been since classified as a weak agonist rather than a true antagonist. It was this partial agonist activity, or, in current terminology, intrinsic sympathomimetic activity (ISA), that apparently precluded it from being considered a useful drug.

The true clinical potential of β-adrenoceptor blocking agents was first recognized by J. W. Black and his colleagues at ICI. Sympathetic stimulation of the heart, whatever its cause, results in increases in heart rate, force, and conductivity, all energy demanding responses. These increases in activity result in a greater oxygen demand, which, unless satisfied, gives rise to anginal pain. Attempts to alleviate this condition by increasing the blood supply to cardiac muscle through the use of coronary vasodilators had not been rewarding, and Black suggested that it might be more rational to improve the oxygen supply and demand relationships by reducing the effects of sympathetic stimulation upon the heart. This would restore balance by decreasing demand. This concept led the project chemist, J. S. Stephenson, to prepare further analogues of DCI and in this program the first clinically useful β-adrenoceptor blocking agent pronethalol [Alderlin * (**7**)] was prepared.[6] Clinical trials showed that the exercise tolerance of patients suffering from angina pectoris was improved and in addition it was found that the drug had an antihypertensive effect. The mechanism of this very useful response was, and still is, a mystery, since although the antianginal effects may be explained by Black's original hypothesis, no single effect seems responsible for the blood-pressure-lowering properties of β-adrenoceptor blocking agents. Unfortunately, during long term toxicity testing of pronethalol, tumors appeared in mice at high dose levels and consequently treatment with pronethanol was terminated.

7

The initial successes achieved with pronethalol led to increased chemical effort and further analogues were synthesized both within ICI and elsewhere in attempts to optimize activity. It was found that the aromatic ring in the

*Trademark of Imperial Chemical Industries P.L.C.

molecule was essential for activity. The 1-naphthyl analogue was as potent a β-adrenoceptor blocking agent as the 2-naphthyl analogue but possessed unacceptably high levels of partial agonist activity. Partially reduced systems, for example, tetralins, indanes, and some heterocyclic analogues also had similar levels of blocking activity, again with the ethanolamine moiety attached at the 2-position being favored, and substitution with simple substituents such as methyl, chloro, and methoxy, did not alter activity significantly.

The next major advance arose from modifications of the ethanolamine side chain. Whereas it could be shown that the ethanolamine group —CH(OH)CH$_2$NHR was essential for activity and could not tolerate further substitution on either the oxygen or the nitrogen atoms, the introduction of spacer groups between it and the aromatic ring could be tolerated; indeed the insertion of an oxymethylene link gave rise to compounds 10-20 times as potent as the corresponding arylethanolamine analogues. Unlike pronethalol, the 1-naphthyl analogue, propranolol (**8**), was more potent than the 2-naphthyl analogue and was devoid of the partial agonist or intrinsic sympathomimetic activity present in so many other analogues.

8

Thus the loss of pronethalol was compensated by a β-adrenoceptor blocking agent of improved potency. The choice of propranolol as opposed to various phenoxy analogues was relatively easy because at that time J. W. Black's concept of reducing cardiac work favored the use of a compound without partial agonist activity. Thus propranolol became the compound of choice and the extent of its clinical usage has since justified that choice. Propranolol is now regarded as the reference drug in the study of β-adrenoceptor blockade and it has stimulated a great deal of clinical and pharmacological research into the use of β-adrenoceptor blockade. However, it is nonselective in its action in that at cardiac effective doses it also affects other organs with β-adrenoceptors, including the peripheral smooth vasculature and the bronchi. This latter property means that it has to be used with caution in patients with obstructive airways disease since blockade of bronchial beta-receptors results in bronchoconstriction. Thus the need for a compound more selective in its action became

$$\overset{\displaystyle OH}{\underset{}{|}}$$

OCH$_2$CHCH$_2$NHCH(CH$_3$)$_2$

NHCOCH$_3$

9

apparent and this objective was achieved when, in 1966, Dunlop and Shanks and their co-workers observed[8] that an analogue blocked the cardiac receptors at lower doses than those at which it blocked the receptors associated with the blood vessels and the bronchi. This observation heralded the discovery of the first cardioselective β-adrenoceptor blocking agent practolol [Eraldin* (9)], which, like propranolol, proved to be a valuable antianginal agent but was in addition much better tolerated in those patients also afflicted with obstructive airways disease. Unfortunately, the occulomucotaneous syndrome, which occurred in a very small number of patients and which the available evidence suggests is quite specific to practolol, caused this potentially valuable compound to be withdrawn from general clinical use.

At this stage it is perhaps of value to digress somewhat to consider what is meant by *specificity* and *selectivity*. The specificity of a β-adrenergic blocking agent refers to its ability to block the effects of stimulation of the β-adrenoceptor and only that receptor. Responses elicited by other mechanisms, for example, α-adrenoceptor stimulation or calcium-mediated increases in cardiac contractility remain unaffected. Further, all β-adrenoceptor blocking agents are intrinsically capable of blocking all β-adrenoceptors, but certain compounds, for example, practolol, exhibit a preference, or *selectivity,* for the β-adrenoceptor of cardiac muscle so that the effects on the peripheral vasculature and bronchial β-adrenoceptors are much reduced. Indications for the existence of such a subpopulation of β-adrenoceptors comes from the work of Lands et al.[9], who subjected the results of a study of 15 sympathomimetic amines used to evoke accepted β-adrenoceptor responses to a thorough statistical analysis. This resulted in a modified classification of β-adrenoceptors in which cardiac receptors were designated β_1 and bronchial and vascular receptors β_2. This means that cardioselective β-adrenoceptor blocking agents are referred to as β_1-adrenoceptor blocking agents. The existence of β-adrenoceptor subpopulations has since received biochemical support, and in certain smooth muscles both may be present.

*Trademark of Imperial Chemical Industries P.L.C.

As with all new concepts, treatment of ischemic heart disease by reduction of sympathomimetic stimulation with β-adrenoceptor blocking agents met with some controversy. In addition to its β-blocking properties propranolol possesses membrane-stabilizing or "quinidine-like" activity and some believed that it was this activity giving a direct depressive action on the heart that gave propranolol its antianginal properties. Not until it was shown that this non-β-adrenoceptor activity manifested itself only at doses far in excess of those required for β-adrenoceptor blockade did support for this theory diminish.

A far more thorny problem, and one that is still not finally resolved, is the role of the intrinsic sympathomimetic activity present in certain β-adrenoceptor blockers. It had been suggested[10] that the presence of ISA in a β-adrenoceptor blocking agent was a significant advantage, since in the clinical situation a compound with such a property would reduce the risk of aggravating heart failure and reduce the degree of bronchospasm in susceptible subjects. This must be regarded as still unproven and the hemodynamic role of ISA is being actively investigated. In the late 1960s we were faced with uncertainties concerning the different hemodynamic effects shown by practolol compared to propranolol, so it seemed desirable to attempt to determine whether partial agonist activity (ISA) reduced blockade of vascular β_2-adrenoceptors or perhaps a combination of these properties was responsible for the differing hemodynamic effects. Therefore, the decision was made to make available for clinical investigation a battery of β-adrenoceptor blocking agents with different combinations of potency, selectivity, ISA and membrane-stabilizing activity. One objective was to find a compound that had as far as was possible only β_1-antagonist properties, since the availability of such an agent would permit studies on the contribution of cardiac sympathetic activity in a wide range of conditions in which propranolol was known to be effective, but whose specificity was in doubt because of its membrane-stabilizing properties and lack of cardioselectivity. Such a compound would be predicted to have the following profile:

1. Possess a potency equivalent to propranolol at the cardiac β-adrenoceptor sites.
2. Possess a greater affinity for cardiac β-adrenoceptors than for the β-adrenoceptors in the bronchial tree, peripheral vasculature, and coronary circulation or those involved in metabolism.
3. Be devoid of partial agonist activity (ISA).
4. Be free of membrane-stabilizing activity.

2. THE BIOLOGICAL TESTING SYSTEM

Scheme 1 shows the reaction sequence for the synthesis of propranolol, a two-step process from α-naphthol. This same chemical sequence can be applied in

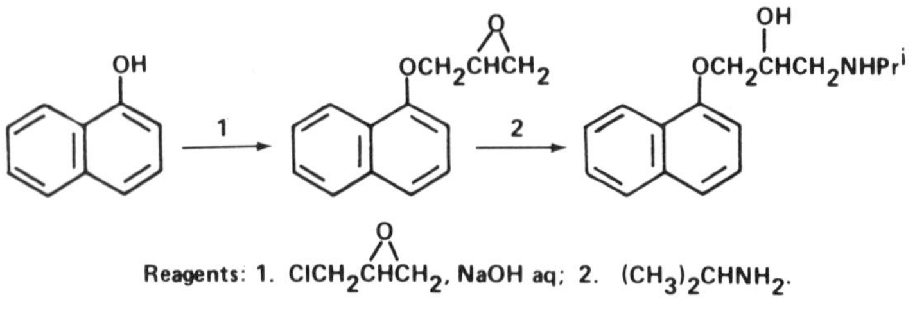
OH
OCH2CHCH2
OH
OCH2CHCH2NHPr^i
1
2
O
Reagents: 1. ClCH2CHCH2, NaOH aq; 2. (CH3)2CHNH2.

Scheme 1. Synthesis of propranolol

principle to any phenol, with a good chance of producing a β-adrenoceptor blocking agent. The relative simplicity of this sequence, at least in the laboratory, is a major reason for the numerous agents now available in the clinic, and one must realize that for every agent available, several hundred analogues have been synthesized and tested. Our own synthetic effort has not been small, nearly 5000 compounds having been investigated. It follows, therefore, that any biological testing system must be capable of screening a large number of compounds and yet furnish data suitable for use in meaningful quantitative structure-activity studies. This is particularly important where activity as a β-adrenoceptor blocking agent is not the sole criterion in compound selection. To enable a large number of compounds to be tested, and substances with desired pharmacological profiles to be selected, the screening sequence shown in Scheme 2 was devised.

Anesthetized rats (β-blocking activity)

↓

Anesthetized cats (β-blocking activity, selectivity)

↓

Guinea pigs (selectivity)

↓

Anesthetized rats (ISA)

↓

Frog sciatic nerve (membrane-stabilizing activity)

Scheme 2. Biological screening sequence

2.1 Pentobarbitone-Anesthetized Rats

This is in effect a prescreen, used to eliminate those compounds possessing little or no activity, and in the case of active compounds, to allow an estimate of a suitable dose range for the following cat screen. In this prescreen the heart rates of pentobarbitone-anesthetized rats are noted before and after an intravenous dose of isoprenaline (isoprenaline is the stimulant of choice since unlike adrenaline and noradrenaline it does not possess any α-adrenoceptor stimulatory activity, therefore, any effect noted arises by stimulation of the β-adrenoceptors only). In this manner a control value for the heart rate increase (tachycardia) produced by isoprenaline is obtained. The animals are then dosed with 10 mg/kg of the test compound followed half an hour later by the same isoprenaline dose given previously. If the tachycardia caused by this isoprenaline dose is below the control value the experiment is repeated at a higher or lower dose, depending on whether reduction of the original isoprenaline-induced tachycardia is less or greater than 50%. In this way it is possible to calculate an approximate ED_{50} (the dose of test substance required to reduce the isoprenaline control tachycardia by 50%), which is used to estimate the dose of that substance required for the following screen. No clinical significance can be attached with certainty to this result, since although there was a good correlation among the activities of closely related structures, the correlation among compounds of different structural classes was sometimes poor compared to that obtained with the more dependable cat screen.

2.2 Chloralose-Anesthetized Cats

In this test a cat is anesthetized with an intravenous injection of chloralose. Catheters are then inserted into both femoral veins, one for isoprenaline injections and the other for test drug infusion. The left femoral artery is cannulated and coupled to a transducer for blood-pressure measurements, and heart rate is measured using ECG lead II connected to a cardiotachometer. Isoprenaline, 0.2 μg/kg i.v., is given at intervals until consistent responses are obtained for both the tachycardia and the lowering of blood pressure.

A solution of the test substance is infused at a constant rate for 30 min, the concentration chosen being indicated by the rat test. During this period isoprenaline challenges are repeated every 10 min. Infusion rates are modified as necessary and the experiment is repeated until the substance under test reduces the isoprenaline-induced tachycardia below 50%. By plotting the percentage blockade against the log of the dose of test compound, the dose of compound infused over 30 min necessary to give 50% blockade can be calculated. In this way it may be shown that the ED_{50} for atenolol is 88 $\pm$ 5 μg/kg. In similar experiments the values for propranolol and practolol were determined to be 62 $\pm$ 10 and 158 $\pm$ 1 μg/kg, respectively.

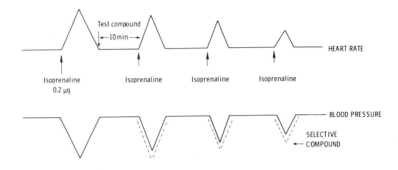

Figure 1. Cat electrocardiogram

In addition to the stimulatory effects on the β-adrenoceptor of the heart, isoprenaline injection results in stimulation of the β-adrenoceptors of the peripheral vasculature, causing vasodilation and a subsequent fall in diastolic blood pressure. Figure 1 shows these effects in diagrammatic form, together with the effects of infusion of a β-adrenoceptor blocking agent. Blockade of the effects of isoprenaline therefore results not only in antagonism of the tachycardia, but also antagonism of the blood pressure response. However, if the β-adrenoceptor blocking drug is selective, then the blood pressure response is proportionately less affected (as indicated by the dotted lines in Figure 1). In this way the first indication of a possible selectivity is obtained. This selectivity is usually expressed by noting the percentage blockade of the blood-pressure response at the heart rate ED_{50}. Table 1 shows the results of experiments with atenolol in such a preparation.

Table 1

β-Adrenoceptor Blocking Activity and Cardioselectivity of Atenolol

Infusion rate (μg/kg/min)	Heart rate (blockade %)	Blood pressure (blockade %)
1.25	25 ± 2	14 ± 7
2.5	49 ± 3	22 ± 7
5.0	63 ± 2	29 ± 8

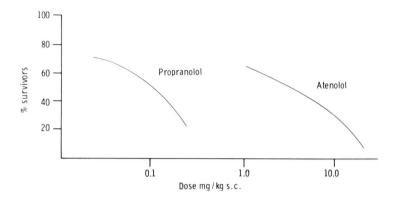

Figure 2.   Cardioselectivity of atenolol (guinea-pig bronchospasm test)

2.3   Guinea-Pig Bronchospasm Test

The cat screen shows that it is relatively easy to determine an eventual differential blockade of cardiac and vascular adrenoceptor. Although the importance of preserving vascular smooth muscle adrenoceptor function is not yet clear, from the clinical point of view it is important that β-adrenoceptor activity be preserved in bronchial smooth muscle to lessen risk of bronchospasm. To detect an action, or perhaps lack thereof, on the bronchial β-adrenoceptors a guinea-pig bronchospasm test is used. Guinea pigs are very susceptible to the bronchoconstrictory action of histamine, an action that may be antagonized by the β-adrenoceptor-mediated bronchodilatory action of isoprenaline.

In this test a group of four animals are pretreated s.c. with isoprenaline (0.1 mg/kg) followed 15 min later by an s.c. injection of the compound under test (at a dose selected on the basis of the ED_{50} of the compound). After a further 15 min induction period the animals are subjected to a 45 sec aerosol spray of histamine prepared from a solution of 200 mg base in 16 ml water. If the animals survive, the test compound is considered to be selective (i.e., it has not blocked the protective effect of isoprenaline). Figure 2 shows the results from a series of such experiments at different doses of both propranolol and atenolol. Although the two compounds are of comparable activity as β_1-adrenoceptor blocking agents the curve for atenolol is shifted significantly to the right, demonstrating its much reduced activity as a β_2-adrenoceptor antagonist.

2.4   Intrinsic Sympathomimetic Activity (ISA)

This test determines the level of partial agonist activity of the compounds by measuring their ability to increase heart rate. To demonstrate this property it is necessary to remove the normal prevailing level of sympathetic stimulation to

Table 2

Partial Agonist Effects (ISA) of β-Adrenoceptor Blocking Agents Relative to Isoprenaline in Catecholamine-depleted Rats, and Their Antagonist Potencies in Anesthetized Cats

Drug	ISA	Antagonist potency
Isoprenaline	1	
D.C.I.	0.73	730 ± 80
Pindolol	0.56	2.5 ± 2
Practolol	0.35	158 ± 11
Oxprenolol	0.29	33 ± 7
Pronethalol	0.28	1260 ± 270
Alprenolol	0.16	60 ± 11
Propranolol	0	62 ± 10
Atenolol	0	88 ± 5

the heart. This is achieved by depleting the natural catecholamine activity in the animal and thus leaving the heart exposed to the partial agonist activity present in the molecule.

Rats are depleted of their natural catecholamine reserves by treatment with 5 mg/kg s.c. syrosingopine (a derivative of reserpine) 24 hours prior to testing. The effects of the β-adrenoceptor blocking agent are tested under nembutal anesthesia by s.c. injection of a standard dose (2.5 mg) and the effects on the heart rate are noted. The presence of partial agonist activity manifests itself in an increase in heart rate, and Table 2 indicates the relative levels of ISA in a number of clinically available β-adrenoceptor blocking drugs.

It is of interest to note that most of the literature quoting the levels of ISA of published drugs relates to this test and that the data from this test are very difficult, if not impossible, to relate to the clinical effect in man.

2.5 Membrane-Stabilizing Properties

Much attention was devoted by both pharmacologists and clinicians to the membrane-stabilizing (local anesthetic or quinidine-like) properties of β-adrenoceptor blocking agents and since one of our objectives was to discover a potent, selective β-adrenoceptor blocking agent without such a property, it was important to determine its presence or absence in the more promising compounds. One of the methods used was the frog sciatic nerve preparation.

In this preparation, frog sciatic nerves with the sheath intact were mounted in 5 ml chambers containing frog Ringer solution. After equilibration the nerves

Table 3
Aromatic Moiety of Some β-Adrenoceptor Blocking Drugs

Ar	Ar-CH$_2$CHCH$_2$NHR OH	Ar

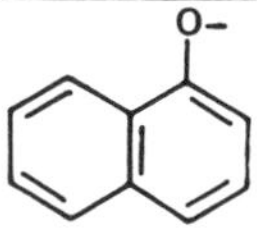

propranolol

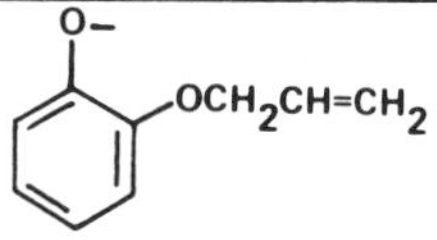

oxprenolol

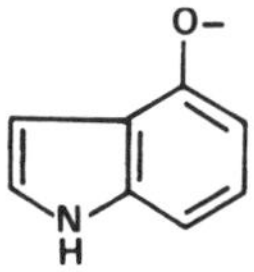

pindolol

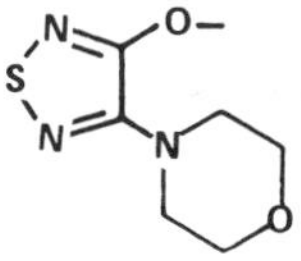

timolol

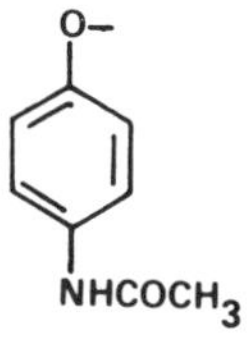

practolol

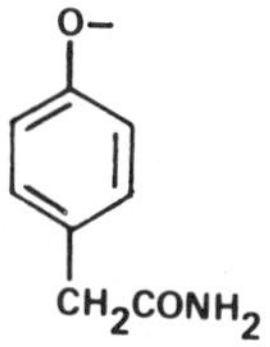

atenolol

were stimulated electrically and the height of the action potential (the spike potential) was read directly from an oscilloscope. The Ringer solution was then exchanged for solutions containing different concentrations of the test substance and, again after equilibration, the experiments were repeated. In this preparation atenolol had no effect on the spike potential at concentrations up to 10 mg/ml, whereas propranolol caused marked depression in the concentrations range 0.01-0.1 mg/ml.

The suitability of this largely *in vivo* testing sequence for β-adrenoceptor blocking agent screening can be judged from the fact that in the search for compounds with different combinations of dose level, ISA, selectivity, and membrane-stabilizing activities, compounds having various combinations of these activities were found using this testing sequence. Following further evaluation only atenolol eventually proceeded to the clinic, and this one drug was sufficient to confirm that for effective and safe treatment of hypertension, selectivity is an important property of a β-adrenoceptor blocking agent. Membrane-stablizing activity is irrelevant for cardioselectivity as is, apparently, partial agonist activity.

3. SYNTHETIC ASPECTS OF ATENOLOL

The realization that the activity of the enthanolamine group of β-adrenoceptor blockers could be improved by insertion of an oxymethylene moiety between the ethanolamine group and the aromatic nucleus provided the impetus for an immense synthetic effort devoted to the synthesis of β-adrenoceptor blocking agents. It is not surprising, therefore, that a wide variety of structural modifications of the aromatic nucleus has emerged, and Table 3 illustrates the diverse nature of some of the more well-known β-adrenoceptor blocking agents synthesized since propranolol. Clearly it is a simple matter to synthesize a molecule that looks like a β-adrenoceptor blocking agent, and not too difficult to synthesize one that is active. Even today, however, there are large gaps in our knowledge of structure-activity relationships, and although the synthesis of a β-adrenoceptor blocking agent had become relatively easy at the time of our research, the structural features responsible for the presence or absence of the other properties of selectivity, ISA, and so on were less obvious. The only difference between the selective practolol and its nonselective relatives was the presence of the acetylamino group in practolol; therefore it was toward this group that our attention turned. Two possibilities were considered as likely to be contributing to the selectivity of practolol:

1. The electron withdrawing effect of the carbonyl group could impart a degree of acidity to the proton of the —NHCO— group, which possibly could be mimicked by a —CH$_2$CO— group;
2. The anilide group present in practolol could be an effective partner in hydrogen bond formation by virtue of the NH moiety, and to incorporate this feature in a new molecule meant extending the new grouping to —CH$_2$CONHR.

The synthetic sequence for the preparation of the parent compound, that is, where R = H, is shown in Scheme 3; subsequent testing of this compound showed that we had indeed synthesized a β-adrenoceptor blocking agent with cardioselective properties. Surprising, however, was the absence in the compound of ISA, since previous experience had led us to believe that the presence of an amide function in the molecule would lead to compounds with this property. In addition, it was found that the compound was devoid of membrane-stabilizing properties.

The discovery of atenolol in this manner was the start of a synthetic effort to optimize activity and to investigate whether the pattern of activity discovered was a general feature of compounds based upon the phenylacetamides. We

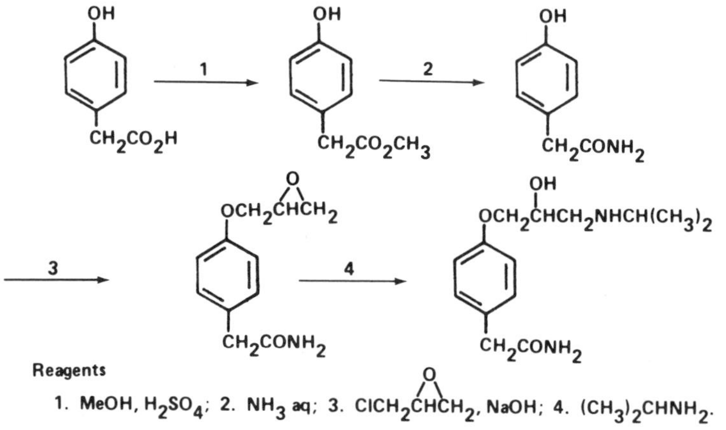

Scheme 3. Synthesis of atenolol

were aided in this work by the large number of hydroxyphenylacetic acids described in the literature. When the compounds actually required were not described, the methods of synthesis for regioisomers were found to be readily acceptable to the desired derivatives. In this manner a collection of acids was built up from which the atenolol analogues in Table 4 were synthesized.

The preferred synthetic route was that shown for propranolol in Scheme 1 and this route required that the acids be converted into their amides. There are, of course, numerous methods known for the conversion of acids into amides, but the method of choice in this case was the little used, but very convenient, method of simply stirring a suspension of the methyl or ethyl ester of the acid in aqueous ammonia at ambient temperatures to obtain quantitative yields of the primary amides (see Scheme 3). The only exception was in the preparation of the amide for **37**, where solubility of the nitro ester in water precluded use of the above convenient method. In this case the more widely known acid chloride route was used. The aqueous amine route was also found to be applicable to the preparation of the *N*-methyl amides, where again quantitative conversion was achieved. However, the method failed in the preparation of the amide for **15**. In this case aqueous *n*-butylamine hydrolyzed the ester and the amine salt of the original acid was produced, causing us to resort to the acid chloride route for the preparation of this analogue. Fortunately **15** and **37** were the only "deviants" of the compounds in Table 4.

4. STRUCTURE-ACTIVITY RELATIONSHIPS

In general terms receptor antagonists may be divided into two groups. One group includes compounds of widely varying structures that often bear little or no obvious resemblance to each other or to the natural agonist, for example, many dopaminergic and α-adrenoceptor antagonists. Their activity may be explained in terms of the compound binding with the receptor in a nonactive conformation, thereby preventing it from assuming an active conformation in the presence of the natural agonist. In contrast, the second group of antagonists bears a strong resemblance to the natural agonists and the β-adrenergic antagonists can be included within this group.

The basic requirement for activity within the β-adrenergic antagonists is the presence of an aromatic ring to which is connected an ethanolamine group, preferably by way of an oxymethylene spacer group. In addition, a further feature is determined from a consideration of the series noradrenaline, adrenaline, isoprenaline, from which emerges the following relative potencies as β-adrenoceptor stimulants:

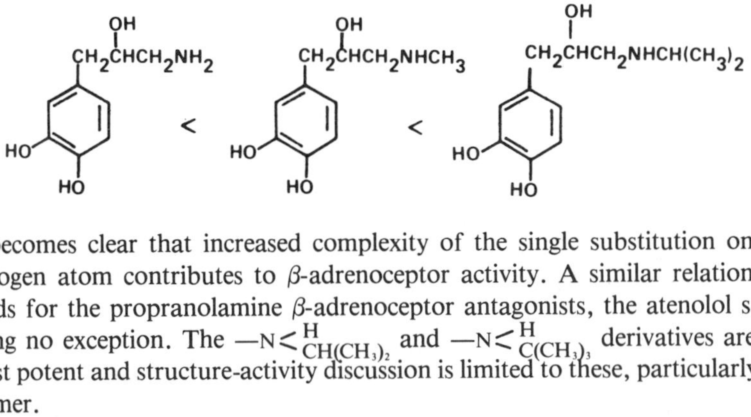

It becomes clear that increased complexity of the single substitution on the nitrogen atom contributes to β-adrenoceptor activity. A similar relationship holds for the propranolamine β-adrenoceptor antagonists, the atenolol series being no exception. The $-N{<}^{H}_{CH(CH_3)_2}$ and $-N{<}^{H}_{C(CH_3)_3}$ derivatives are the most potent and structure-activity discussion is limited to these, particularly the former.

The effects of substitution on the phenyl ring are less straightforward, but certain patterns of activity do emerge. First and foremost is the p-acetamido substituent. As was envisaged, this substituent gives rise to a cardioselective β-adrenoceptor blocking agent with the amide $-NH-$ group apparently playing an important role in this activity. Tertiary amides of this series are of such low activity that they may be regarded as inactive. In these cases the amido group is merely another large p-substituent with a steric requirement incompatible with β-adrenoceptor activity. The amide proton also permits the formation of hydrogen bonds with the solvent, particularly when the molecule is in an aqueous environment. In this context it is interesting to note that the log P value (octanol-water) of atenolol is 0.23, compared to 0.79 for practolol and

Table 4
Structural Analogues of Atenolol

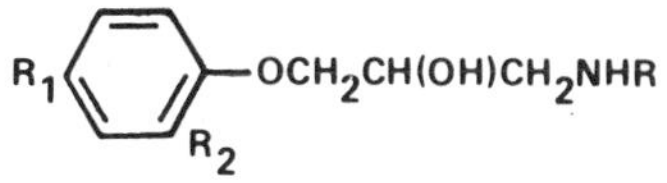

$$R_1 \langle \bigcirc \rangle \text{—OCH}_2\text{CH(OH)CH}_2\text{NHR}$$
$$R_2$$

No.	R	R_1	R_2	m.p. (°C)	ED_{50}
10	$i\text{-}C_3H_7$	CH_2CONH_2	H	146-148	88
11	$t\text{-}C_4H_9$	CH_2CONH_2	H	129-130	136
12	$i\text{-}C_3H_7$	$(CH_2)_2CONH_2$	H	102-104	681
13	$i\text{-}C_3H_7$	$(CH_2)_3CONH_2$	H	85-87	682
14	$i\text{-}C_3H_7$	$CH_2CONHCH_3$	H	87-89	335
15	$i\text{-}C_3H_7$	$CH_2CONHC_4H_9\text{-}n$	H	115-117	606
16	$i\text{-}C_3H_7$	$CH=CHCONH_2$	H	135-137	995
17	$i\text{-}C_3H_7$	CH_2CONH_2	OCH_3	118-120	72
18	$t\text{-}C_4H_9$	CH_2CONH_2	OCH_3	87-89	153
19	$i\text{-}C_3H_7$	$(CH_2)_2CONH_2$	OCH_3	108-109	154
20	$t\text{-}C_4H_9$	$(CH_2)_2CONH_2$	OCH_3	148-149	125
21	$i\text{-}C_3H_7$	$CH=CHCONH_2$	OCH_3	138-140	245
22	$i\text{-}C_3H_7$	CH_2CONH_2	F	97-100	310
23	$t\text{-}C_4H_9$	CH_2CONH_2	F	92-95	151
24	$i\text{-}C_3H_7$	CH_2CONH_2	Cl	101-102	118
25	$t\text{-}C_4H_9$	CH_2CONH_2	Cl	100-101	24
26	$i\text{-}C_3H_7$	CH_2CONH_2	Br	105-107	40
27	$i\text{-}C_3H_7$	$(CH_2)CONH_2$	Br	102-104	370
28	$i\text{-}C_3H_7$	CH_2CONH_2	I	126-128	88
29	$i\text{-}C_3H_7$	CH_2CONH_2	CH_3	126-127	49
30	$i\text{-}C_3H_7$	CH_2CONH_2	$n\text{-}C_3H_7$	116-117	50
31	$i\text{-}C_3H_7$	$CH_2CONHCH_3$	$n\text{-}C_3H_7$	125-127	87
32	$i\text{-}C_3H_7$	CH_2CONH_2	$(CH_3)_2\text{-}^{2,3}$	213-215	352
33	$i\text{-}C_3H_7$	CH_2CONH_2	$(CH_3)_2\text{-}^{2,5}$	111-113	300
34	$i\text{-}C_3H_7$	CH_2CONH_2	$CH_2CH=CH_2$	101-102	30
35	$i\text{-}C_3H_7$	$(CH_2)_2CONH_2$	$CH_2CH=CH_2$	93-95	382
36	$i\text{-}C_3H_7$	$(CH_2)_3CONH_2$	$CH_2CH=CH_2$	78-80	622
37	$i\text{-}C_3H_7$	$(CH_2)_2CONH_2$	NO_2	130-132	431

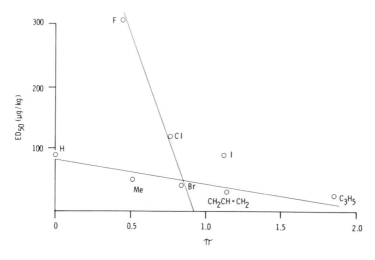

Figure 3. ED_{50} as a function of π for the series

$$H_2NCH_2C \overset{\text{O}}{\underset{\text{II}}{}} \hspace{-2mm} \overbrace{}^{R} \hspace{-2mm} OCH_2CH(OH)CH_2NHCH(CH_3)_2$$

3.56 for the nonselective propranolol, an indicator that hydrophilicity and selectivity are not unconnected. The presence of a hydrophilic group alone, however, is insufficient in itself for cardioselectivity, since the compound sotalol, an ethanolamine-based antagonist, is nonselective in spite of its sulfonamide substituent, whereas its propranolamine analogue is selective.

From the above discussion it would appear that the methylene group of the acetamido substituent plays little or no part in either the antagonistic activity or the cardioselectivity, but it has one important property, namely it reduces ISA to negligible levels. These and subsequent researches[11] have confirmed this property. Antagonists with a *para*-amidic substituent, with either the nitrogen or carbonyl group attached to the aromatic nucleus, have varying levels of ISA that are significantly reduced when a methylene group separates the phenyl ring and amidic substituent. There are, however, constraints on this property. Extension of the spacer group beyond one methylene group leads to a decreased activity.

An additional feature of the atenolol series is that a further substituent can be tolerated, but preferably when the extra substituent is *meta* to the amide substituent. A further substituent *ortho* to the amide group results in reduction of potency, most probably because of steric factors. An increase in the lipophilic character of the *meta* substituent results in increased potency, but this is not immediately obvious from a simple ranking of the lipophilicity coefficient π.

However, if activity is plotted against π for a number of derivatives (Figure 3), two orders of potency are observed, one containing the halogen substituents and the other, of much shallower slope, containing the alkyl substituents. The reason for this is found in the Hammett factor σ_m, which is higher for the halogen substituents. Thus in addition to the positive lipophilic effect of the substituents there is a negative electronic effect on activity that is counteracted by increasing the lipophilicity of the substituent (the iodo substituent deviates somewhat, possibly for steric reasons).

Table 4 contains no information on the selectivity of the compounds. It is stated earlier that for a quantitative estimation, selectivity may be recorded as the percentage blockade of the depressor response to isoprenaline at the cardiac ED_{50}. Unfortunately, most of the compounds tested caused a progressive fall in blood pressure during the experiment so that it became impossible to do more than judge in a qualitative manner whether a compound was selective or not. What does emerge, however, is that the compounds that displayed qualitative cardioselectivity lie on the "alkyl line" of Figure 3 and include the bromo derivative. It appears that electronic effects not only act against activity, but also against cardioselectivity!

It had been proposed that the N-H group of the amide substituent is in part responsible for the receptor binding by acting as a proton donor, but the results shown in Figure 3 offer an alternative explanation for the contribution of the amide substituent to the activity of the atenolol series. The reduced electron availability caused by the halogen substituent could exert itself through to the carbonyl group, thus decreasing its potential as a proton *acceptor* and thereby causing a reduction in activity, an effect counterbalanced by an increase in lipophilicity. Our knowledge of receptor binding is insufficient to differentiate between the two possibilities, but whichever effect is responsible, the presence of the acetamido group *para* to the propanolamine side chain gives atenolol, a β-adrenoceptor blocking drug, which is the closest yet to a pure β_1-adrenoceptor antagonist.

ACKNOWLEDGMENTS
The discovery of a drug depends not on the efforts of an individual, but on effective team work, and I would like to take this opportunity to mention the other members of our team who contributed toward the discovery of atenolol. It was with Dr. Roy Hull that the original concept was devised and it was Chris Squire upon whom the majority of the synthetic effort fell. No matter how good a compound is, it must be tested, and it was Professor M. Barrett and Mr. J. Carter who set up the biological sequence described in this chapter. Finally, I would like to thank Dr. Barry Cox for his helpful criticism in the preparation of the manuscript.

REFERENCES

1. H. H. Dale, *J. Physiol.,* **34,** 163 (1906).
2. G. Barger and H. H. Dale, *J. Physiol.,* **51,** 19 (1910).
3. R. P. Ahlquist, *Am. J. Physiol.,* **153,** 586 (1948).
4. H. Konzett, *Arch. Exp. Path. Pharmacol.,* **197,** 27 (1940).
5. J. Mills, U.S. Patent 2,938,921 (1960).
6. J. W. Black and J. S. Stephenson, *Lancet,* 711 (1962).
7. J. W. Black, A. F. Crowther, R. G. Shanks, L. H. Smith, and A. C. Dornhorst, *Lancet,* 1081 (1964).
8. A. M. Barrett, A. F. Crowther, D. Dunlop, R. G. Shanks, and L. H. Smith, *Arch. Pharmakol. Exp. Pathol.,* **259,** 152 (1968).
9. A. M. Lands, A. Arnold, J. P. McAuliff, F. P. Luduena, and T. G. Brown, *Nature,* **214,** 597 (1967); A. M. Lands, F. P. Luduena, and H. J. Buzzo, *Life Sci.,* **6,** 2241 (1967).
10. B. Ablad, *Acta Pharmacol. Toxicol.,* Suppl. 2, 25:5 (1967).
11. L. H. Smith, *J. Med. Chem.,* **20,** 1254 (1977).

Bumetanide

Peter W. Feit

6

Work in medicinal chemistry, like that in other sciences, can be compared to the building of a complicated mosaic of unlimited dimensions. No master drawing is available and pieces are added to existing parts of the mosaic by continuous trial and error, using a variety of theoretical and experimental approaches. Progress is made in a series of steps and requires the cooperation of many scientists. The shape, size, and color, as well as the position of every single piece in the mosaic is of importance and when a small area of the mosaic is filled in, for example, when a new drug with valuable therapeutic properties is found, it often initiates the completion of further parts. Consequently, the starting point of the process that eventually leads to the development of a particular drug is situated somewhere in the mosaic. Thus the sulfamoyl diuretic bumetanide (3-*n*-butylamino-4-phenoxy-5-sulfamoylbenzoic acid) (**1**) has its real origin in the antibacterial sulfanilamide (**2**). The diuretic effect of this *p*-aminobenzoic acid antagonist is a side effect due to inhibition of the enzyme carbonic anhydrase in the kidney. Though weakly effective, even at massive

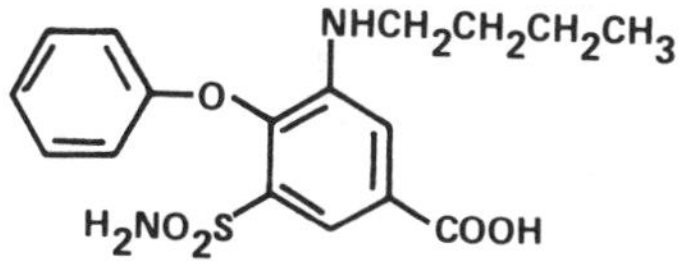

1

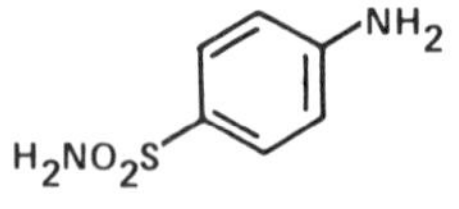

2

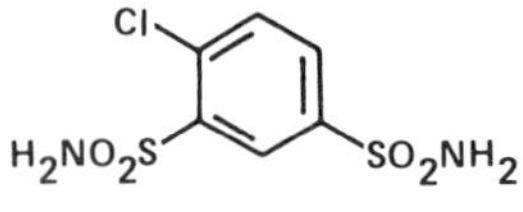

3

doses, **2** was the first sulfamoyl compound used as a diuretic in the treatment of patients.[1] I have summarized earlier the ways in which chemical alterations of this basic model have led to three different types of diuretic drugs,[2] from the carbonic anhydrase inhibitors by way of clofenamide (4-chloro-1,3-benzenedisulfonamide) (**3**) in an intermediate position, to the thiazide-type diuretics, and finally to the "high ceiling" or loop diuretics, including bumetanide (**1**).

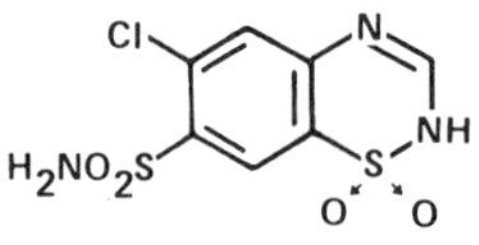

4

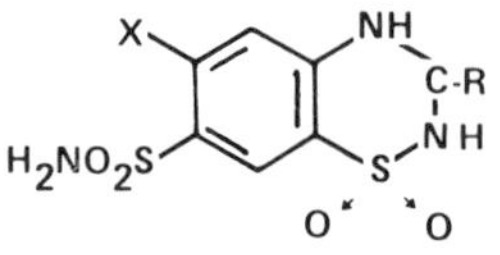

5, X = Cl, R = H
6, X = CF$_3$, R = H
7, X = CF$_3$, R = C$_6$H$_5$CH$_2$

In connection with the present account the period following the synthesis of chlorothiazide (6-chloro-7-sulfamoyl-2H-1,2,4-benzothiadiazine 1,1-dioxide) (**4**)[3] is of special interest. The valuable diuretic properties of **4**, discovered in the late fifties,[4] and quite different from those of carbonic anhydrase inhibitors, had initiated worldwide interest in sulfamoyl compounds as potential diuretics. A tremendous amount of chemical and pharmacological research resulted in a large number of diuretically active sulfamoyl compounds, many of which were introduced into clinical practice. The pharmacological characteristics of these new drugs resembled those of chlorothiazide (**4**). They caused an increased urinary excretion of nearly equivalent amounts of sodium and chloride accompanied by an osmotic equivalent of water. Furthermore, they all showed the same degree of maximal sodium excretion, namely, about 8% of the ultrafiltrate, the latter being produced in the glomeruli of the nephrons of the human kidney. Interestingly, with respect to chemical structure they were all related either to clofenamide (**3**) or to the bicyclic structure of chlorothiazide (**4**) and its dihydro derivative, hydrochlorothiazide (**5**).[5] Although structural alterations of the thiadiazine ring and its replacement by various cyclic systems had been performed, and the structure of clofenamide (**3**) had been extensively modified as well, it became evident that certain common structural features contributed to a high order of potency in this type of diuretic. Consequently, in the mid-sixties it was generally held that the diuretic activity of the above mentioned compounds depended on the presence of:

1. An unsubstituted sulfamoyl group.
2. A chlorine atom or a CF_3-group.
3. A SO_2 or CO electronegative group, either as a substituent or incorporated in a cyclic structure.
4. The same mutual position of these groups as indicated in 3 and 4.

Since then, these empirical rules have been stated in a more definite way,[6] and they still hold for the thiazide-type of action.

Since the mid-sixties, these various thiazide-type diuretics have served as valuable tools in the management of clinical situations accompanied by edematous states, and in the treatment of hypertension, alone or in concomitant adminsitration with other antihypertensive drugs. They are fairly well absorbed from the gastrointestinal tract and are generally well tolerated. Many of them are interchangeable since they differ clinically only in two major respects: their milligram potency in the context of activity per weight unit varies over a range of 1 to 2000, and their duration of action varies from 6 to more than 24 hours. Since the well-known side effects, such as a tendency to decrease serum potassium levels, were apparently common features of these diuretics and partly a physiological consequence of their particular mechanism of action, and since these side effects could be handled in clinical practice, the medicinal chemist would not have been interested in further variations on the same structural theme if it had not been for a drug named furosemide [4-chloro-N-(2-furylmethyl)anthranilic acid](8). Since the priority date (December 1959) of the appropriate patent application[7] revealed that this diuretic was synthesized in the period following the synthesis of chlorothiazide, it was probably not by chance that the former compound had the structural characteristics of the thiazide-type diuretics, which are discussed above. Even more remarkable, therefore, were the diuretic properties of this drug, since they differed substantially from those of other sulfamoyl diuretics known in the sixties. Both animal studies[8] and the first clinical investigations in volunteers and patients had shown furosemide (8)

8

$$H_5C_2-\overset{\overset{\displaystyle CH_2}{\|}}{C}-\overset{\overset{\displaystyle O}{\|}}{C}$$

[chemical structure with Cl, Cl, and OCH$_2$COOH substituents on benzene ring]

9

to be superior to the thiazide-type drugs with respect to maximal diuretic and saluretic effect[9-11]. Furthermore, a more rapid onset of action and a steeper dose-response curve had been demonstrated, as well as effectiveness when given either orally or parenterally. All these properties were similar to those that had been reported for ethacrynic acid [2,3-dichloro-4-(2-methylenebutyryl)-phenoxyacetic acid] (9), a nonsulfamoyl diuretic of unrelated structure[12-14]. It is well known now, that both drugs have their major site of action in the same section of the nephron, the ascending limb of the loop of Henle. The fact that a chemical variation of the thiazide-type structure had provided a drug with high ceiling action in terms of total quantity of urinary sodium chloride and water excretion, quite different in this respect from the remaining sulfamoyl diuretics, gave the impetus to our laboratories to perform further structural alterations to find new structures with "high ceiling" or "loop diuretic" activity.

As for myself, on one hand I was thoroughly convinced that such new structures should exist, but on the other hand, I had no idea what they should look like. Consequently, the only thing to do was to keep free from prejudice and start synthetic work. Screening for diuretic effect had been performed continuously in our laboratories since the late fifties, when chemical variation of chlorothiazide (4) led to two of our drugs, hydroflumethiazide (6-trifluoro-methyl-3,4-dihydro-7-sulfamoyl-2H-1,2,4-benzothiadiazine 1,1-dioxide) (6) and its 3-benzyl derivative, bendroflumethiazide (7).[15,16] Fortunately, there has never been any doubt about the validity of the diuretic screening procedure used in the work being described. Our pharmacologist at that time, Professor H.-H. Frey, suggested that the dog assay should be used since both ethacrynic acid (9) and furosemide (8) were active in this species. The parameters to be measured were, of course, the urinary volume and the excreted amount of Na$^+$, K$^+$, and Cl$^-$. To be independent of the degree of absorption after oral administration and, furthermore, to be able to detect compounds with only marginal activity, all candidates were screened intravenously in a dose of 10 mg/kg bodyweight.

To begin with, it was natural to consider the structure of furosemide (8) as a starting point for structural alteration and, because of tradition, to retain both the sulfamoyl group and the chloro substituent in the molecule. Consequently, our first efforts were directed to (a) an exchange of the carboxylic group and (b)

10, R = C$_6$H$_5$CH$_2$NH
11, R = OH
12, R = SH
13, R = C$_6$H$_5$CH$_2$O
14, R = C$_6$H$_5$CH$_2$S

an alteration of the substituted amino function. As to *a*, it is worth mentioning that replacement of the carboxylic group by various other groups in both furosemide (**8**) and its corresponding *N*-benzyl anthranilic acid derivative (**10**),[7-17] resulted in diuretically inactive compounds. Thus, within the limits of our knowledge at that time, we gained the false impression that the carboxylic group might be a prerequisite for potent high ceiling diuretic activity. The decision relating to alternative *b* had a greater influence on our further work. We investigated the 4-chloro-5-sulfamoylsalicylic and thiosalicylic acids **11** and **12**, as well as some of their derivatives, among them the benzyloxy and benzylthiobenzoic acids **13** and **14**. Benzyl substitution instead of furylmethyl substitution, as seen in furosemide (**8**), was chosen for synthetic reasons, although **10** was shown in the dog experiment to be only one-tenth as potent as **8**. Compound **11** was synthesized from 4-chlorosalicylic acid by chlorosulfonation and subsequent amidation.[18] Reaction of **11** with diazotoluene followed by saponification of the carboxylic ester simultaneously formed provided **13**. Compound **12** was prepared from 4-chloro-5-sulfamoylanthranilic acid by way of its diazonium salt and the corresponding disulfide, while **14** was at first made available by reaction of 2,4-dichloro-5-sulfamoylbenzoic acid with benzylmercaptan under alkaline condition and was then separated from the diuretically completely inactive isomeric 2-chloro-4-benzylthio-5-sulfamoylbenzoic acid by means of fractional crystallization of the sodium salts. The diuretic screening results of **11-14** revealed only marginal activity for **12-14** at the screening dose of 10 mg/kg, while, remarkably, the salicylic acid **11** was almost equal in potency to the anthranilic acid derivative **10**. We had a temporary interest in **11** and its diuretically similarly effective CF$_3$- analogue, 5-sulfamoyl-4-trifluoromethylsalicylic acid.[18] In a preclinical study, **11** was shown to have the pharmacological picture of a high ceiling diuretic, but with a potency one-tenth that of furosemide.[19] A few months after we had prepared (**11**) for our experiments, a Dutch patent application was published[20] in which **11** was used as an intermediate in the synthesis of some of its esters and amides, including xipamide [4-chloro-5-sulfamoylsalicylic acid (2′,6′-dimethyl)anilide]. The pharmacological effects[21] and the first clinical investigation[22] of the latter diuretic have been published with 9 and 4 years delay, respectively, while the comparatively less potent diuretic activity of **11** has not been described.

15, R = [structure with CH₃, N—NH, CH₃]

16, R = OH

One finding came from the above mentioned studies: the unsubstituted phenolic hydroxyl group could replace the benzylated aromatic amino function in the anthranilic acid derivatives without loss of potency, while the corresponding benzyloxy, mercapto, and benzylthio groups could not. I do not remember how many speculations were made on the importance of spatial arrangements and pK_a values, but the question arose of whether a substituent in the position *ortho* to the carboxylic group was required at all. In connection with the tailoring of the thiazide-type diuretic, clopamide [4-chloro-3-sulfamoylbenz(N-cis-2,6-dimethylpiperidino)amide] (15), it had been stated that in the 4-chloro-3-sulfamoylbenzhydrazide series substitution in the corresponding position decreased potency.[23] Although we were searching for structures with loop diuretic activity, we felt that it would be informative to have a look at 4-chloro-3-sulfamoylbenzoic acid (16). In fact this compound, which might be considered to be a simple parent compound of both the chlorosulfamoylanthranilic acid and benzhydrazide diuretics, had escaped my notice prior to that time. A British patent specification[24] told us that 16 should be of value on account of its diuretic and/or natriuretic properties. Its effectiveness was confirmed in our laboratories. Compound 16 shared the diuretic profile of the anthranilic acid derivative 10 and was rather short acting but almost as potent as 10 and the salicylic acid derivative 11. Although the individual compounds were not investigated in more detail, the sum of these studies could be interpreted in only one way, namely, that substitution in positions *ortho* to the carboxylic function was not mandatory for loop diuretic activity.

There was then no question as to where to concentrate our chemical efforts. How would the diuretic potency of 4-chloro-3-sulfamoylbenzoic acid (16) be influenced when various substituents were introduced in the position *meta* to the carboxylic group, which would amount to moving the *ortho*-substituent in the anthranilic, salicylic, and thiosalicylic acid derivatives to this particular position. Our first step was to synthesize 3-amino-4-chloro-5-sulfamoylbenzoic acid (17)[25] as an intermediate for numerous N-alkylated compounds and as a potential starting material for the introduction of other 3-substituents. Years later, when I wrote the first manuscript on the aminobenzoic acid diuretics, the name metanilic acid (i.e., 3-aminobenzenesulfonic acid) came to mind, and was, much to my subsequent chagrin, used erroneously throughout the publication[25] for 3-aminobenzoic acid, the mistake strangely enough being overlooked through all proofreading. Be that as it may, as biological activity is fortunately independent of nomenclature, let me return to the more crucial points. When 3-amino-4-chloro-5-sulfamoylbenzoic acid (17) was tested in our screening pro-

17, R = NH$_2$
18, R = C$_6$H$_5$CH$_2$NH
19, R = CH$_3$CH$_2$CH$_2$CH$_2$NH
20, R = C$_6$H$_5$CH$_2$S
21, R = CH$_3$CH$_2$CH$_2$CH$_2$S

cedure, its effect resembled, both qualitatively and quantitatively, that seen with 16. Consequently, for a period of time we forgot our ideas regarding the corresponding mercapto and hydroxy compounds and yielded to the temptation to deal more extensively with the impact of N^3 alkylation on the diuretic potency of 17. The outcome has been reported previously.[25] With respect to the structure-activity relationship, there was one observation of special interest. When intravenously administered to dogs, several of the prepared N^3-alkylated 3-amino-4-chloro-5-sulfamoylbenzoic acids had a diuretic potency similar to that of furosemide (8), while in the anthranilic acid series only the N-2-methylfuryl substitution, present in 8, afforded outstanding activity. Two selected compounds, namely, the 3-benzylamino-4-chloro-5-sulfamoylbenzoic acid (18) and the corresponding 3-n-butylamino analogue (19) were found to be suitable for a preliminary comparison with furosemide in four volunteers. When given orally as the crystalline substance in gelatin capsules both 18 and 19 were found to be about one-half as potent as furosemide as judged by dosage, but appeared essentially similar in diuretic profile and length of action. Since the scope of this rather limited study was only to confirm activity in human beings, the results did not allow more precise statements.

Although our initial plan was to provide the corresponding 3-hydroxy-, 3-alkoxy-, 3-mercapto-, and 3-alkylthio-4-chloro-5-sulfamoylbenzoic acids as well, we postponed this again in 1968 because of other interesting leads. However, some years later, we became interested anew in which way the shift from 2- and 3-alkylamino and 2- and 3-alkylthio in various 4-substituted 5-sulfamoylbenzoic acids influenced diuretic activity and potency.[26,27] We were able to show that 3-benzylthio-4-chloro-5-sulfamoylbenzoic acid (20) and the corresponding 3-n-butylthiobenzoic acid (21) were active diuretics in our dog assay, **21** apparently being more potent than the corresponding *n*-butylamino derivative **19**.[26]

An honest assessment of the results obtained thus far revealed, however, that no impressive progress had yet been made. Although from a structure-activity point of view we had gained the interesting knowledge that loop diuretic activity of sulfamoyl compounds was not dependent on the anthranilic acid structure represented by furosemide, we still had not found a more potent compound nor had we abandoned those structures that were generally accepted to be a requirement for diuretic activity of sulfamoyl compounds at that time, which I mention earlier when describing the background of our research. As often happens, for too long a time we had enjoyed getting compounds that were diuretically active and so we had been less inclined to run the risk of preparing a series of biologically inactive compounds by making more drastic structural changes. However, remembering that our initial goal was to search for new specific structures leading to high ceiling diuretic activity, the decision was made to alter the 4-substituent, which hitherto had been kept as Cl or CF_3. Within the limits of our knowledge at that time it was difficult to argue for any particular new substituent to be introduced into that position in the molecule and in such circumstances, I prefer to let the synthetic possibilities have a predominant influence on the first choice. It is clearly understood that although this approach is the easiest way to provide compounds for screening, it should, however, only be applied until the first sign of activity.

Actually, in 4-chloro-3-nitro-5-sulfamoylbenzoic acid (**22**) we had available an appropriate starting material, which we had used previously as an intermediate in the synthesis of the above discussed 3-substituted 4-chloro-5-sulfamoylbenzoic acid series.[25] The halogen in **22** is highly activated for nucleophilic substitution and consequently its reactivity could be expected to be suitable for the introduction of various groups as outlined in Scheme 1. Reduction of the resulting nitro compounds **23** to the corresponding aminobenzoic acids **24** and a subsequent alkylation should provide the desired 3,4-disubstituted 5-sulfamoylbenzoic acids **25** for diuretic screening. In any event, R^1 in **25** should include $C_6H_5CH_2$ to facilitate comparison. Although a few other synthetic attempts were made simultaneously, the rather uncomplicated sequence outlined in Scheme 1 turned out to be adjustable to many desired final compounds of type **25** with respect to synthetic details.[28]

Beginning with the reaction of **22** with several simple aliphatic and cycloaliphatic amines we started parallel preparations of various compounds of type **25**. By chance, the very first compound of this new series ready for diuretic screening was 3-benzylamino-4-*n*-butylamino-5-sulfamoylbenzoic acid (**25**; $R^1 = C_6H_5CH_2$, A = $CH_3CH_2CH_2CH_2NH$). The reader can imagine my

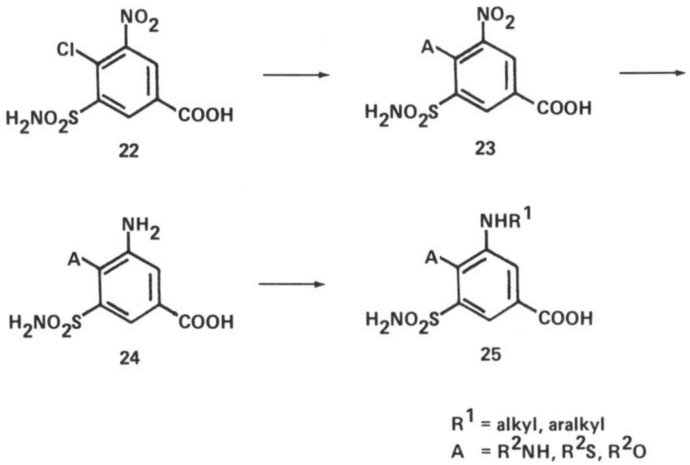

Scheme I.

enthusiastic feelings and expectations for future work when this compound at the screening dose of 10 mg/kg intravenously was shown to have a similar diuretic potency and profile as that of the corresponding 4-chlorobenzoic acid derivative **18**. In the light of this result, the closest we had come to what we wanted, we intensified the work on this particular series. However, essentially the same results were obtained subsequently with the 4-benzylamino, 4-morpholino-, and 4-piperidine-3-benzylamino-5-sulfamoylbenzoic acids **25**. This outcome was disappointing, since one would expect such variations in the substituent to be reflected in great differences in potency. Nevertheless, a final judgment required more compounds to be investigated.

My close collaboration with Professor Frey, whom I not only joined at lunch, but also met regularly to discuss the details of the diuretic screening, soon led to an event that, retrospectively, may be regarded as an important step on the way to the structure of bumetanide. I recall being at an informal meeting one day discussing with Professor Frey the results obtained with 4-anilino-3-benzylamino-5-sulfamoylbenzoic acid (**25**, $R^1 = C_6H_5CH_2$, $A = C_6H_5NH$). The values of urinary volume and electrolyte excretion following the screening dose of 10 mg/kg intravenously appeared to be almost similar to those seen with the previously tested compounds of this series. However, as the urine samples had been collected hourly in the screening procedure, an impression of the duration of action could be obtained, and in this particular case the results could be interpreted as an indication of a prolonged effect. This was indeed a speculation, on the basis of one single test, but, nevertheless, we became interested in whether such an effect could be real and still present at a lower dose and, furthermore, whether or not the dose-response curve was a steep one like that of furosemide (8) and 3-*n*-butylamino-4-chloro-5-sulfamoylbenzoic acid (16). An experiment was set up. The next day at lunch Professor Frey told me that a mistake must have been made when dosing the dog, because although the analysis of the electrolyte excretion had not yet been performed, the response in urinary output of water at the scheduled dose of 4 mg/kg had been found to be subtantially greater than seen after the screening dose of 10 mg/kg. We soon learned that the dosing in the study had been performed correctly and that the diuretic effect was even more pronounced when the dose was lowered to 0.5 mg/kg, where the maximal effect of loop diuretic activity in terms of volume and electrolyte excretion was obtained. If this reduction in dose had not been employed as a second-line investigation, the high potency of this particular compound might have been missed. We then reduced the screening dose to 0.25 mg/kg and continued to synthesize the various other compounds of the general formula 25 as planned. As reported,[28] we soon substantiated the high potency of many ofthe 4-substituted-3-amino-5-sulfamoylbenzoic acid derivatives (25). In preliminary experiments several compounds of this new series were shown to be 50-100 times as potent as furosemide when given intravenously or orally to trained conscious dogs. With respect to N substitution (R^1 in 25), benzyl, 2-furylmethyl, and *n*-butyl were found to contribute equally to high potency, a similar situation having been observed by us[25] in the corresponding 3-amino-4-chloro-5-sulfamoylbenzoic acid series discussed above.

Since we were in the position of having compounds showing high ceiling diuretic activity of hitherto unknown potency in dogs, we wanted, of course, to select one candidate for clinical assessment. For various reasons, such as similar potency in dogs, simple structure and fairly good synthetic availability, the first two compounds on the short list were 3-benzylamino-4-phenylthio-5-sulfamoylbenzoic acid (25, R^1 = $C_6H_5CH_2$, A = C_6H_5S) and the corresponding 4-anilino compound (25, R^1 = $C_6H_5CH_2$, A = C_6H_5NH), the latter of which is mentioned earlier. The pharmacology of the two compounds appeared to be similar and neither had toxicological effects. A pilot volunteer study revealed that the oral administration of 4 mg of either compound in an aqueous solution produced a response over 6 hours, similar to 40 mg of furosemide. Although we had not presumed that results in the dog and man would be the same, the fact that the potency ratio between furosemide and these compounds had changed from about 1:50 in dogs to about 1:10 in man required further consideration. Assuming that the renal response was dependent on urinary excreted drug, the results in man could be due to unfavorable pharmacokinetics, for example, the metabolism and extrarenal excretion of the compounds or, perhaps, their impaired absorption from the gastrointestinal tract. Excellent absorption after oral administration was, however, a prerequisite for a potential diuretic. Of course, the proper way to investigate the bioavailability and excretion patterns of our compounds would have been to determine drug levels in serum and urine after both oral and parenteral administration. However, in 1969 the analytical methods available for these compounds, although adequate for the concentrations obtained in pharmacological investigations, were not sensitive enough to measure the low drug levels expected in man. One way to obtain additional information on the compounds was to look at the time course of the renal response. Volunteer studies involving restriction of food and fluid intake for several days and frequent collections of urine are not easy to organize, so I decided to design a very simple study in one man, namely, myself. Furthermore, I wanted to include not only the two compounds already studied in volunteers, but also a third one of the general formula **25**, which pharmacodynamically and toxicologically appeared similar to the former ones. This particular compound was 3-*n*-butylamino-4-phenoxy-5-sulfamoylbenzoic acid (bumetanide) (**1**). I felt it would be interesting to see whether the simultaneous change to the phenoxy moiety and to the *n*-butylamino group in the 4- and 3-positions of the molecule, respectively, would have any influence on the diuretic behavior. I carried out the study over 5 days, carefully keeping the diet and the fluid intake constant. On days 1, 3, and 5, 1 mg of the respective compounds was taken as a solution in 50 ml of dilute sodium bicarbonate, while the vehicle only was administered on days 2 and 4, as a control. The response was determined by measuring the renal water output in collection periods of 30 minutes for 6 hours following administration. The original histograms depicting the results, which were hand drawn by me on March 1, 1969, are still available and are reproduced as Figure 1. The reader who is familiar with the Danish language might even detect some spelling errors reflecting that Danish is not my native tongue. It will be seen from the histogram of bumetanide, which is indicated by an arrow in Figure 1, that this compound appeared to distinguish itself from the other two benzoic acid derivatives in showing a quicker onset of action and by far the greatest diuretic response. Knowing the response to furosemide, a potency ratio of about 40 could be suggested for bumetanide/furosemide. Shortly afterward a volunteer study proved that this ratio was correct with respect to both urinary volume and electrolyte excretion.[29]

These results encouraged us to select bumetanide for further evaluation. Basic pharmacological investigations confirmed the loop diuretic activity in dogs, but showed that rather high doses were required to obtain a diuretic

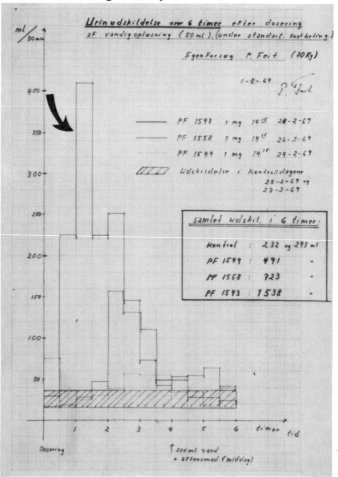

Figure 1. Reproduction of the original hand-drawn histograms showing the excretion of urine following oral administration of 1 mg to one single volunteer of three different compounds: 4-anilino-3-benzylamino-5-sulfamoylbenzoic acid (laboratory code: PF 1549), 3-benzylamino-4-phenylthio-5-sulfamoylbenzoic acid (laboratory code: PF 1558), and 3-n-butylamino-4-phenoxy-5-sulfamoylbenzoic acid (bumetanide, laboratory code: PF 1593). The arrow indicates the histogram of bumetanide. The ordinate gives the volume of urine in ml/30 min. The hours following administration are shown on the abscissa (dose given at zero-time). The excretion over the 30 min periods on two control days were found to be inside the hatched area. The 6 hour cumulative excretion on the control days was 232 and 292 ml, respectively, while the corresponding values for PF 1549, PF 1558, and PF 1593 (bumetanide) were found to be 491, 723, and 1538 ml, respectively.

effect in rats.[30] It has since been shown that the lowest effective doses in the dog, rabbit, mouse, and rat are 0.005, 0.1, 0.5, and 30 mg, respectively, a difference that correlates with variations in the metabolism of bumetanide in these species.[31] Once a suitable GLC method for measuring bumetanide had been developed and ^{14}C-labeled bumetanide had been synthesized, a parallelism between urinary recovery of bumetanide and its diuretic/saluretic action over the total period of response was demonstrated in volunteers too.[32,33]

In this type of work, processes often turn out to be more complicated than initially expected. Thus, for example, the original GLC method used in the above study for the determination of bumetanide (1) in biological fluids, comprising a methylation in the injection part of the gas chromatograph by means of tetramethylammonium hydroxide and trimethylanilinium hydroxide, was expected to simply transform the drug to methyl 3-*n*-butylamino-5-dimethylsulfamoyl-4-phenoxybenzoate (26). However, it turned out that the flash heater methylation leads to a sequence of reactions ending up in methyl 3-(*N*-*n*-butylanilino)-5-dimethylsulfamoyl-4-methoxybenzoate (28) as shown in Scheme 2. The formation of 28 involves a Smiles rearrangement and subsequent methylation of the phenolic hydroxyl in the intermediate 27.[32]

It is not within the scope of this account to detail how we met our own requirements and those of the regulatory agencies of various countries with respect to preclinical and clinical assessment. On the basis of numerous

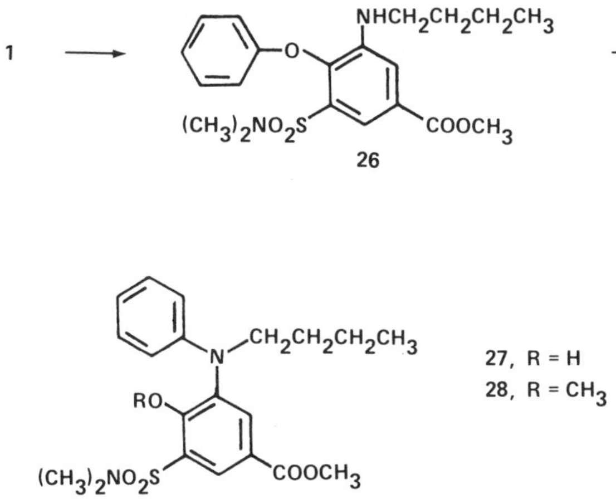

1 ⟶

NHCH$_2$CH$_2$CH$_2$CH$_3$

(CH$_3$)$_2$NO$_2$S   COOCH$_3$

26

⟶

CH$_2$CH$_2$CH$_2$CH$_3$

RO

(CH$_3$)$_2$NO$_2$S   COOCH$_3$

27, R = H
28, R = CH$_3$

Scheme 2.

investigations, including the original studies on human pharmacokinetics and others on the therapeutic use of bumetanide[33-37] the diuretic was approved for oral and parenteral administration by the health authorities in Denmark on September 11, 1972. Since then, pharmacological and clinical investigations have continued and approval has been given for the clinical uses of bumetanide in many countries.

Once the high potency loop diuretic activity of the 4-substituted 3-amino-5-sulfamoylbenzoic acid derivatives of the general formula **25**, including bumetanide, had been discovered, several new and interesting questions concerning structure-activity relationships of sulfamoyl diuretics emerged. Of most relevance to bumetanide was the question of investigating whether or not the phenoxy group or related groups, which apparently contributed to high potency, were specific for loop diuretic activity, or in other words, whether, with this new series, a distinction could be made between the structural requirements for the thiazide type and loop diuretic type of sulfamoyl compounds. This question was answered unequivocally when it was shown that introduction of phenoxy or phenylthio moieties in the place of Cl in selected thiazide type diuretics led to diuretically inactive compounds,[38] while, on the contrary, exchange of Cl in the loop diuretic furosemide (**8**) and the related anthranilic acid derivatives drastically increased diuretic potency.[39] Following these observations, we carried out further alterations of the substituents in both the 2,4- and 3,4-disubstituted 5-sulfamoylbenzoic acids by various synthetic routes. As reported previously,[26,27,40,41] many of these compounds showed high potency, high ceiling diuretic activity, among them 3-(3-thenyloxy)-4-benzoyl-5-sulfamoylbenzoic acid, which exhibited activity in the dog when given intravenously at a dose as low as 1 μg/kg,[27] and consequently was about five times as potent as bumetanide per weight unit. Another remarkable finding was that neither the sulfamoyl group nor the carboxylic acid group was a prerequisite for high ceiling diuretic activity.[42-44] However, since their pharmacodynamic profile was very similar to that of bumetanide, none of these compounds could be expected to have any advantages over this drug with respect to clinical usefulness.

ACKNOWLEDGMENT

In closing this account on bumetanide I would like to address my thanks to all members of the team who contributed to the discovery and development of bumetanide. I am indebted to Dr. Marian Rasbridge, Leo Laboratories, Ltd., United Kingdom, for linguistic corrections of the manuscript.

REFERENCES

1. W. Schwarz, *N. Engl. J. Med.,* **240,** 173 (1949).
2. P. W. Feit, "Structure-Activity Relationships of Sulfamoyl Diuretics," in *Bumetanide,* B.I. Hoffbrand and G. Jones, Eds., *Postgraduate Med. J.,* **51,** Suppl. 6, 1975, p. 9.
3. F. C. Novello and G. M. Sprague, *J. Am. Chem. Soc.,* **89,** 2028 (1957).
4. K. H. Beyer, *Ann. N.Y. Acad. Sci.,* **71** (4), 363 (1958).
5. G. deStevens and co-workers, *Experientia,* **14,** 463 (1958).
6. J. M. Sprague, "Diuretics" in *Topics in Medical Chemistry,* Vol. 2, J. L. Rabinowitz and R. M. Myerson, Eds., Wiley, Inc. New York, 1968, p. 41.
7. K. Sturm, W. Siedel, and R. Weyer, Deutsch Bundes Patent 1,122,541, *Chem. Abstr.* **56,** 14032e (1962), corresponding to U.S. Patent 3,058,882 (Oct. 16, 1962).
8. R. Muschaweck and F. Hajdu, *Arzneim.-Forsch..,* **14,** 44 (1964).
9. H. Kleinfelder, *Deutsch Med. Wochensch.,* **88,** 1965 (1963).
10. R. J. Timmerman, F. R. Springman, and R. K. Thoms, *Curr. Ther. Res.,* **6,** 88 (1964).
11. W. Stokes and L. C. A. Nunn, *Br. Med. J.,* **2,** 910 (1964).
12. E. M. Schultz, E. J. Cragoe, J. B. Bicking, W. A. Bolhofer, and J. M. Sprague, *J. Med. Pharm. Chem.,* **5,** 660 (1962).
13. K. H. Beyer, J. E. Baer, J. K. Michaelson, and H. F. Russo, *J. Pharmacol. Exp. Ther.,* **147,** 1 (1965).
14. P. J. Cannon, R. P. Ames, and J. H. Laragh, *J. Am. Chem. Assoc.,* **185,** 854 (1963).
15. W. Kobinger and F. J. Lund, *Acta Pharmacol. Toxicol.,* **15,** 265 (1959).
16. F. J. Lund and W. Kobinger, *Acta Pharmacol. Toxicol.,* **16,** 297 (1960).
17. K. Sturm, W. Siedel, R. Weyer, and H. Ruschig, *Chem. Ber.,* **99,** 328 (1966).
18. Løvens Kemiske Fabrik, Produktionsaktieselskab, French M. Patent 6090 (1968); *Chem. Abstr.,* **72,** 12382a (1970).
19. Personal communication from Professor, Dr. K. H. Olesen, Medical Department B, Rigshospital, University of Copenhagen, Medical School.
20. P. Beiersdorf and Co. A.G., Dutch Patent Application 6,607,680 (Dec. 20, 1966) *Chem. Abstr.,* **67,** 21706h (1967).
21. F. Leuschner, W. Neumann, and H. Bahrman, *Arzneim.-Forsch.,* **25,** 245 (1975).
22. McO. Hammer and U. Dembowski, *Med. Klin.,* **64,** 1862 (1969).
23. E. Jucker, A. Lindemann, E. Schenker, E. Fluckiger, and M. Taescher, *Arzneim.-Forsch.,* **13,** 269 (1963).
24. V. Petrow, O. Stephenson, and A. M. Wild, The British Drug House Ltd., British Patent 896,137 (May 9, 1962), *Chem. Abstr.,* **58,** 2409b (1963).
25. P. W. Feit, H. Bruun, and C. Kaergaard Nielsen, *J. Med. Chem.,* **13,** 1071 (1970).
26. P. W. Feit, O. B. T. Nielsen, and H. Bruun, *J. Med. Chem.,* **17,** 572 (1974).
27. O. B. T. Nielsen, H. Bruun, C. Bretting, and P. W. Feit, *J. Med. Chem.,* **18,** 41 (1975).
28. P. W. Feit, *J. Med. Chem.,* **14,** 432 (1971).
29. K. Roholt, personal communication.
30. E. H. Østergaard, M. P. Magnussen, Chr. Kaergaard Nielsen, E. Eilertsen, and H.-H. Frey. *Arzneim.-Forsch.,* **22,** 66 (1972).
31. M. P. Magnussen and E. Eilertsen, *Arch. Pharmacol.,* Suppl. to **282,** R61 (1974).
32. P. W. Feit, K. Roholt, and H. Sørensen, *J. Pharm. Sci.,* **62,** 375 (1973).

33. D. L. Davies, A. F. Lant, N. R. Millard, A. J. Smith, J. W. Ward, and G. M. Wilson, *Clin. Pharm. Ther.,* **15,** 141 (1974).

34. K. H. Olesen, B. Sigurd, E. Steiness, and A. Leth, *Acta Med. Scand.,* **193,** 199 (1973).

35. M. J. Asbury, P. B. B. Gatenby, S. O'Sullivan, and E. Bourke, *Br. Med. J.,* **22,** 211 (1972).

36. K. J. Berg, K. G. Gisholt, and T. Widerϕe, *Tidskr. Norske Laegeforen.,* **93,** 843 (1973).

37. P. I. Hoffbrand and G. Jones, Eds., *Bumetanide, Postgrad. Med. J.,* **51,** Suppl. 6 (1975).

38. P. W. Feit, O. B. T. Nielsen, and H. Bruun, *J. Med. Chem.,* **15,** 437 (1972).

39. P. W. Feit and O. B. T. Neilsen, *J. Med. Chem.,* **15,** 83 (1972).

40. P. W. Feit, O. B. T. Nielsen, and N. Rastrup-Andersen, *J. Med. Chem.,* **16,** 127 (1973).

41. O. B. T. Nielsen, C. K. Nielsen and P. W. Feit, *J. Med. Chem.,* **16,** 1170 (1973).

42. P. W. Feit, and O. B. T. Nielsen, *J. Med. Chem.,* **19,** 402 (1976).

43. P. W. Feit, and O. B. T. Nielsen, *J. Med. Chem.,* **20,** 1687 (1977).

44. O. B. T. Nielsen and P. W. Feit, "Structure-Activity Relationships of Aminobenzoic Acid Diuretics and Related Compounds," in *Diuretic Agents,* E. J. Cragoe, Jr., Ed., ACS Symposium Series 83, American Chemical Society, 1978, Chap. 2.

Ibuprofen

7

John S. Nicholson

1. INTRODUCTION

Some aspects of the development of (±)-2-(4-isobutylphenyl)propionic acid
(1), ibuprofen (BTS 13 621, Brufen, The Boots Company; U 18 573, Motrin,
The Upjohn Company), have already been described,[1-3] but it is hoped that this
chapter will provide a more detailed insight into its development within the context of the medicinal chemical aspects of the research. Ibuprofen was introduced into therapy as an anti-inflammatory agent for the treatment of
rheumatic and allied conditions in the United Kingdom in February 1969 by
The Boots Company and in the United States by the Upjohn Company in
August 1974. It is now being marketed in over 120 countries.

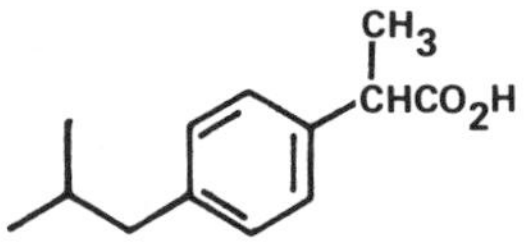

1

During the 1950s the Research Department of The Boots Company com-
menced work on nonsteroidal anti-inflammatory agents. This decision followed from an appreciation of the problems that had arisen from the long term
use of the corticosteroids in rheumatoid arthritis. During this period Stewart
Adams, then project pharmacologist and later project leader, was active in pro-
posing new hypotheses to explain the anti-inflammatory nature of aspirin and

149

other compounds such as pyrazoles.[4] Our initial objective, therefore, was to find anti-inflammatory compounds more potent than aspirin and with very much reduced side effects. The principal side effects of aspirin are gastrointestinal complications, ranging from mild dyspepsia to ulceration and bleeding in severe cases. Adams and Cobb[4,5] successfully modified the ultraviolet erythema test of Wilhelmi[6] so that large numbers of compounds could be screened for their anti-inflammatory effect. In this test, guinea pigs received an oral dose of either the drug in acacia suspension or acacia suspension alone 30 min before irradiation of the depilated backs. Two hours later the degree of erythema was estimated visually using a score of 0-4. Sodium salicylate, aspirin, and phenylbutazone were all active in this test in doses that could be approximately related to their clinical antirheumatic dose.

2. PHENOXYALKANOIC ACIDS

Numerous compounds selected for various specific reasons were examined in the UV- erythema model. Earlier studies on aspirin and its analogues had already indicated the importance of a carboxylic acid group and therefore we were particularly interested in our finding that a number of phenoxyalkanoic acids, originally made as potential herbicides and available in the files of the Boots Co., were more active than aspirin. One such compound was 2-(4-ethyl-phenoxy)propionic acid (2) with an activity twice that of aspirin. As Shen[2] has

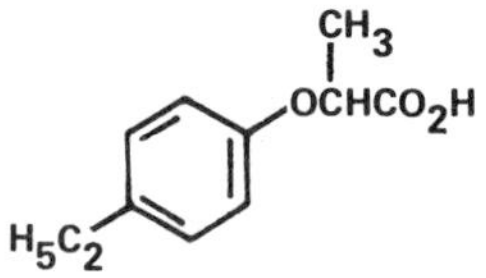

2

pointed out, it is interesting that two plant growth regulators, namely, indolyl-acetic acid and the phenoxyalkanoic acids, served as the basic lead compounds for anti-inflammatory studies at both Merck and Boots. After the synthesis and testing of more than 600 phenoxyalkanoic acids, 2-(4-phenylphenoxy)propionic acid (3), with a UV-erythema activity of 6-10 times that of aspirin, was selected as one of the most active members of the series.

Not surprisingly, the major urinary metabolite of 3 in rabbits was the 4 '-hydroxy compound 4. As this metabolite was dextrorotatory, it alerted us to the possibility of stereospecific changes occurring during the metabolism of propionic acids. In contrast, the same metabolite (4) from man was only slight-ly dextrorotatory. In view of these findings the resolution of 3 was attempted; it

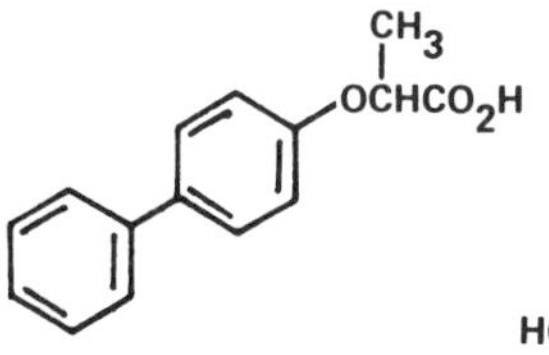

3 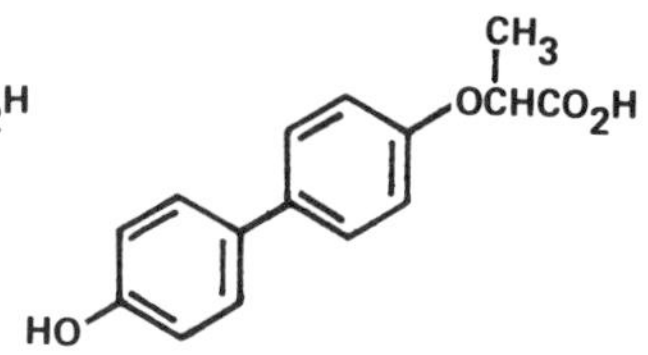   4

failed with both (-)-α-methylbenzylamine and cinchonine but was achieved with strychnine. The enantiomers were each as active as the racemate in the UV-erythema test.

Because it was felt that the ethyl ester of **3**, with a UV-erythema activity 2-8 times that of aspirin, might cause less gastric intolerance than the acid, it was submitted for clinical trial but was inactive in rheumatoid arthritis at 1.8 g daily.[5] This clinical inactivity of ethyl 2-(4-phenylphenoxy)propionate caused a drastic reassessment of our approach. It was subsequently found that the ester showed low analgesic activity, as measured by a modification of Randall and Selitto's rat foot test,[7] and low antipyretic activity. Adams[5,8] concluded that all three properties, namely, anti-inflammatory, analgesic, and antipyretic activity, were necessary for a clinical nonsteroidal antirheumatic effect. This concept was quite novel in 1960 and our search was then directed toward compounds with this full pharmacological spectrum.

3. PHENYLALKANOIC ACIDS

Even before the demise of the phenoxyalkanoic acids in 1960, a transition into the phenylalkanoic acids had been taking place. In particular, we first examined 4-alkylphenylalkanoic acids and 4-biphenylylalkanoic acids and were very encouraged to find that these compounds possessed the type of pharmacological spectrum that we were seeking. We found that the 4-biphenylylalkanoic acids were a highly potent group of anti-inflammatory compounds and for some time we proceeded simultaneously with these and the other phenylalkanoic acids. The decision was made to proceed in detail with the less potent phenylalkanoic acids at first because it seemed, in view of the toxicological data then available, more likely that a product candidate could be selected from this less potent group. The 4-biphenylylalkanoic acids were not discarded and we returned to an intensive study of this area in the years after 1963. In 1957 Cavallini[9] suggested that some alkanoic and alkenoic acids derived from biphenyl, stilbene, and diphenylethane had potential antirheumatic and hypocholesterolemic properties, but no biological results were presented to substantiate these suggestions.

Table 1
Potencies of 4-Alkylphenylacetic Acids
in Pharmacological Tests

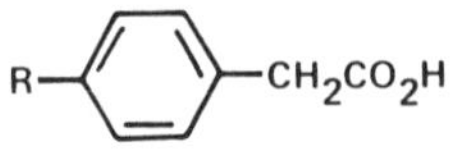

R—⟨benzene ring⟩—CH$_2$CO$_2$H

R	UV-erythema[a]	RFA[b]	AP[c]
Me	0.5	NA 240[d]	
Et	1	≯ 1	< 0.5
Pr	2-4		
i-Pr	2		
n-Bu	2	1	
i-Bu	2-4	2-4	4
s-Bu	2-4	2	2-4
t-Bu	4	≮ 4	2-4
n-pentyl	NA 160	NA 120	
i-pentyl	1	≯ 1	
t-pentyl	4	2-4	2

[a]Aspirin = 1.
[b]Rat foot analgesia. Aspirin = 1.
[c]Antipyresis. Aspirin = 1.
[d]Not active at 240 mg/kg.

3.1 Structure-activity Relationships

Excluding the 4-biphenylylalkanoic acids, approximately 450 compounds were synthesized and tested in this project. The main conclusions to be drawn from this work are summarized in sections 3.1.1 to 3.1.6.

3.1.1 4-Alkylphenylalkanoic Acids   We examined a series of 4-alkylphenyl-acetic acids (Table 1) after initial results had been obtained indicating that the 3-alkyl compounds were less effective than the 4-alkylphenylacetic acids. 2-Alkylphenylacetic acids were inactive in the UV-erythema test; this was also true for a number of other 2-substituted compounds, but more recently some active compounds in this category, such as sodium 2-(2,6-dichloroanilino)-phenylacetate (diclofenac sodium)[10] and 2-(2,4-dichlorophenoxy)phenylacetic acid (fenclofenac)[11] have been identified. Phenylacetic acid is a totally inactive compound; on increasing the size of the alkyl group in the *para* position a gradual increase in potency occurs until the 4-butyl compounds are reached,

Table 2
Potencies of 2-(4-Alkylphenyl)propionic Acids in Pharmacological Tests

R—⟨benzene ring⟩—CHCO$_2$H (with Me on the CH)

R	UV-erythema[a]	RFA[b]	AP[c]
Me	NA 160[d]	NA 120	
Et	2	< 2	
Pr	8-16	8-16	
i-Pr	4	2	
n-Bu	4-8	8-16	
i-Bu	16-32	8-16	20
s-Bu	8	4-8	
t-Bu	4	2-4	2
n-pentyl	≱ 2	2	
i-pentyl	8		
t-pentyl	4-8	4	
n-hexyl	NA 160		

[a]Aspirin = 1.
[b]Rat foot analgesia. Aspirin = 1.
[c]Antipyresis. Aspirin = 1.
[d]Not active at 160 mg/kg.

with 4-*tert*-butylphenylacetic acid showing the maximum response. 4-Isobutyl-phenylacetic acid (ibufenac) is also one of the more active compounds in this series. With increasing alkyl chain length beyond butyl, activity falls away again with a tendency for retention of activity in the more highly branched alkyl compounds, such as the 4-*tert*-pentyl compound, but even this declines in the higher homologues. Additional substitution by such groups as aryl, cycloalkyl, hydroxy, and carbonyl on the alkyl moiety led in many cases to loss of activity. Ring substitution, especially by a halogen in the 3-position, can lead to an enhanced anti-inflammatory response.[12]

Our first results with the 2-(4-alkylphenyl)propionic acids were not very promising. Experience with the phenoxy acids had suggested that the propionic acids might be more active than the acetic acids. However, the first compound

Table 3
Potencies of 4-Cycloalkylphenylalkanoic Acids
in Pharmacological Tests

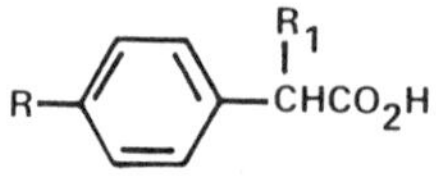

$$R \!\!-\!\!\left\langle\!\!\!\bigcirc\!\!\!\right\rangle\!\!-\!\!\overset{\overset{\displaystyle R_1}{|}}{CHCO_2H}$$

R	R_1	UV-erythema[a]	RFA[b]	AP[c]
Cyclopentyl	H	4	4	
Cyclopentyl	Me	≮ 8		
Cyclohexyl	H	4	10	4
Cyclohexyl	Me	32-64	32-64	20
Cycloheptyl	H	1	2	
Cycloheptyl	Me	4-8		

[a]Aspirin = 1.
[b]Rat foot analgesia. Aspirin = 1.
[c]Antipyresis. Aspirin = 1.

to be made, the 4-methyl derivative, was completely inactive, as was the parent 2-phenylpropionic acid (hydratropic acid). In view of the good activity of 4-*tert*-butylphenylacetic acid, it was also surprising to find that the propionic acid was no more potent. It was only after other compounds in the series had been synthesized that the true picture of activity emerged.[13] Activity with the 2-(4-alkylphenyl)propionic acids is more widely spread and at higher levels (Table 2) than in the corresponding acetic acids, but the general pattern is the same. Again a maximum response is shown by some of the 4-butyl compounds with ibuprofen (**1**), clearly the outstanding compound.

3.1.2 Cycloalkylphenylalkanoic Acids These compounds were prepared concurrently with the alkyl derivatives. Of the relatively small number of compounds examined (Table 3), cyclohexyl gave the maximum activity. The outstanding compound in this group was 2-(4-cyclohexyl)phenylpropionic acid (hexaprofen), and although it had anti-inflammatory activity at a higher level than ibuprofen, this alone did not elevate it above ibuprofen in our overall assessment. Further substitution by alkyl in the cycloalkyl moiety invariably lowered activity.

Table 4
Potencies of 4-Substituted Phenylalkanoic Acids in Pharmacological Tests

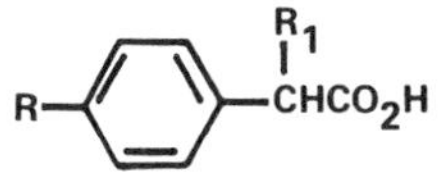

$$R-\text{⟨⟩}-\overset{\overset{R_1}{|}}{C}HCO_2H$$

R	R_1	UV-erythema[a]	RFA[b]
HO	H	NA 160[c]	NA 120
HO	Me	NA 160	
MeO	H	≯ 0.5	NA 120
MeO	Me	NA 80	
EtO	H	2	
PrO	H	2	2
PrO	Me	4-8	
i-PrO	H	2	4
i-PrO	Me	8	4
n-BuO	H	NA 180	< 1
n-BuO	Me	1-2	2
t-BuO	H	NA 160	
Allyloxy	H	2-4	2
Allyloxy	Me	8-16	16
2-Butenyloxy	H	NA 160	NA 240
2-Butenyloxy	Me	2-4	
PhO	H	≯1	4
PhO	Me	32	16
PhS	H	≯1	2
PhS	Me	8-16	8
EtS	H	2-4	2
PrS	H	1-2	
PrS	Me	4-8	
i-PrS	H	2	
n-BuS	H	< 0.5	

[a]Aspirin = 1.
[b]Rat foot analgesia. Aspirin = 1.
[c]Not active at 160 mg/kg.

Table 5
Potencies of 2-(4-Isobutylphenyl)alkanoic Acids in Pharmacological Tests

$$^{i}Bu\!-\!\!\bigcirc\!\!-\!\!CHCO_2H \quad (R)$$

R	UV-erythema[a]	RFA[b]	AP[c]
H	2-4	2-4	4
Me	16-32	8-16	20
Et	2	≯ 1	
Pr	< 1		

[a]Aspirin $= 1$.
[b]Rat foot analgesia. Aspirin $= 1$.
[c]Antipyresis. Aspirin $= 1$.

3.1.3   Miscellaneous 4-Substituted Phenylalkanoic Acids   A large number of 4-substituted phenylalkanoic acids[13,14] have been prepared and tested and a selection of the more interesting results is recorded in Table 4. For convenience this 4-substituent has been limited to hydroxy, alkoxy, alkenyloxy, phenoxy, phenylthio, and alkylthio. No activity is shown by the hydroxy compounds and anti-inflammatory response in the 4-alkoxyphenylalkanoic acids gradually builds up in a manner somewhat reminiscent of the 4-alkyl compounds, giving maximum activity in the 4-isopropoxy compounds. There is then a sharp decline in activity on moving up to the 4-butoxy compounds; neither 4-n-butoxyphenylacetic acid nor 4-tert-butoxyphenylacetic acid show any response in the UV-erythema test. 4-Allyloxyphenylalkanoic acids show useful activity, but always at a level below that of the corresponding 4-isobutylphenyl-alkanoic acids.4-Alkylthio- compounds are very similar to the 4-alkoxyphenylalkanoic acids in their activity in the UV-erythema test.

3.1.4   Side-Chain Variants   It was important to establish at an early stage in our investigations whether a 2-propionic acid group was the optimum size for maximum anti-inflammatory activity. Although this had been found to be true for the phenoxyalkanoic acids, there was no certainty that the same relationship would apply to the 4-alkylphenylalkanoic acids. In practice, the 2-propionic acid proved to be the most effective substituent. Table 5 shows the

Table 6

**Potencies of 2-(4-Substituted phenyl)butyric Acids
in Pharmacological Tests**

R	UV-erythema[a]	RFA[b]
Pr	1	
i-Bu	2	⧺ 1
s-Bu	1-2	
t-Bu	1	1
t-pentyl	1-2	
Cyclopentyl	2-4	
Cyclohexyl	2-4	8
Cycloheptyl	1-2	

[a]Aspirin = 1.
[b]Rat foot analgesia. Aspirin = 1.

results for a number of 2-(4-isobutylphenyl)alkanoic acids, where it can be seen that the 2-butyric acid is less potent than 4-isobutylphenylacetic acid (ibufenac). It has been claimed, however, that 2-(4-isobutylphenyl)butyric acid (butibufen)[15,16] is comparable to ibuprofen in the usual animal tests. The generally low potency of a number of other 2-butyric acids is shown in Table 6; in each case the butyric acids are less active than the corresponding acetic acids. Activity declines still further in the higher homologues (Table 5). Subsequent studies by other workers in numerous other series have confirmed that, with few exceptions, maximum response is shown by the 2-propionic acids. One of the better known exceptions is provided by the indomethacin series, in which the acetic and propionic acids are of comparable activity.[17]

Further substitution in the propionic acid moiety usually lowers activity; this is true for methyl, since the isobutyric acids show very little anti-inflammatory activity, and for other 2-substituents, such as amino, hydroxyl, and aryl. Unsaturation in the side chain also lowers potency, as exemplified by 2-(4-isobutylphenyl)acrylic acid, which is approximately half as active as ibuprofen, and by other unsaturated analogues.[18]

In contrast to the results obtained with the branched-chain alkanoic acids, those obtained with straight-chain analogues were disappointing. 3-Arylpropionic acids were inactive, but a slight response could be detected in higher homologues with an uneven number of methylene groups. Presumably these compounds can be degraded by β-oxidation to the corresponding phenylacetic acid derivatives.

3.1.5   Side-Chain Terminal Groups   A carboxyl appears to be the best terminal group for the side chain, probably because it is one of the necessary features to fit the hypothetical receptor site, now equated to the prostaglandin synthetase active site.[19] Other groups that are capable of metabolic conversion into carboxyl *in vivo* give some response. Thus, lower alkyl esters are approximately half as active as the corresponding acids in the UV-erythema test, whereas 2-arylethanols and 2-arylpropanols are almost as potent as the acids. Whitehouse and Famaey[20] have suggested that these alcohols may be active in their own right. We have found that acetamides show a little activity, whereas *N*-unsubstituted propionamides can be as much as half as active as the related propionic acids. In contrast, *N*-substituted propionamides have weak activity; a similar finding has been made by Spickett et al.[21] Although hydroxamic acids have been claimed to be useful anti-inflammatory agents,[23,23] we have always found them to be less effective than the corresponding carboxylic acids. 2-(4-Isobutylphenyl)propionhydroxamic acid (ibuproxam) (5) is said to progressively release ibuprofen into the circulatory system and to be better tolerated than ibuprofen.[24,25] Though tetrazoles are often equivalent biologically to carboxylic acids, replacement of the carboxyl by an acidic tetrazole moiety as in 6 leads to a sharp decline in anti-inflammatory activity. The 2-oxazoline 7, which contains a masked carboxyl group,[26] is less effective than ibuprofen in the UV-erythema test.

5

6

7

3.1.6   The Aromatic Ring   The aromatic ring of ibuprofen appears to be another essential feature of its structure and the 2-phenylpropionic acid moiety has been retained in many later analogues.[27] In general, it is more correct to say that an aromatic system in the widest sense of the term, is a necessary structural feature. Total or partial hydrogenation of the aromatic system leads to elimination of anti-inflammatory activity. 2-(4-Isobutylcyclohex-1-yl)propionic acid (8)[28] had no activity in the carrageenin edema test but retained the fibrinolytic activity of ibuprofen. The pyridine analogue (9)[29] had approximately the same platelet aggregation inhibitory activity as ibuprofen.

3.2   Product Candidates
In our phenylalkanoic acid series, four product candidates were selected and submitted for clinical trial in a period of only 4 years. It should be remembered that part of this work was carried out before the establishment of drug regulatory authorities, so it is now unlikely that similar rapid progress could occur again.

3.2.1   4-*Tert*-Butylphenylacetic Acid (BTS 10335)   In the middle of 1961, 4-*tert*-butylphenylacetic acid was one of the most active compounds then available with a low toxicity. It was a known compound and its preparation was very straightforward. Clinical trials showed that BTS 10 335 was active in rheumatoid arthritis at a daily dose of 2-4 g, but unfortunately a significant number of patients developed a skin rash.[3] Of course this was disappointing, but clinical activity had been confirmed in the series and it was felt that the pharmacological basis of the project was correct. The problem was to select other compounds that would be free from side effects, especially the skin rashes that had not been detected in animal tests.

3.2.2   4-Isobutylphenylacetic Acid (Ibufenac)   This was the next compound to be chosen for clinical trial on the basis of its pharmacological spectrum (Table 1).[30,31] It was assessed as two to four times as potent as aspirin and twice as potent as aspirin in suppressing the development of adjuvant-induced arthritis in the rat.[31] Ibufenac proved to be active in man at a daily dose of 2 g;[32-35] it did not give rise to a skin rash and was largely free from gastric irritation. In a small proportion of patients it caused a reversible liver dysfunction on prolonged dosage,[33,34,36] but further clinical studies carried out in Japan showed no such effects and the clinical results were very good. Ibufenac was marketed in the United Kingdom in 1966 as Dytransin, but was withdrawn in 1968 owing to the problem of hepatotoxicity. This occurred in only a small proportion of patients and certainly not in chronic toxicity studies in animals. Surprisingly, hepatotoxicity was not encountered with ibufenac in the Japanese and the drug proved to be a useful and well-tolerated antirheumatic agent for several years in Japan.

3.2.3 4-Cyclohexylphenylacetic Acid (BTS 10 499) Although BTS 10 499 appeared to be a more potent analgesic agent than ibufenac in man,[3] early trials were terminated because it produced a rash in 20% of the patients. Long-term toxicological studies in dogs indicated an effect on the adrenals in this species,[37] but there was no evidence of similar effects in man following short term dosage.

3.2.4 2-(4-Isobutylphenyl)propionic Acid (Ibuprofen) Ibuprofen was the fourth compound in the series to be selected for clinical trial after a detailed pharmacological and toxicological evaluation. This was the first of our 2-phenylpropionic acids to be studied in depth clinically.

3.2.4.1 Pharmacology. The anti-inflammatory, analgesic, and antipyretic activities of ibuprofen are recorded in Table 2; it is the most potent of the 4-alkyl series, with an antierythemic activity approximately 16-32 times that of aspirin.[38,39] In carrageenin-induced edema in the paw of the rat the potency of ibuprofen was similar to that of phenylbutazone but less than that of indomethacin; similar findings have since been reported by other groups.[15,40,41] Acetylcholine-induced writhing in mice showed that ibuprofen had an analgesic potency 28 times as great as that of aspirin. It had no effect on the response to the application of pressure to the noninflamed foot of the rat, demonstrating that the analgesic activity is of a mainly peripheral rather than central nature. Although ibuprofen showed relatively low potency in established adjuvant arthritis in the rat compared with phenylbutazone or indomethacin, it was nevertheless three to four times as potent as aspirin.[39] The low potency in this test system may be due in part to the rapid metabolism of ibuprofen in the rat.

It is believed that the principal mode of action of ibuprofen, in common with a number of other anti-inflammatory agents, is through the inhibition of prostaglandin biosynthesis.[42]

3.2.4.2 Toxicology. Ibuprofen has a very low toxicity; in mice the acute oral LD_{50} was 800 mg/kg and in rats 1600 mg/kg.[43] Although there was a little accumulation of radioactivity in the adrenals, ovaries, skin, thyroid, and fat following repeated dosing with [¹⁴C]ibuprofen, structures or functions of these organs were not affected.[44] An early problem with the propionic acids was the appearance of ulcerogenicity in dogs. Later it was established that this was caused by slow metabolic clearance, leading to high plasma levels on multiple dosing. Gastric ulceration is probably largely a systemic rather than a local effect and therefore can be produced by high plasma levels. In the chronic toxicity studies in rats, gastric ulceration was the only consistent pathological finding; however, it occurred at only high dose levels.

3.2.4.3 Metabolism.   Absorption of ibuprofen is rapid in man, with maximum serum concentrations attained 1-2 hours after a single dose. Elimination from the circulation is also rapid, giving a half-life of ibuprofen in serum of approximately 2 hours in the period up to 9 hours after a single oral dose.

The stereochemical aspects of the metabolism of ibuprofen and other propionic acids have proved to be important in their development; the nature of these stereochemical changes has provided some unusual features of academic interest. The Merck group found that the anti-inflammatory activity of 2-(3-chloro-4-cyclohexylphenyl)propionic acid resides almost completely in the (S)-(+) form,[45] and they were the first to recognize the relevance of configuration to the activity of 2-phenylpropionic acid derivatives. Ibuprofen can readily be resolved with (-)-α-methylbenzylamine,[38] and the resulting (+)-enantiomer, believed to have the (S)-configuration, was highly active in the inhibition of a prostaglandin synthetase system *in vitro,* whereas the (-)-enantiomer was only slightly active. This large difference in potency between the enantiomers was not, however, found *in vivo* when they were compared side by side with the racemate in anti-inflammatory and analgesic tests. It was concluded by Adams et al.[46] that in the rat, the mouse, and the guinea pig, there is almost complete inversion of the poorly active (-)-enantiomer into the much more active (+)-enantiomer. Previously, during a study of the metabolism of ibuprofen and its enantiomers in animals and in man, it had been suggested that inversion of the (-)-enantiomer might occur.[47] Recently Wechter and Kaiser[48,49] demonstrated unequivocally that the (R)-(-)-enantiomer is converted into the (S)-(+)-enantiomer in man. This conversion process has been characterized by the Upjohn workers as a sequential dehydrogenation and stereospecific hydrogenation of only the (R)-(-)-enantiomer by lipid-associated enzymes. A similar stereospecific inversion of the (-)-enantiomer of α-methylfluorene-2-acetic acid (cicloprofen) to the (+)-enantiomer has been reported in rats and monkeys.[50]

When ibuprofen was administered to man, two principal urinary metabolites, (+)-2-[4-(2-hydroxy-2-methylpropyl)phenyl]propionic acid **(10)** and

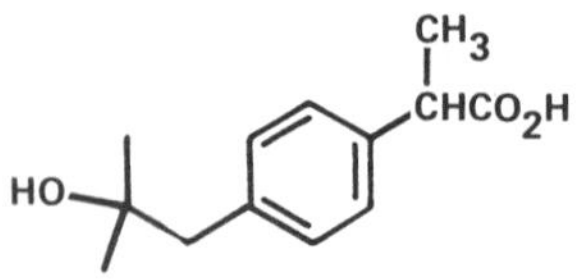

(+)-2-[4-(2-carboxypropyl)phenyl]propionic acid (**11**),[47] were isolated. Both of these metabolites were dextrorotatory and both were inactive in UV-erythema.[38] The structures of the metabolites were elucidated by NMR and confirmed by the more recent studies of Wechter and co-workers[49]; Brooks and Gilbert,[51] using gas-liquid chromatography-mass spectrometry (GLC-MS), also showed the presence of two minor metabolites, **12** and **13**, the latter being the precursor of **11**. The inversion of R-(-)-ibuprofen accounts for the isolation of dextrorotatory metabolites **10** and **11** when either the racemate or the (R)-(-)-enantiomer is administered to man.[47] Previously, we had established that the isobutyl group in ibufenac gave the acetic acid analogues of **10** and **11** in man, and Pettersen,[52] using GLC-MS, has confirmed these findings with the addition of the acetic acid analogue of **12** as a minor metabolite. Analogously, the isobutyl group in the hypoglycemic agent 2-p-methoxybenzenesulfon-amido-5-isobutyl-1,3,4-thiadiazole is metabolized by hydroxylation at the three possible sites, followed by oxidation of the primary alcohol to the correspond-ing 2-carboxypropyl compound.[53] 2-(4-Carboxyphenyl)propionic acid was pre-sent in substantial amounts in the dialysis fluid of a nephrectomized patient following the ingestion of ibuprofen. This acid is regarded by Petterson et al.[54] as an end product of metabolism, possibly by the β-oxidation of **11**. It is in-teresting that although the propionic acid moiety can undergo a stereo-specific change involving biochemical transformations, it seems to be inert to other biochemical processes, such as hydroxylation or oxidation.

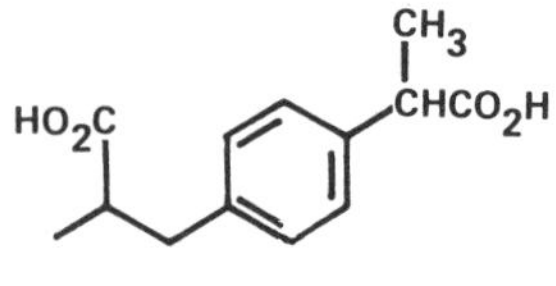

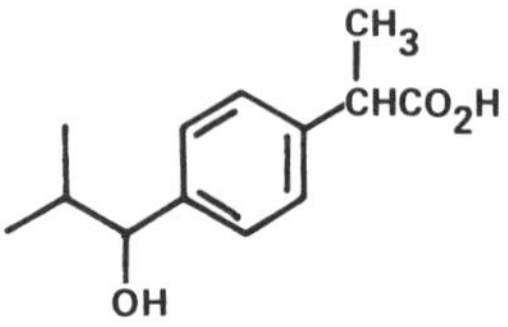

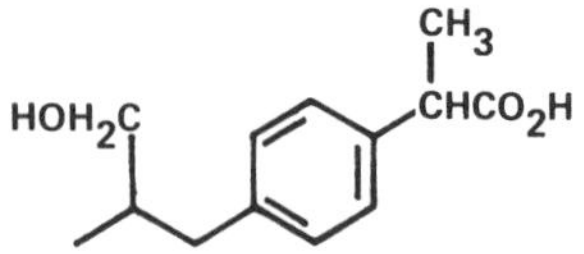

3.2.4.4   Clinical Studies.   As ibuprofen has been in clinical use for 15 years, a very considerable amount of data has been acquired. Davis and Avery[55] have reviewed the earlier literature, Buckler and Adams,[3] have described some of

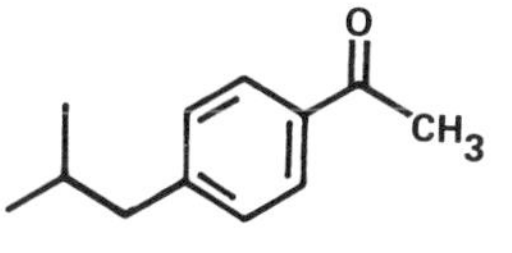

14

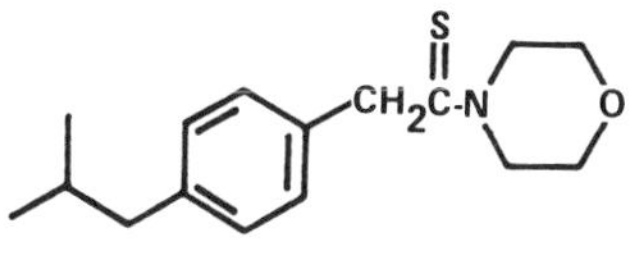

15

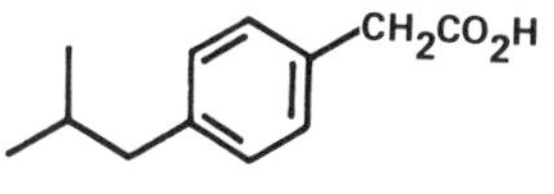

16

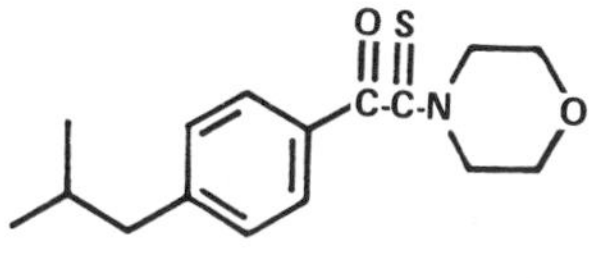

17

the first trials, and a recent review by the same authors[56] has brought the clinical position up to date. The early trials established the effective anti-inflammatory and analgesic nature of ibuprofen in a wide range of the rheumatic diseases. An analysis by Hall[57] of a long-term study with 1200 patients in rheumatoid arthritis and osteoarthritis and allied conditions has shown the benefit of ibuprofen in 70% of the cases. This study also showed that little gastrointestinal irritation was associated with long-term therapy. For some years ibuprofen has been found to be effective in the treatment of nonarticular rheumatic conditions and soft-tissue injuries and its clinical indications are now widening still further. Recently ibuprofen was approved in the United States for the treatment of primary dysmenorrhea and as an analgesic in postoperative pain and other conditions.[58] The normally recommended daily dose of ibuprofen for adults is 1.2-1.6 g, but in certain countries, including the United States, higher doses are regularly prescribed.

3.3 Synthetic Routes

This chemistry section is limited to phenylacetic acids and a selection of methods for the synthesis of ibuprofen.

3.3.1 Phenylacetic Acids One of the reasons for our initial choice of 4-*tert*-butylphenylacetic acid (BTS 10 335) as a candidate for clinical trial was the accessibility and low cost of *tert*-butylbenzene. At that time isobutylbenzene was not commercially available and was made in pilot plant quantities either by the reduction of isobutyrophenone or by the isopropylation of benzyl sodium. Eventually isobutylbenzene became a commercial product manufactured by the catalyzed addition of propylene to toluene.

Methods of synthesis of phenylacetic acids are legion, but 4-alkylphenyl-acetic acids are most readily available by the Kindler modifiction of the Willgerodt reaction. 4-Isobutylphenylacetic acid (ibufenac) was therefore synthesized from isobutylbenzene, which was acetylated by the Perrier modifica-

tion[59] of the Friedel–Crafts reaction to give a high yield of
4′-isobutylacetophenone (14) containing small amounts of 3′-isobutyl-
acetophenone. The ketone (14) on refluxing with sulfur and morpholine in the
Kindler-Willgerodt reaction afforded the thiomorpholide 15, which was
hydrolyzed to ibufenac (16)[13] under either acidic or alkaline conditions. The
formation of the oxothiomorpholide 17, produced to some extent under normal reaction conditions, can lead to a reduced yield of ibufenac, but this can be
suppressed by carrying out the Kindler-Willgerodt reaction in a closed vessel at
130°C. 4-Cyclohexylphenylacetic acid was prepared by the same procedure.

3.3.2 Ibuprofen   A considerable number of different routes are now known
for the synthesis of 2-arylpropionic acids and the Japanese patent literature has
a prolific number of disclosures in this area. Of necessity, this selection of
methods for the preparation of ibuprofen is far from comprehensive.

3.3.2.1 From 4′-Isobutylacetophenone.   Because of its ready availability
and the variety of reactions it can undergo, 4′-isobutylacetophenone is a widely
used intermediate for many syntheses of ibuprofen. Ibuprofen was originally
synthesized from ibufenac (Scheme 1). Esterification gave ethyl 4-isobutyl-
phenylacetate (18), which on heating with diethyl carbonate and sodium ethoxide with concurrent distillation of ethanol afforded the sodio derivative of
diethyl 4-isobutylphenylmalonate (19). Methylation of 19 produced 20;
hydrolysis afforded 21, which gave ibuprofen (1) on decarboxylation. The intermediate 19 allowed a variety of other substituents to be introduced into the
molecule. The more direct methylation of 18, with, for example, sodamide in
liquid ammonia and methyl iodide, gave ethyl 2-(4-isobutylphenyl)propionate
and on hydrolysis ibuprofen, but it was difficult to avoid undue contamination
of the product with ibufenac and 2-(4-isobutylphenyl)isobutyric acid.

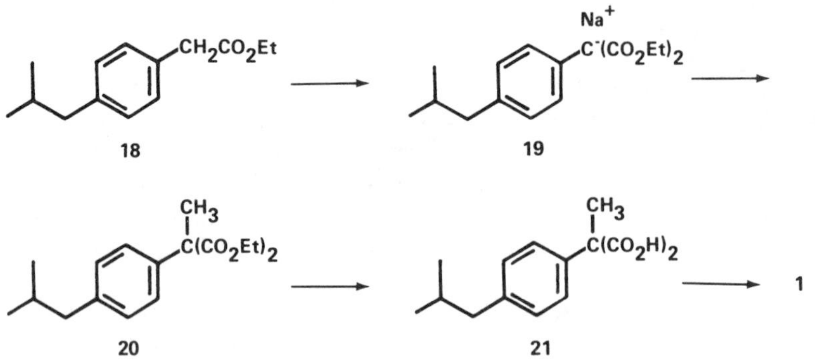

Scheme 1.

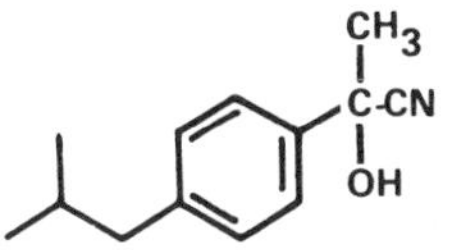

22

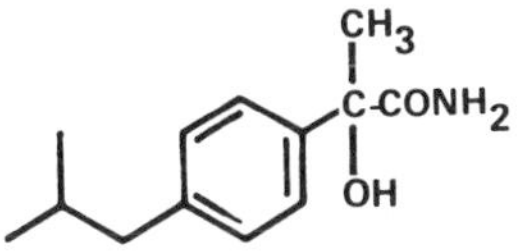

23

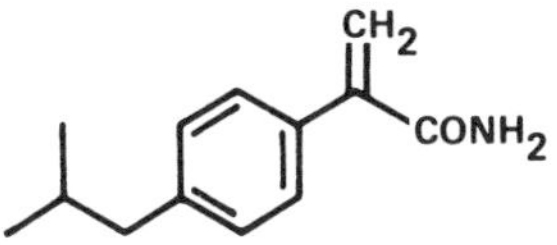

24

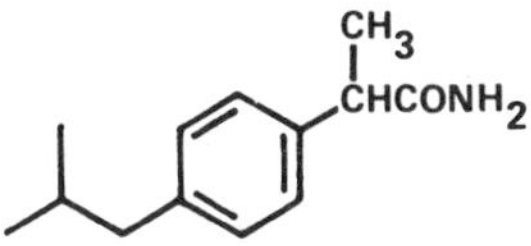

25

The reaction of 4′-isobutylacetophenone (14) with either anhydrous hydrogen cyanide and piperidine or with aqueous hydrogen cyanide gave a surprisingly low yield of the cyanohydrin 22, with at least 50% of the ketone unreacted. Alkaline hydrolysis of the crude cyanohydrin (22) afforded the hydroxy-amide 23, accompanied by the acrylamide 24; 24 on catalytic hydrogenation gave 2-(4-isobutylphenyl))propionamide (25) and then on hydrolysis, ibuprofen. Alternatively, the hydroxy-amide 23 on hydrolysis produced the hydroxy-acid 26, dehydration of which afforded the acrylic acid 27, and on hydrogenation, ibuprofen. Another synthesis of the hydroxy-acid (26) can be effected by the acylation of isobutylbenzene with ethyl oxalyl chloride to give 28 followed by reaction with methylmagnesium iodide and hydrolysis to 26.

The poor yields experienced in the cyanohydrin reaction prompted a search for alternative methods. 4′-Isobutylacetophenone (14) with potassium cyanide

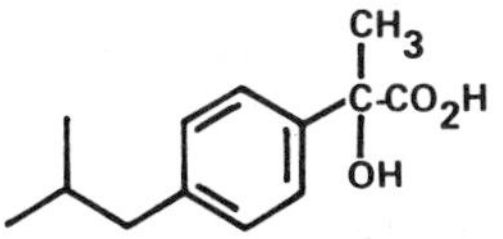

26

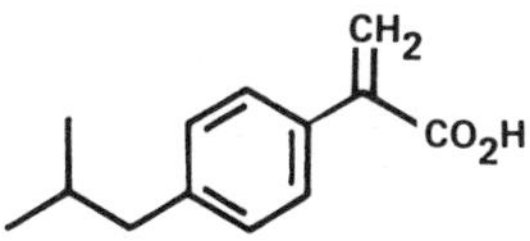

27

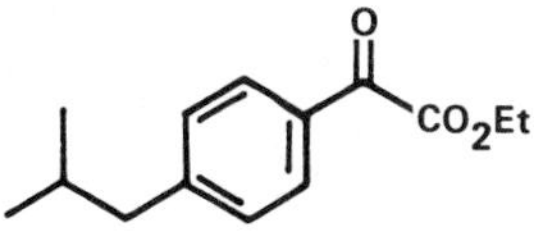

28

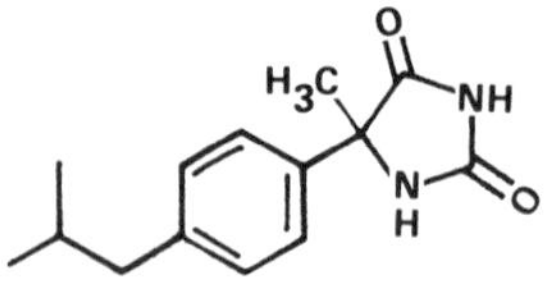

29

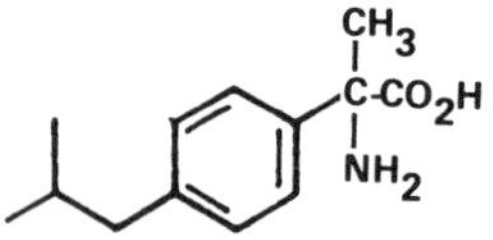

30

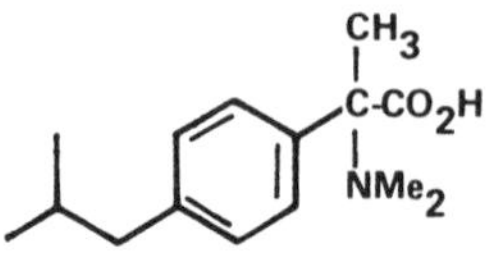

31

and ammonium carbonate in a Bucherer-Bergs reaction produced a good yield of the hydantoin (29), which on alkaline hydrolysis furnished an almost quantitative yield of the amino-acid 30. Treatment of 30 with nitrous acid again afforded the hydroxy-acid 26. A more satisfactory route was methylation with formaldehyde and formic acid to give 31, followed by catalytic hydrogenolysis to ibuprofen.[60]

The Darzens glycidic ester synthesis with 4′-isobutylacetophenone (14) and ethyl chloroacetate with a sodium alkoxide gave a good yield of the glycidic ester 32, which on alkaline hydrolysis and acidification produced 2-(4-isobutylphenyl)propionaldehyde (33). Oxidation, typically with silver oxide, then gave ibuprofen.[61] This route can produce some unusual impurities arising from oxidative coupling, such as the hydroxybutanolide 34, which is

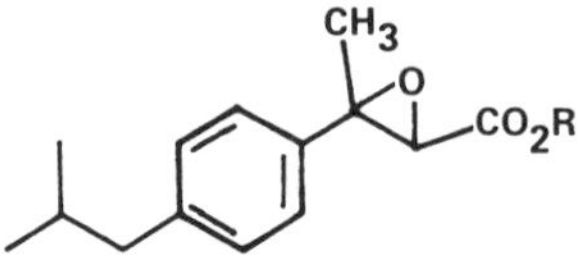

32, R = alkyl

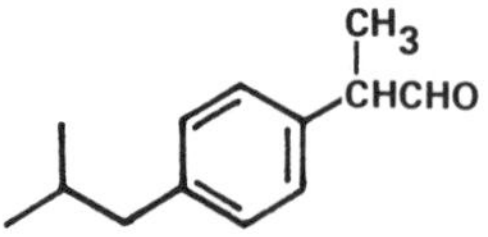

33

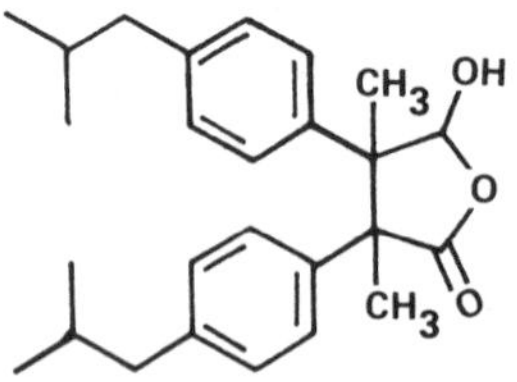

34

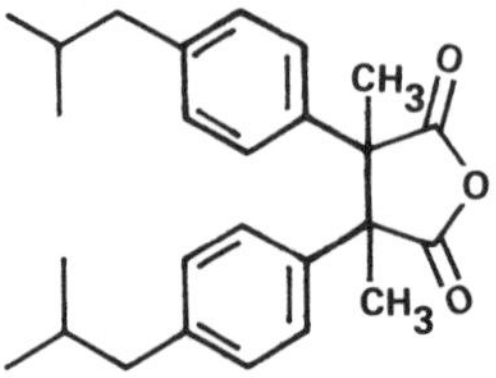

35

formed as a complex mixture of isomers. Chromatography separated the *cis* isomers from the *trans* isomers as demonstrated by the NMR spectra and these butanolides were individually oxidized with chromium (III) oxide to the pure *cis* and *trans* forms of the anhydride **35**. The *trans* anhydride (**35**) was synthesized by an Ivanov reaction involving isopropyl magnesium iodide and ibuprofen followed by coupling with iodine. An equivalent series of reactions from the glycidate (**32**) to ibuprofen has been described by the Nisshin Company. In one approach the glycidate (**32**) was rearranged to the hydroxybutenoate ester **36** with a Lewis acid such as boron trifluoride etherate, treated with sodium methoxide, hydrolyzed to the pyruvic acid **37**, and oxidized with alkaline hydrogen peroxide to ibuprofen.[62]

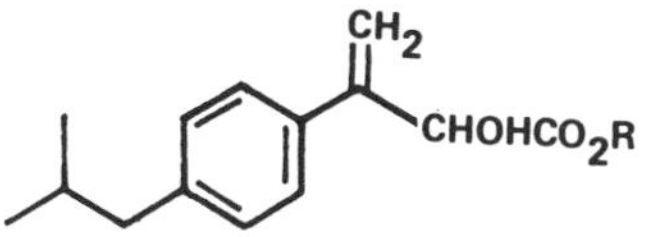

36, R = alkyl

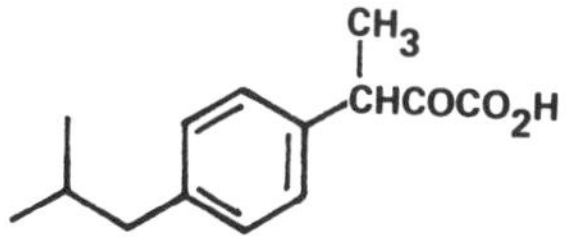

37

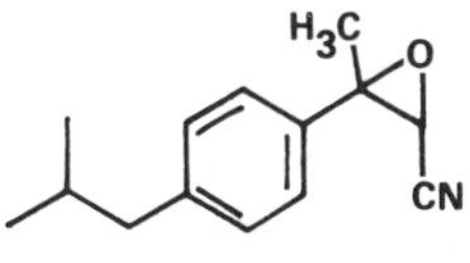

38

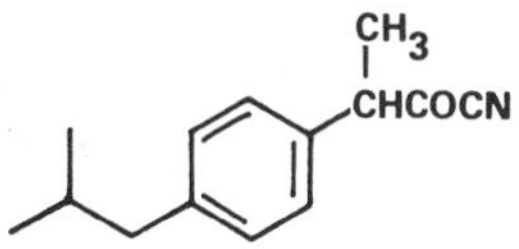

39

The Upjohn Company has investigated a process in which the glycidonitrile **38** is produced from 4'-isobutylacetophenone (**14**) and chloroacetonitrile in the presence of a sodium alkoxide in a modified Darzens reaction. Lewis acid rearrangement of **38**, preferably with lithium perchlorate afforded the α-ketonitrile **39**, largely in a dimeric form, which on hydrolysis in aqueous base gave ibuprofen.[63] Hydrogen cyanide is evolved during the formation of **39** and its dimer.

3.3.2.2 From 4'-isobutylpropiophenone.

An alternative starting point for a number of syntheses is provided by 4'-isobutylpropiophenone (**40**), readily available by acylation of isobutylbenzene. Thallium(III)nitrate (TTN) oxidation of propiophenone in trimethyl orthoformate (TMOF)-methanol gave a quantitative yield of methyl 2-phenylpropionate,[64] and Walker and Pillai[65] have found that the enol ether **41** generated *in situ* from **40** with TMOF-methanol and TTN·3H$_2$O can rapidly give a high yield of methyl 2-(4-isobutylphenyl)pro-

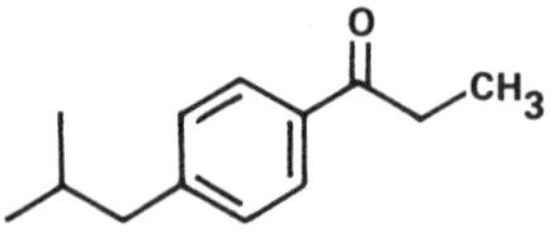

40

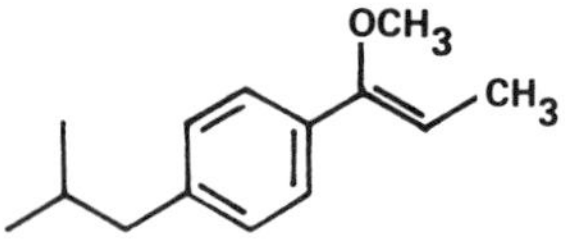

41

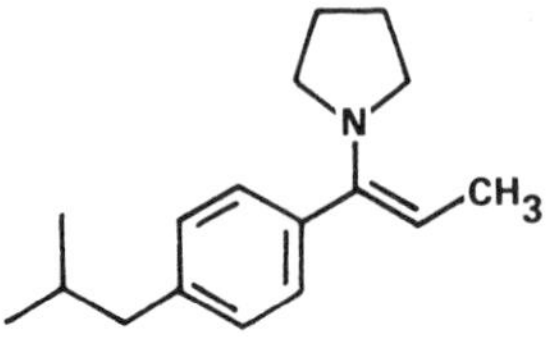

42

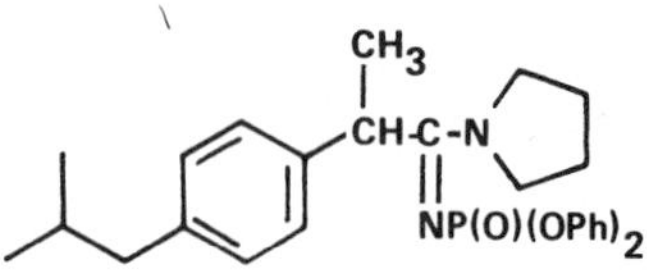

43

pionate. As thallium salts are highly toxic, the potential of this route for ibuprofen is in some doubt. In another approach[66] from **40**, the pyrrolidine enamine **42** underwent a 1,3-dipolar cycloaddition with diphenyl phosphorazidate [(PhO)$_2$P(O)N$_3$] followed by aryl migration and nitrogen evolution to give the *N*-phosphorylated amidine **43** in 78% overall yield. Ibuprofen was produced in 79% yield by the hydrolysis of **43** with potassium hydroxide in ethylene glycol.

3.3.2.3 *From Isobutyl Vinyl Ketone.*   A number of companies, including The Boots Company, have investigated routes to ibuprofen starting from nonbenzenoid precursors such as isobutyl vinyl ketone (**44**). This can either be obtained as such, or generated by quaternization of the Mannich base 2-di-

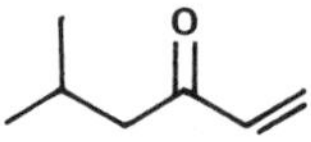

44

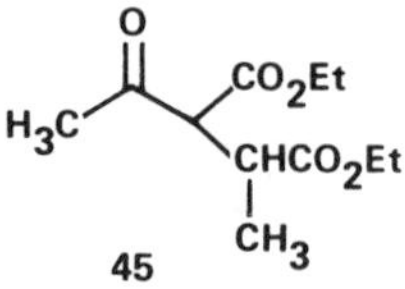

45

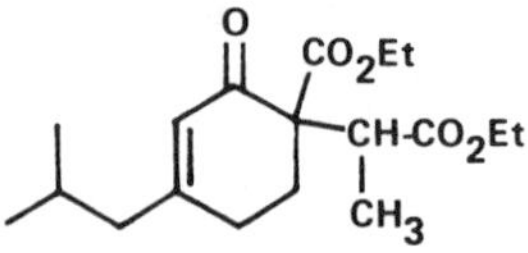

46

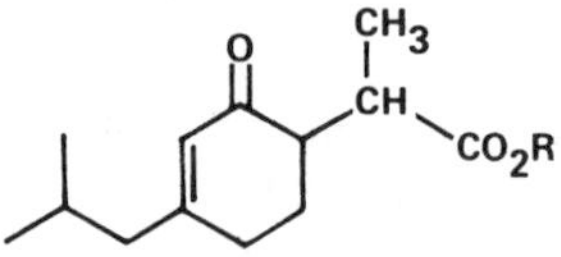

47, R = Et

48, R = H

ethylaminoethyl isobutyl ketone with dimethyl sulfate, followed by treatment with alkali. Diethyl 2-aceto-3-methylsuccinate (45) and 44 underwent a Michael addition to give largely a mixture of the two esters 46 and 47. Alkaline hydrolysis of the mixture of esters furnished the keto-acid 48 as a mixture of stereoisomers separable by preparative-layer chromatography. Aromatization of the keto-acid (48) with pyridine hydrochloride afforded ibuprofen.[67] Pyridine hydrochloride has been used by Palazzo and Baiocchi[68] for the aromatization of 2-oxocyclohexen-3-ylacetic acid. Baiocchi et al.[69] could only isolate the butenolide 49 in low yield from 44, generated from the quaternized

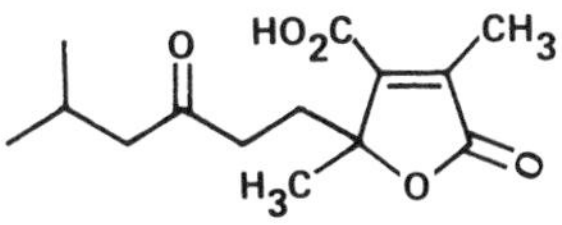

49

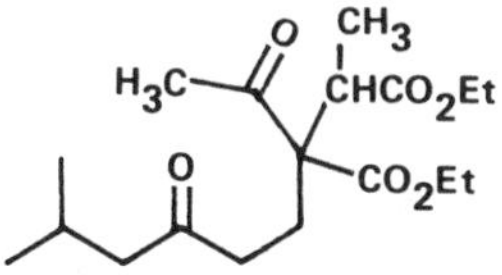

50

Mannich base, and 45. The Angelini workers have reported that 44 and 45 in the presence of small amounts of sodium ethoxide gave the open chain ester diethyl 2-acetyl-3-methyl-2-(5-methyl-3-oxohexyl)succinate (50) as a mixture of stereoisomers, which on treatment with pyridine hydrochloride afforded ibuprofen.[70] It seems very probable that aromatization proceeds through structures such as 46, 47, and 48. The Upjohn Company has investigated alternative aromatizing agents such as succinic anhydride for use with this series of compounds, but good yields have not been achieved.[71]

4. CONCLUSIONS

The extent of activity in 2-phenylpropionic acid derivatives is more diverse than could have been imagined at the outset of these investigations. Our studies now represent only a small proportion of the total work that has since been carried out with phenylalkanoic acids, but whether anything fundamentally different is still emerging from this approach seems debatable. Looking back over our own contribution we recognize the successes and the frustrations of the program. A small project group that was set up at an early stage proved to be invaluable in providing the majority of the ideas and was the driving force of the research operation. It also managed by its enthusiasm to be self-sustaining during difficult periods. The international success of ibuprofen is a matter of satisfaction to us all, and even if the ultimate goal of curative agents for the rheumatic diseases is reached, there will still be a place for effective anti-inflammatory agents in therapy.

ACKNOWLEDGMENTS

Thanks are expressed to all those who over many years have made a contribution to ibuprofen research and especially to those in the original project group, which included Professor S. S. Adams, Dr. J. Warwick Buckler, Dr. E. E. Cliffe, Dr. B. Lessel, and Dr. D. A. Peak, and members of the Boots' Patent Section led by Mr. T. S. Simpson.

REFERENCES

1. P. F. Juby, in *Anti-inflammatory Agents, Chemistry and Pharmacology,* R. A. Scherrer and M. W. Whitehouse, Eds., *Medicinal Chemistry,* Vol. 13-1, Academic Press, New York, 1974, p. 91.

2. T. Y. Shen, *Angew. Chem., Int. Ed. Engl.,* **11,** 460 (1972).

3. J. W. Buckler and S. S. Adams, *Med. Proc.,* **14,** 574 (1968).

4. S. S. Adams and R. Cobb, *Nature (Lond.),* **181,** 773 (1958).

5. S. S. Adams and R. Cobb, in *Salicylates,* A. St. J. Dixon, B. K. Martin, M. J. H. Smith, and P. H. N. Wood, Eds., Churchill, London, 1963, p. 127.

6. G. Wilhelmi, *Schweiz. Med. Wochenschr.,* **79,** 577 (1949).

7. L. O. Randall and J. J. Selitto, *Arch. Int. Pharmacodyn. Ther.,* **111,** 409 (1957).

8. S. S. Adams, *J. Pharm. Pharmacol.,* **12,** 251 (1960).

9. G. Cavallini, E. Massarani, D. Nardi, and R. D'Ambrosio, *J. Am. Chem. Soc.,* **79,** 3514 (1957).

10. A. Sallmann and R. Pfister, U. S. Patent 3,558,690 (1971).

11. D. C. Atkinson, K. E. Godfrey, B. J. Jordan, E. C. Leach, B. Meek, J. D. Nichols, and J. F. Saville, *J. Pharm. Pharmacol.,* **26,** 357 (1974).

12. T. Y. Shen, *Chim. Ther.,* **1967,** 459.

13. J. S. Nicholson and S. S. Adams, British Patent 971,700 (1964).

14. J. S. Nicholson and S. S. Adams, British Patent 1,012,480 (1965).

15. L. Aparicio, *Arch. Int. Pharmacodyn. Ther.,* **227,** 130 (1977).

16. J. M. Carretero, J. L. Martin, and A. Ron, *Eur. J. Med. Chem.,* **13,** 77 (1978).

17. T. Y. Shen, in *Topics in Medicinal Chemistry,* Vol. 1, J. L. Rabinowitz and R. M. Myerson, Eds., Wiley-Interscience, New York, 1967, p. 29.

18. P. De Witt and M. T. Ramacci, *Farmaco, Ed. Sci.,* **27,** 897 (1972).

19. P. Gund and T. Y. Shen, *J. Med. Chem.,* **20,** 1146 (1977).

20. M. W. Whitehouse and J. P. Famaey, *Agents Actions,* **3/4,** 217 (1973).

21. R. G. W. Spickett, A. Vega, J. Prieto, J. Moragues, M. Marquez, and D. J. Roberts, *Eur. J. Med. Chem.,* **11,** 7 (1976).

22. N. P. Buu-Hoi, G. Lambelin, C. Gillet, C. Lepoivre, J. Thiriaux, and G. Mees, *Nature (Lond.),* **211,** 752 (1966).

23. G. Lambelin, N. P. Buu-Hoi, H. Bronilhet, M. Gautier, C. Gillet, J. Roba, and J. Thiriaux, *Arzneim.-Forsch.,* **18,** 1404 (1968).

24. G. Orzalesi, R. Selleri, O. Caldini, I. Volpato, F. Innocenti, J. Colome, A. Sacristan, and G. Varez, *Arzneim.-Forsch.,* **27,** 1006 (1977).

25. G. Orzalesi, R. Selleri, O. Caldini, I. Volpato, F. Innocenti, J. Colome, A. Sacristan, G. Varez, and G. Pisaturo, *Arzneim.-Forsch.,* **27,** 1012 (1977).

26. A. I. Meyers, D. L. Temple, D. Haidukewych, and E. D. Mihelich, *J. Org. Chem.,* **39,** 2787 (1974).

27. J. G. Lombardino, in *Annual Reports in Medicinal Chemistry,* Vol. 13, F. H. Clarke, Ed., Academic Press, New York, 1978, p. 167.

28. M. Vincent, G. Remond, P. Desnoyers, and J. Labaume, *J. Med. Chem.,* **16,** 710 (1973).
29. R. H. Rynbrandt, B. D. Tiffany, D. P. Balgoyen, E. E. Nishizawa, and A. R. Mendoza, *J. Med. Chem.,* **22,** 525 (1979).
30. S. S. Adams, E. E. Cliffe, B. Lessel, and J. S. Nicholson, *Nature (Lond.),* **200,** 271 (1963).
31. S. S. Adams, P. Hebborn, and J. S. Nicholson, *J. Pharm. Pharmacol.,* **20,** 305 (1967).
32. T. M. Chalmers, *Ann. Rheum. Dis.,* **22,** 358 (1963).
33. M. Thompson, P. Stephenson, and J. S. Percy, *Ann. Rheum. Dis.,* **23,** 397 (1964).
34. F. D. Hart and P. L. Boardman, *Ann. Rheum. Dis.,* **24,** 61 (1965).
35. J. B. Dick-Smith, *Med. J. Aust.,* **263,** (1966).
36. T. Hargreaves, *Nature (Lond.),* **208,** 1101 (1965).
37. B. Lessel, E. E. Cliffe, and J. E. Hall, *Br. J. Pharmacol.,* **29,** 121 (1967).
38. S. S. Adams, E. E. Cliffe, B. Lessel, and J. S. Nicholson, *J. Pharm. Sci.,* **56,** 1686 (1967).
39. S. S. Adams, K. F. McCullough, and J. S. Nicholson, *Arch. Int. Pharmacodyn. Ther.,* **178,** 115 (1969).
40. K. F. Swingle, G. G. I. Moore, and T. J. Grant, *Arch. Int. Pharmacodyn. Ther.,* **221,** 132 (1976).
41. J. G. Lombardino, I. G. Otterness, and E. H. Wiseman, *Arzneim.-Forsch.,* **25,** 1629 (1975).
42. R. J. Flower, H. S. Cheung, and D. W. Cushman, *Prostaglandins,* **4,** 325 (1973).
43. B. Lessel, in *Symposium on Ibuprofen,* supplement to *Rheumatol. Phys. Med.,* **14,** (1970).
44. S. S. Adams, R. G. Bough, E. E. Cliffe, B. Lessel, and R. F. N. Mills, *Toxicol. Appl. Pharmacol.,* **15,** 310, (1969).
45. T. Y. Shen in *Annual Reports in Medicinal Chemistry,* Vol. 2, C. K. Cain, Ed., Academic Press, New York, 1967, p. 217.
46. S. S. Adams, P. Bresloff, and C. G. Mason, *J. Pharm. Pharmacol.,* **28,** 256 (1976).
47. R. F. N. Mills, S. S. Adams, E. E. Cliffe, W. Dickinson, and J. S. Nicholson, *Xenobiotica,* **3,** 589 (1973).
48. W. J. Wechter, D. G. Loughhead, R. J. Reischer, G. J. Van Giessen, and D. G. Kaiser, *Biochem. Biophys. Res. Commun.,* **61,** 833 (1974).
49. D. G. Kaiser, G. J. Van Giessen, R. J. Reischer, and W. J. Wechter, *J. Pharm. Sci.,* **65,** 269 (1976).
50. S. J. Lan, K. J. Kripalani, A. V. Dean, P. Egli, L. T. Difazio, and E. C. Schreiber, *Drug Metab. Dispos.,* **4,** 330 (1976).
51. C. J. W. Brooks and M. T. Gilbert, *J. Chromatogr.,* **99,** 541 (1974).
52. J. E. Pettersen, *Biomed. Mass Spectr.,* **5,** 488 (1978).
53. H. W. Ruelius, D. C. De Jongh, and S. R. Schrader, *Arzneim.-Forsch.,* **20,** 115 (1970).
54. J. E. Pettersen, G. A. Ulsaker, and E. Jellum, *J. Chromatogr.,* **145,** 413 (1978).
55. E. F. Davies and G. S. Avery, *Drugs,* **2,** 416 (1972).
56. S. S. Adams and J. W. Buckler in *Clinics in Rheumatic Diseases,* Vol. 5, E. C. Huskisson, Ed., Saunders, London, 1979, p. 359.
57. J. E. Hall, J. Agar, J. W. Buckler, P. G. Dodsworth, and A. A. J. Goldberg, *Therapiewoche,* **37,** 3293 (1973).
58. Anonymous, *Chem. Eng. News,* **57** (37), 25 (1979).
59. D. T. Mowry, M. Renoll, and W. F. Huber, *J. Am. Chem. Soc.,* **68,** 1105 (1946).
60. J. S. Nicholson, British Patent 1,167,192 (1969).
61. R. A. Dytham, British Patent 1,160,725 (1969).
62. Nisshin Flour Milling Co. Ltd., British Patent 1,445,211 (1976).
63. D. R. White and D. K. Wu, *J. Chem. Soc., Chem. Commun.,* **1974,** 988.
64. E. C. Taylor, R. L. Robey, K.-T. Liu, B. Favre, H. T. Bozimo, R. A. Conley, C.-S. Chiang, A. McKillop, and M. E. Ford, *J. Am. Chem. Soc.,* **98,** 3037 (1976).

65. J. A. Walker and M. D. Pillai, *Tetrahedron Lett.*, **1977**, 3707.
66. T. Shioiri and N. Kawai, *J. Org. Chem.*, **43**, 2936 (1978).
67. M. W. Partridge, H. J. Vipond, J. Urwin and J. S. Nicholson, British Patent 1,265,800 (1972).
68. G. Palazzo and L. Baiocchi, *Tetrahedron Lett.*, **1968**, 4739.
69. L. Baiocchi, M. Giannangeli, and M. Bonanomi, *Tetrahedron,* **34**, 955 (1978).
70. L. Baiocchi, British Patent 1,462,407 (1977).
71. D. R. White, U.S. Patent 4,008,270 (1977).

Piroxicam

8

Edward H. Wiseman
and Joseph G. Lombardino

1. INTRODUCTION

When piroxicam (Feldene) became available to the medical profession in Europe in 1979, it represented the culmination of more than 15 years of collaborative research between the authors of this chapter and their colleagues. The properties of piroxicam (Figure 1) represent not simply desirable qualities elaborated after pharmacological and clinical evaluation, but rather the rational design and selection of a compound believed to have a high likelihood of possessing qualities ideally suited for treating chronic inflammation.

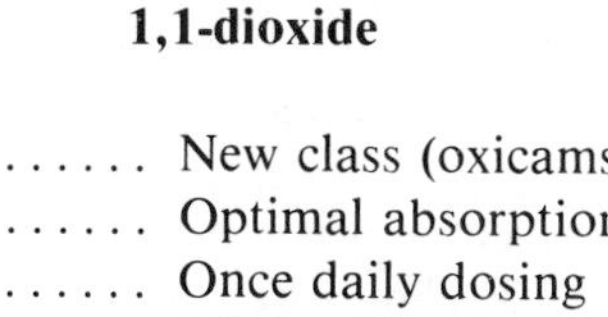

4-Hydroxy-2-methyl-*N*-(2-pyridyl)-2*H*-1,2-benzothiazine-3-carboxamide 1,1-dioxide

Structurally novel	....	New class (oxicams)
Acidic and lipophilic	....	Optimal absorption, distribution
Long plasma half-life	....	Once daily dosing
High potency	....	Minimal load on gastrointestinal tract, liver and kidneys

Figure 1. Piroxicam (Feldene) — a designed drug.

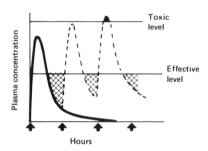

Figure 2. Plasma drug concentrations after multiple administration.

In the early 1960s, there were three nonsteroidal anti-inflammatory drugs (NSAID) widely used to treat human articular and musculoskeletal disease — aspirin, phenylbutazone, and indomethacin. To these was soon added ibufenac (quickly withdrawn and eventually replaced by ibuprofen), the first example of what was to be an ever-increasing number of agents from a series of arylalkanoic (carboxylic) acids. In general, these carboxylic acids are all of low or moderate potency in animals and man and have a short plasma half-life. Thus despite multiple daily administration, the plasma concentrations of these agents frequently fall below those associated with efficacy and occasionally rise to levels associated with toxicity (Figure 2). Such characteristics obviously are undesirable for the treatment of a chronic disease such as rheumatoid arthritis.

By inspection of the then existing drugs, important physicochemical properties associated with anti-inflammatory activity could be discerned. Structurally, the molecules seemed capable of assuming a planar form, which was envisaged as conducive to a proper fit on the receptor site of an enzyme (unknown at that time).* Their acidity was such that at physiological pH, the molecules were largely ionized [pK_a ranged from 3 to 6 in an aqueous titration system; solubility considerations usually dictated measurement of acidity in 2:1 dioxane/water (v/v) where pK_a' was about 1-2 units higher than that in fully aqueous systems] and thus were essentially confined to plasma and extracellular water, and their lipophilicity was such that they would be expected to readily cross biological membranes (partition coefficients in the range of 1-100, between octanol and pH 7.4 buffer). All these properties are possessed by the known anti-inflammatory carboxylic acids; however, such compounds are generally susceptible to facile elimination from the body, usually by conjuga-

---

*In retrospect, most likely arachidonic acid cyclooxygenase.

tion of the carboxylic acid as a glucuronide and/or sulfate and subsequent renal excretion. Almost without exception, therefore, carboxylic acids have relatively short (1-4 hours) plasma half-lives.[†] There also appeared to be little chance that the relatively high potency of the carboxylic acid indomethacin, itself a product of a massive structure-activity screening program in animal models, was likely to be exceeded by another representative of one of the arylalkanoic acid series.

The decision was made, therefore, to concentrate efforts to seek other structural classes possessing the desired biological and physicochemical properties — high anti-inflammatory potency, suitable acidity, and long plasma half-life — and to conduct a classical structure-activity search to optimize these properties. Since the ionizable hydrogen on the β-diketone functional group offered the

$$
\begin{array}{ccc}
& \overset{H}{\underset{|}{}} & \\
-\underset{\underset{O}{\|}}{C} - \underset{\underset{R}{|}}{C} - \underset{\underset{O}{\|}}{C} - & \rightleftharpoons & -\underset{\underset{O}{\|}}{C} - \underset{\underset{R}{|}}{C} = \underset{\underset{O^- H^+}{|}}{C} -
\end{array}
$$

possibility of achieving the appropriate acidity, attention was turned to a variety of cyclic β-diketones[1] with the aim of enhancing acidity so as to achieve the acidic range exhibited by the carboxylic acids (i.e., pK_a' about 4-7). Concurrently, appropriate laboratory animal pharmacology procedures were streamlined to support the structure-activity search efforts.

2. PHARMACOLOGIC/PHARMACOKINETIC PROCEDURES

In the early 1960s, it was well recognized that NSAID could inhibit edema formation induced by the injection of carrageenan into the food-pad of the rat [the rat-foot edema (RFE) test]. Later it was shown that the potencies of NSAID in the RFE test bear rank order correlation to their clinical potency.[2] However, to permit careful ordering of potency within analogues, and to allow high compound throughput, a standardized and systematic procedure was needed. Statistical bounds were placed upon normal day-to-day and animal-to-animal variation, the performance of a standard drug was defined, and the RFE operation was optimized to permit testing of up to 65 compounds weekly, with all results[*] calculated and displayed by computer (Figure 3).

[†]Such was the case in 1963 when this research began. Recently naproxen (half-life 14 hours) and benoxaprofen (half-life 35 hours) have been reported.

[*]In structure-activity tables (Tables 1, 2, 4, 5, 7) anti-inflammatory activity is reported as a mean inhibition of edema in the treated animals within the range of 0.5-1.5 times that of the mean inhibition of concurrently treated animals receiving aspirin (100 mg/kg p.o.); +, drug given at 100 mg/kg; + +, drug given at 33 mg/kg; + + +, drug given at 10 mg/kg p.o. Compounds with anti-inflammatory activity (at 100 mg/kg) of less than 0.5 times aspirin reported as -.

COMPOUND	LOT NUMBER	WGT	DOSE MG/KG	SOLN	DRUG FORM	PCENT INHIB	P	MIN	MAX	EVALUATION	PAW VOLUMES
CP 0 0	CONTROL	178	0.0			0.77 ••••••••••				::	5380 5582 5582 5882 5479 / 5480 5384 5384 5378 5789 / 5466 5666 5666 5265 5672
P 05618	STANDARD	178	100.0	NAOH	SOLN	55.76 ••••••••••				::	5766 5971 / 5478 5378 5378 5469 5777
CP 16160	6077 55 6	178	3.3	NAOH	SOLN	20.33	0.53	0.3	0.8	1 S	5771 5269 5269 5071 5480
CP 16172	6090 9 5	178	3.3	NAOH	SOLN	6.60	0.12	0.0	0.3	1 S	5377 5688 5688
CP 16171	6090 4 9	179	3.3	NAOH	SOLN	50.23	0.90	0.7	1.1	2 S	5985 5679 5679 5868 5469
CP 16158	6077 43 21	179	3.3	NAOH	SOLN	26.88	0.48	0.3	0.7	1 S	4859 5873 5873 / 5268 5872 5872 / 5169 5173 5173 5776 5474
CP 16218	3848 177 1	178	10.0	NAOH	SOLN	25.52	0.38	0.2	0.8	2 S	5278 5973 5973 / 5470 5468 5468 5072 5173
CP 16110	6086 26 2	178	10.0	POIL	SUSP	-6.29 ••••••••••				1 :*	5885 / 5382 5489 5489 5481 5678
CP 16048	3970 130 2	179	1.0	NAOH	SOLN	5.49	0.11	0.0	0.3	1 S	5687 5988 5988 / 4973 5384 5384 5173 5477
CP 16071	3919 272 30	178	0.3	NAOH	SOLN	-2.61 ••••••••••				1 :*	5580 5684 5684 / 5580 4874 4874 5170 4985
CP 16070	3919 771 29	179	1.0	NAOH	SOLN	12.74	0.23	0.0	0.5	1 S	5893 5278 5278 / 5479 5488 5488 5269 5472
CP 16118	3919 786 11	179	0.1	NAOH	SOLN	10.90	0.20	0.0	0.5	1 NS	5782 5578 5578 / 5672 5275 5275 5376 5287
CP 16119	3919 787 11	178	0.3	NAOH	SOLN	28.72	0.52	0.2	0.9	1 NS	5474 5583 5583 / 5376 5364 5364 5267 5468
CP 16090	3593 232 29	179	0.3	NAOH	SOLN	5.99	0.11	0.0	0.3	1 S	5987 5277 5277 / 5379 5182 5182 5381 5276
CP 16214	6077 92 6	178	10.0	NAOH	SOLN	26.26	0.47	0.3	0.8	1 S	5477 5374 5374 / 5375 5079 5079 5070 5164
CP 15847	3955 120 C	178	33.0	POIL	SUSP	-22.88 ••••••••••				1 :*	6280 5472 5472 / 4665 5895 5895 5891 5789 / 5290 5698 5698

1 = LESS THAN

Dec. 26 1967

Figure 3. Computer printout of carragenan edema screening data.

176

For operational ease of specimen collection, pharmacokinetic studies were performed in mongrel dogs. Compounds were administered intravenously and serial blood samples were drawn and analyzed by spectrophotometric assays developed for each agent. These results were analyzed to obtain plasma half-life. Structure-activity relationships were then pursued on the basis of both antiedema activity in rats and plasma half-life in dogs.[3] Methods and analytical procedures developed for kinetic studies in dogs were adapted for other species (rat, monkey, human) as needed.

3. ARYL INDANDIONES

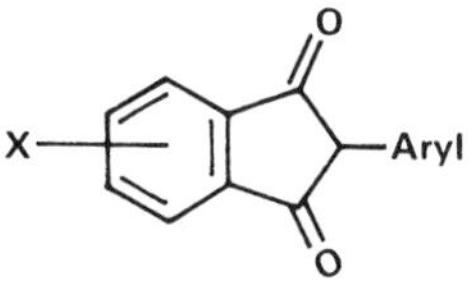

Aryl indandiones

Our initial probes of β-diketones of enhanced activity involved the cyclic diketones of the indandione series.[4] Anti-inflammatory activity in both laboratory animals and man had previously been reported[5] for 2-phenyl-1,3-indandione (1-1; pK_a' 5.4), but this compound had not been developed for treatment of arthritis, probably because of coexisting anticoagulant activity. We proceeded on the basis that separation of anti-inflammatory and anticoagulant activity might be achieved by molecular modification. Results showed most nuclear unsubstituted 2-aryl-1,3-indandiones (1-1 to 1-13; Table 1) to be inhibitors of both inflammation and coagulation (as measured by prothrombin time measurements*). However, fairly large *meta* substituents on the 2-aryl function (e.g., 1-2, 1-9) diminished anticoagulant activity. Combination of a *meta*-substituted 2-aryl group with a 5-substituent on a 1,3-indandione produced a group of compounds with no measurable prothrombin effects in rats but with useful anti-inflammatory activity (e.g., compounds 1-16, 1-18, 1-20, 1-23).

---

*In structure-activity tables (Tables 1 and 2) effects on prothrombin time are reported as follows: +, prolongation of prothrombin time 16 hours after administration of nine oral doses, 8 hours apart (100 mg/kg p.o.); + + +, prolongation of prothrombin time 16 hours after administration of nine oral doses, 8 hours apart (100 mg/kg p.o.); + + +, prolongation of prothrombin time 16 hours after administration of two oral doses, 8 hours apart (100 mg/kg p.o.); -, no prolongation of prothrombin time after nine oral doses (100 mg/kg p.o.).

Table 1
2-Aryl-1,3-Indandiones

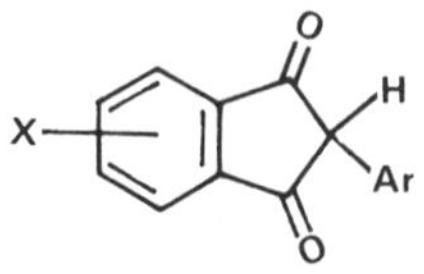

No.	A	X	pK_a'	Anti-inflammatory activity	Prothrombin effects
1-1	C_6H_5	H	5.4	+ +	+ +
1-2	3-BrC_6H_4	H	4.6	+ +	+
1-3	4-BrC_6H_4	H	4.7	+ +	+ +
1-4	2-$CH_3OC_6H_4$	H	7.6	−	−
1-5	4-$CH_3OC_6H_4$	H	5.6	+ + +	+ +
1-6	4-$(C_6H_5)C_6H_4$	H	5.2	+	+ +
1-7	4-ClC_6H_4	H	4.8	+ + +	+ +
1-8	3-ClC_6H_4	H	4.7	+ +	+ +
1-9	3-IC_6H_4	H	4.7	+	+
1-10	$(C_2H_5)_2NCH_2CH_2OC_6H_4$	H	8.5	−	−
1-11	4-$NH_2C_6H_4$	H	6.2	−	−
1-12	3-$CH_3C_6H_4$	H	5.7	+ +	+ +
1-13	2-ClC_6H_4	H	6.1	+ +	+ +
1-14	C_6H_5	5-CH_3	5.9	+ +	+ +
1-15	3-$CF_3C_6H_4$	5-CH_3	4.7	+ +	+
1-16	2-BrC_6H_4	5-CH_3		+	−
1-17	C_6H_5	5-Br		+	+
1-18	2-Naphthyl	5-Br		+ +	−
1-19	C_6H_5	4-NO_2	3.5	+ +	+ +
1-20	3-$CF_3C_6H_4$	5-NO_2		+ +	−
1-21	C_6H_5	5-CF_3	4.0	+ + +	+ +
1-22	3-$CF_3C_6H_4$	5-CF_3	3.5	+	−
1-23	3-$CH_3C_6H_4$	5-CF_3	4.2	+ + +	−

A further requirement for useful anti-inflammatory activity was deduced after determining the apparent acidities (pK_a') of the 2-aryl-1,3-indandiones. Generally, active compounds exhibited a pK_a' of 5.9 or less. Two examples (1-**19**, and 1-**22**) with pK_a' as low as 3.5 were also active anti-inflammatory agents. When coplanarity in the conjugate base was prevented by a large 2-aryl group (e.g., 1-**4**) or a basic amine function was introduced (e.g., 1-**10**, 1-**11**), pK_a' was increased and anti-inflammatory activity was abolished.

Since none of the compounds with anti-inflammatory activity had a plasma half-life of greater than 2 hours in the dog, the desired profile of properties could not be achieved in this series.

4. ARYL BENZO(b)THIOPHENES

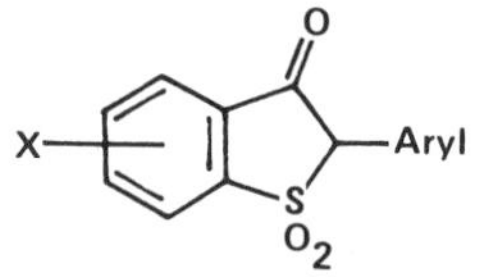

Aryl benzo(b)thiophenes

Encouraged by the successful separation of anti-inflammatory and anticoagulant activities in the arylindandiones, the related benzo(b)thiophene structure was explored.[6] 2-Phenylbenzo(b)thiophen-3(2H)-one 1,1-dioxide (2-**1**; Table 2) was found to be both an anticoagulant and an anti-inflammatory agent. Similarly, other 2-arylbenzo(b)thiophen-3(2H)-one 1,1-dioxides unsubstituted at the 5-position (2-**2** to 2-**4**) were found to have anticoagulant activity. Introduction of a substituent at the 5-position in combination with a 2-*meta*-substituted aryl group (e.g., 2-**6**) produced compounds with anti-inflammatory activity but free of anticoagulant (prothrombin) effects. With a few exceptions (e.g., 2-**12** and 2-**13**), compounds exhibiting anti-inflammatory activity fell within an acidity range of pK_a' 4.8-6.2. The most potent anti-inflammatory activity was seen with compounds having a 5-trifluoromethyl substituent (i.e. 2-**16**, 2-**17**). Comparing dose-response curves for 2-**16** and phenylbutazone in the RFE test indicated a relative potency of 1.24. Compound 2-**8** had a plasma half-life in dogs of 7-9 hours; however, the desired combination of high potency and extended half-life did not appear to be attainable in this series. Interestingly, in animal safety evaluation studies, compound 2-**8** caused nephrotoxicity in rats and dogs, a phenomenon now well associated with other nonsteroidal anti-inflammatory agents.[7]

Table 2
2-Arylbenzo[b]thiophene-3(2H)-one 1,1-Dioxides

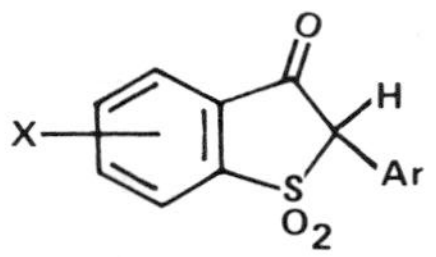

No.	Ar	X	pK_a'	Anti-inflammatory activity	Prothrombin effects
2-1	C_6H_5	H	6.2	+	++
2-2	$4-ClC_6H_4$	H	5.6	+	++
2-3	$3-CF_3C_6H_4$	H	5.2	+	++
2-4	1-Naphthyl	H	—	—	++
2-5	C_6H_5	5-Cl	5.5	+	++
2-6	$3-CF_3C_6H_4$	5-Cl	4.3	+	—
2-7	$3-NO_2C_6H_4$	5-Cl	3.8	+	—
2-8	C_6H_5	$5,6-(CH)_4$	5.7	—	—
2-9	$3-CF_3C_6H_4$	$5,6-(CH)_4$	4.9	+	—
2-10	$4-ClC_6H_4$	$5,6-(CH)_4$	5.2	+	—
2-11	C_6H_5	$5-(CH_3)_2NSO_2$	4.8	+	—
2-12	$3-CF_3C_6H_5$	$5-(CH_3)_2NSO_2$	3.5	—	—
2-13	$3-CH_3C_6H_5$	$5-(CH_3)_2NSO_2$	4.7	—	—
2-14	$3-CF_3C_6H_4$	$5,6-(OCH_3)_2$	6.4	+	—
2-15	$3-CH_3C_6H_4$	$5-NO_2$	4.3	+	—
2-16	C_6H_5	$5-CF_3$	5.0	+++	—
2-17	$3-CH_3C_6H_4$	$5-CF_3$	5.2	++	—
2-18	$3-CF_3C_6H_4$	$5-CF_3$	4.1	+	—

5. DIOXOISOQUINOLINE CARBOXANILIDES

Isoquinoline carboxanilides

Efforts were expanded at this time to a series of 1,3-dioxoisoquinoline-4-carboxanilides in collaboration with Dr. Saul Kadin and furnished the next advance.[8] In this series, anti-inflammatory potency in the range of that of phenylbutazone was seen in association with extended plasma half-life in laboratory animals. The unexpectedly enhanced acidic properties of these cyclic β-diketones may partially be ascribed to a hydrogen bonded stabilization of a planar enolate anion (shown in Table 3).

A most striking finding in these studies was the exquisite sensitivity of the dog's basal metabolism to those compounds carrying a methyl moiety at position 2 of the isoquinoline nucleus (Class 1).[9] In the conscious dog, emesis and rapid respiration rate were noted within 1 or 2 hours after administration, the animals becoming progressively cyanotic. In the anesthetized dog, the increased respiration rate was accompanied by an increased oxygen consumption rate, tachycardia, and elevation of body temperature. The syndrome was not elicited in the rat, monkey, or man, even upon chronic administration of high doses. In no species was the syndrome elicited by administration of these isoquinolinecarboxanilides bearing a hydrogen in place of the methyl moiety at position 2 of the isoquinoline nucleus (Class 2). A perfect correlation was observed between effects on basal metabolism and displacement of thyroxine binding to plasma globulins *in vitro*. The most important thyroxine-binding proteins in the blood of the rat, dog, monkey, and man are α-globulins. Isoquinolinecarboxanilides of Class 1 interfered with the thyroxine binding to α-globulin in dog plasma only, corresponding to their species-specific effect on basal metabolism. Compounds in Class 2, which showed no effect on basal metabolism in the rat, dog, or monkey, did not interfere with thyroxine-protein binding in the respective plasmas.

The pharmacokinetics of these isoquinoline carboxanilides reflected their metabolic vulnerability and lipophilicity. Thus in Class 2, plasma half-life was increased by blocking the metabolically vulnerable 4′-position in the carboxanilide moiety (3-2b). A further increase in half-life was seen in 3-1c, presumably reflecting the increased facility of tubular resorption due to increased lipophilicity. Of greater interest was the marked difference in the

Table 3
Properties of Isoquinolinecarboxanilides

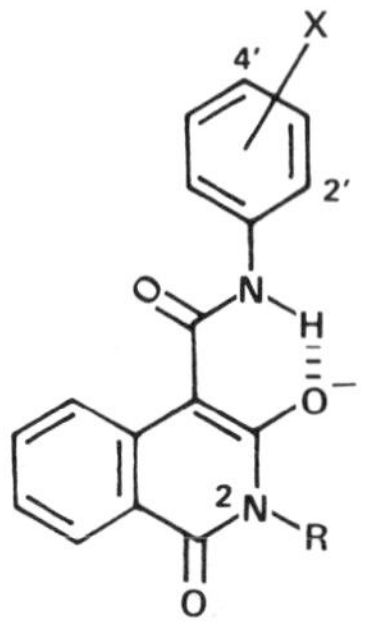

X	Class 1 (R = CH₃)	Class 2 (R = H)
H	a	a
4'-Cl	b	b
2',4'-diCl	c	
4'-OH	d	

	3-1a	3-1b	3-1c	3-1d	3-2a	3-2b Tesicam
Partition: octanol-buffer	12.9	58.1	138.0	2.4	2.4	20.6
pK_a'	5.7	5.2	4.2	5.9	4.8	4.6
Plasma half-life (hours)						
Rat	1.0		6.0			1.5
Dog	6.0	10.0	35.0	0.2	2.0	19.0
Monkey	6.0	10.0	6.5	0.7		
Man	8.5			15.0		22.0

plasma half-life of 3-**1d** in laboratory animals and man. This compound was the major human metabolite of 3-**1a** and, because of its longer half-life, accumulated to concentrations above that of the parent drug upon chronic administration of the latter. In laboratory animals, the plasma half-life of 3-**1d** was extremely short, and indeed 3-**1d** proved to be almost undetectable in the plasma of animals receiving 3-**1a**. It is interesting to speculate that the difference between animals and man may be due to man's inability to conjugate 3-**1d**; in subjects receiving 3-**1a** chronically, up to 70% of the daily dose could be recovered in the urine as free 3-**1d**. In contrast, little free 3-**1d** could be recovered in the urine of animals receiving either 3-**1a** or 3-**1d**.

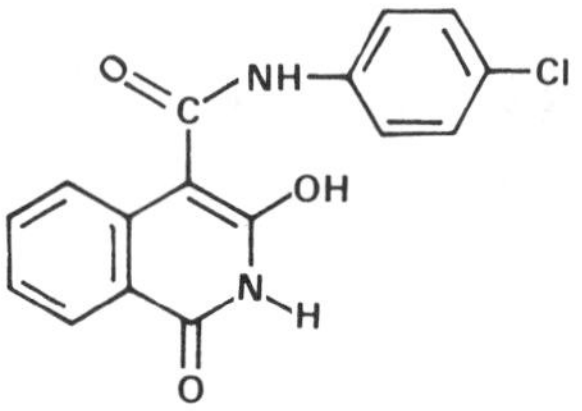

Tesicam

The site of metabolism in 3-**1a** was blocked in compound 3-**2b** (tesicam), and, as expected, a significant increase in plasma half-life was seen. In normal man, tesicam produced a marked hypouricemia (Figure 4), as predicted from the prolongation of phenol red half-life in the rat. In patients with rheumatoid arthritis and osteoarthritis, tesicam (250 mg, twice daily) improved clinical symptoms of the arthritis. Thus tesicam marked the first successful step in the search for a long half-life, high potency, nonsteroidal anti-inflammatory agent. However, potency was not believed to be fully sufficient to satisfy the original aims of the research.

6. CARBOXAMIDES OF BENZOTHIAZINE 1,1-DIOXIDE

Concurrently with synthesis in the dioxoisoquinoline carboxanilide series, explorations in an isosteric heterocyclic series were undertaken. Based on the sulfone-carbonyl bioisosterism previously described in the literature,[10] it was decided that the then unknown 1,2-benzothiazine-3(4H)one 1,1-dioxides would be made as possible bioisosteres of the dioxoisoquinolines. Carboxamides of 3-oxo-2H-1,2-benzothiazine 1,1-dioxide (Table 4) were synthesized from o-toluenesulfonamides in four steps (Figure 5) and many had good antiedema activity in the RFE model.[11] A dose-response comparison of 4-**9** (pK_a' 5.6) with indomethacin showed 4-**9** to be 1.5 times as potent. The half-life of 4-**9** was greater than 14 hours in the dog and 9 hours in the monkey. It was

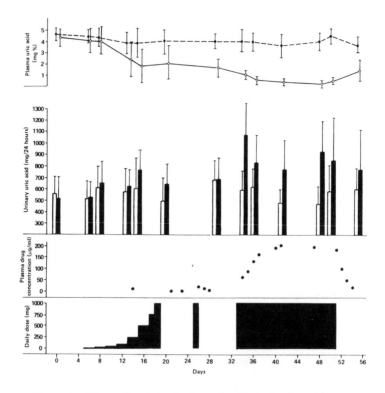

Figure 4. Hypouricemic and uricosuric effect of tesicam in man.

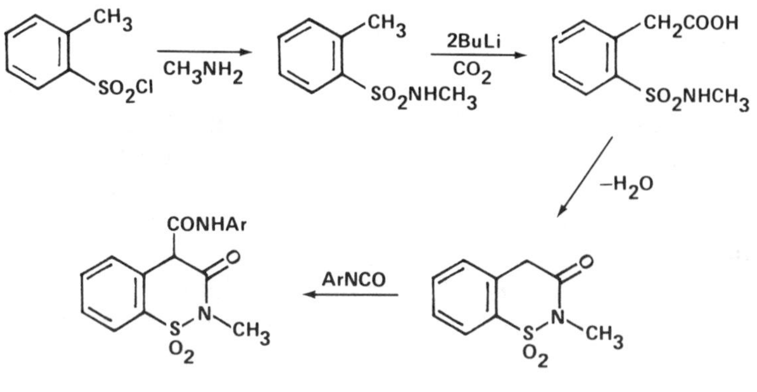

Figure 5. Synthesis of 3-oxo-2*H*-1,2-benzothiazine-4-carboxamide 1,1-dioxides.

Table 4
3,4-Dihydro-2-Methyl-3-oxo-2H-1,2-Benzothiazine-4-Carboxamide 1,1-dioxides

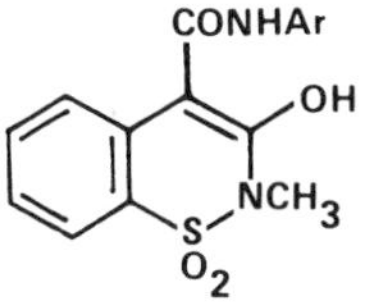

No.	Ar	Anti-inflammatory activity
4-1	C_6H_5	+ +
4-2	$2\text{-}ClC_6H_4$	+ +
4-3	$4\text{-}FC_6H_4$	+ + +
4-4	$4\text{-}ClC_6H_4$	+ +
4-5	$3\text{-}CF_3C_6H_4$	+ + +
4-6	$4\text{-}CH_3C_6H_4$	+ +
4-7	$4\text{-}CH_3OC_6H_4$	+ +
4-8	$2,4\text{-}Cl_2C_6H_3$	+ + + +
4-9	$4\text{-}BrC_6H_4$	+ + + + +
4-10	$4\text{-}NO_2C_6H_4$	+ + + + +
4-11	1-Naphthyl	+
4-12	$3\text{-}CH_3C_6H_4$	+ +
4-13	$3\text{-}ClC_6H_4$	+ + +
4-14	$2,5\text{-}Cl_2C_6H_3$	+ + + +
4-15	$2\text{-}CH_3OC_6H_4$	+ +
4-16	$3,4\text{-}Cl_2C_6H_3$	+ +
4-17	$CH_2CH = CH_2$	+ + +
4-18	COC_6H_5	+ +
4-19	$4\text{-}CF_3C_6H_4$	+ +
4-20	$CH_2C_6H_5$	+ + + +
4-21	C_6H_{11}	+ + +
4-22	$CH_2CH_2C_6H_5$	+

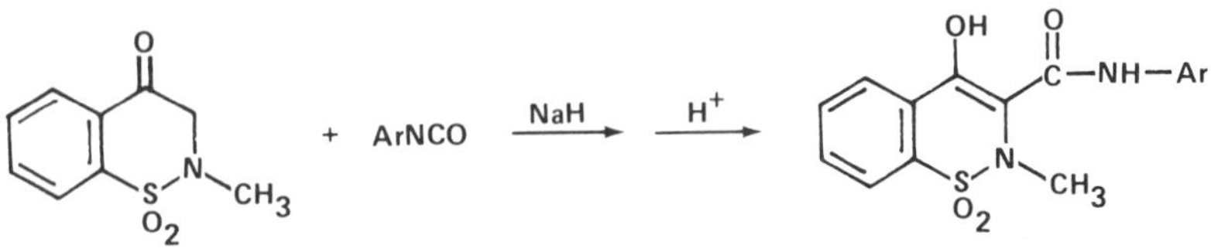

Figure 6. Synthesis of 4-hydroxy-2H-1,2-benzothiazine-3-carboxamide 1,1-dioxides (route 1).

well tolerated in animal safety evaluation studies, although at autopsy the usual low incidence of renal papillary necrosis was noted in the rodents. Compound 4-9 was, however, the only representative of the series with these attributes; in fact structure-activity relationships were difficult to discern.

Our interest then shifted to the isomeric carboxamides of the 4-hydroxy-2H-1,2-benzothiazine 1,1-dioxide series.[12] Although 3-benzoyl-[13] and 3-acetyl-4-hydroxy-2H-1,2-benzothiazine 1,1-dioxide[14] were known in the literature, only the successful preparation of the 3-carboxamides[12] of this series produced compounds with enhanced acidity and significant anti-inflammatory activity. The experience with the anti-inflammatory dioxoisoquinoline carboxamides provided a strong motivation to develop the specific reaction conditions necessary to prepare the 4-hydroxy-1,2-benzothiazine-3-carboxamides. Although the known 2-methyl-2H-1,2-benzothiazine-4(3H)-one 1,1-dioxide in the presence of base was known to rapidly self-condense and to fail to condense with esters,[14] conditions were found[12] to cause this compound to condense with isocyanates using NaH as a base (Figure 6). The resultant carboxamides proved to have good anti-inflammatory activity in animals (Table 5), enhanced acidity, and extended plasma half-lives in dogs.

After anti-inflammatory activity was demonstrated for the initial 3-carboxamides of 1,2-benzothiazines, a more versatile approach for preparing a wide variety of 3-carboxamides was developed (Figure 7). Gabriel-Colman type rearrangement of methyl 1,2-benzisothiazol-3(2H)one 1,1-dioxide 2-acetate gave a 1,2-benzothiazine 3-carboxylic ester. NaOMe was used in a variety of solvents in an effort to maximize yields of this rearrangement and it was eventually found that the best results were obtained in DMSO. N-Alkylation of this ester yielded 4-hydroxy-2-methyl-2H-1,2-benzothiazine-3-carboxylic acid 1,1-dioxide, methyl ester. This ester was then caused to react with amines under forcing conditions (18 hour in DMF at 130 °C or 22 hours in refluxing xylene) to provide the desired 3-carboxamides of 4-hydroxy-2H-1,2-benzothiazines.[12] This more versatile route, which did not require the use of an isocyanate, allowed the preparation of many novel carboxamides simply by using the 1,2-benzothiazine-3-carboxylic ester and the appropriate primary or

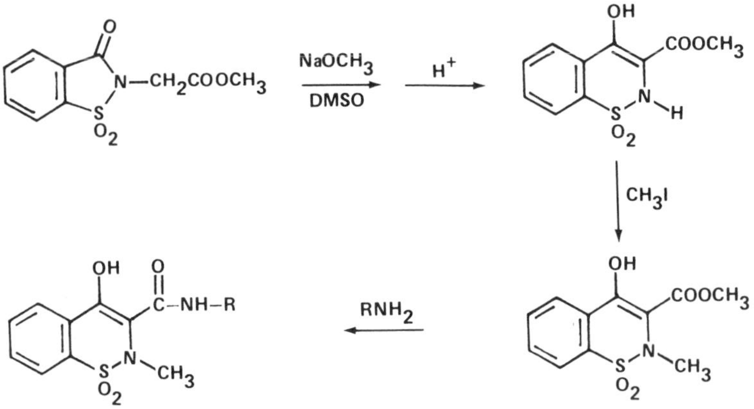

Figure 7. Synthesis of 4-hydroxy-2H-1,2-benzothiazine-3-carboxamide 1,1-dioxides (route 2).

secondary amine. This synthetic approach was to prove critically important for the later preparation of N-heterocyclic carboxamides of 4-hydroxy-2H-1,2-benzothiazine 1,1-dioxide.

Structure-activity relationships among the 3-carboxamides (Table 5) were developed by the preparation of over 50 analogues. It was clearly shown that 2-CH$_3$ substitution produced compounds (e.g., 5-1, 5-3, and 5-8) with excellent anti-inflammatory activity. Carboxanilides such as 5-1 were generally superior anti-inflammatory agents to alkylamides such as 5-17 and 5-18. The *meta*-substituted carboxanilides (5-6, 5-8, and 5-15) were generally superior to *para*-substituted carboxanilides (5-7 and 5-2). No correlation was observed among anti-inflammatory activity and acidity, partition coefficient, electronic, and spatial factors.[12] As observed with other analogues from the 4-hydroxy-1,2-benzothiazine series, compound 5-1 was found to be active in the antiedema model using adrenalectomized rats, ruling out an adrenal-mediated mechanism of action. Dose-response regression lines determined for 5-1 (ID$_{50}$ 37 mg/kg, p.o.) and phenylbutazone in the antiedema model were parallel, with 5-1 being 2.1 times as potent as phenylbutazone.

While some of these carboxanilides exceeded tesicam in potency and duration, it was of importance to learn if the clinical properties and metabolic susceptibility in man resembled those of the dioxoisoquinoline carboxanilides.

The metabolic fates of the carboxanilides of the two series are compared in Table 6. Half-lives in laboratory animals were generally long for the parent benzothiazine 1,1-dioxide (5-1, pK_a' 7.3).[15] For this series, all four species hydroxylated the 3-carboxanilide moiety, and metabolites related to 5-19 (pK_a'

Table 5
3-Carboxamides of 4-Hydroxy-2-Alkyl-2H-1,2-Benzothiazine 1,1-Dioxide

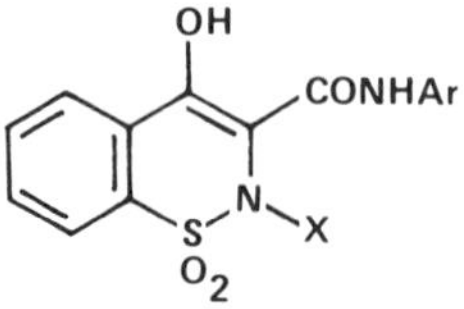

No.	Ar	X	Anti-inflammatory activity
5-1	C_6H_5	CH_3	+ + + +
5-2	$4\text{-}ClC_6H_4$	CH_3	+ +
5-3	$2\text{-}CH_3OC_6H_4$	CH_3	+ + +
5-4	$2,5\text{-}Cl_2C_6H_3$	CH_3	+
5-5	$2\text{-}CH_3OC_6H_4$	CH_3	+ +
5-6	$3\text{-}CF_3C_6H_4$	CH_3	+ + +
5-7	$4\text{-}CH_3C_6H_4$	CH_3	+
5-8	$3\text{-}ClC_6H_4$	CH_3	+ + + +
5-9	$3,4\text{-}Cl_2C_6H_3$	CH_3	+
5-10	$2\text{-}ClC_6H_4$	CH_3	+
5-11	$4\text{-}NO_2C_6H_4$	CH_3	−
5-12	$4\text{-}FC_6H_4$	CH_3	+ +
5-13	1-Naphthyl	CH_3	+ +
5-14	$4\text{-}BrC_6H_4$	CH_3	−
5-15	$3\text{-}CH_3C_6H_4$	CH_3	+ + +
5-16	$4\text{-}EtOC_6H_4$	CH_3	−
5-17	$CH_2CH=CH_2$	CH_3	+ +
5-18	$n\text{-}C_4H_9$	CH_3	+
5-19	$4\text{-}HOC_6H_4$	CH_3	−
5-20	$2,5\text{-}F_2C_6H_3$	CH_3	+ +
5-21	$2,4\text{-}F_2C_6H_3$	CH_3	+ +
5-22	$2\text{-}FC_6H_4$	CH_3	+ + +
5-23	$3\text{-}NO_2C_6H_4$	CH_3	+ +
5-24	C_6H_5	$CH_2CH=CH_2$	−
5-25	C_6H_5	CH_2CH_3	+
5-26	C_6H_5	$CH_2CH_2CH_3$	+
5-27	C_6H_5	$CH_2C_6H_5$	+ +
5-28	C_6H_5	H	+ +

Table 6
Plasma Half-Lives in Various Species of Carboxanilides of the 1,2-Benzothiazine 1,1-Dioxide and Dioxisoquinoline Ring Systems

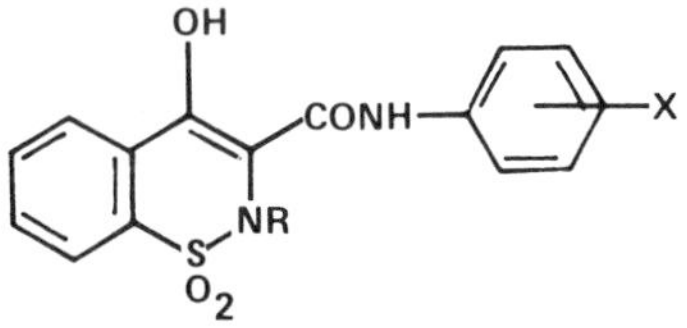

5-1, R = CH$_3$; X = OH
5-19, R = CH$_3$; X = OH

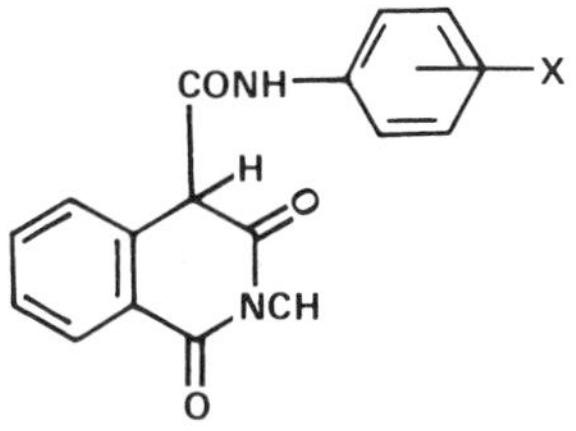

3-Ia, X = H
3-Id, X = OH

| Species | Plasma half-life (hours) | | | |
	5-1	5-19	3-1a	3-1d
Rat	6	7	1	
Dog	30	14	6	0.2
Monkey	4.5	11	6	0.7
Man	21	37	8.5	15

7.4) accounted for about 70% of a single dose in man, about 50% in the rat and monkey, and about 10% in the dog. In the last species, about 70% of administered drug was excreted in the urine as a conjugate of the 4-OH function of the parent drug; a further 10% was excreted unchanged. Differences in the pharmacokinetics of 5-1 and its major metabolite 5-19 in the four species studied reflected the metabolic dispositions. In the dog the plasma half-life of 5-1 was twice as long as that of 5-19 (Table 6). The average plasma concentration of 5-1 24 hours after the ninety-sixth daily dose (10 mg/kg, oral) was 25 μg/ml; the average plasma concentration of 5-19 was 11 μg/kg. Thus the difference in plasma half-life between 5-1 and 5-19 in the dog was reflected in the plateau plasma concentrations achieved during multiple dosing. During human toleration studies, after 30 days of repeated administration (300 mg, daily) concentrations of 5-1 averaged 34 μg/ml and those of 5-19 averaged 40 μg/ml. These data were consistent with the longer half-life in man of the metabolite 5-19 compared with that of the parent drug 5-1. Almost without exception, drug metabolites have lower oil-water partition coefficients than the parent drug. It is generally accepted that this increased hydrophilicity aids the process of excretion by the kidney (urine) and/or liver (bile). It is therefore of interest that the metabolite 5-**19** of the carboxanilide 5-**1**, has a longer plasma half-life (37 hours) in man than its parent drug (21 hours). The same phenomenon was noted in the earlier series of anti-inflammatory isoquinolinedione carbox-anilides. In the former series, the parent drug 3-**1a** had a plasma half-life of 8.5 hours in man, whereas the major metabolite 3-**1d** had a plasma half-life of 15 hours.

Thus the knowledge of the metabolic behavior of these simple carboxanilides was much advanced by this study. A subsequent study of 5-**1** in rheumatoid arthritis, at a mean dose of 170 mg/day for 23 days, showed modest anti-inflammatory activity, but not hypouricemic activity. We were concerned that the metabolite plasma concentrations were markedly above those of the parent drug, especially in an agent given in doses of about 200 mg daily, a dose still somewhat higher than the expressed aims of the project. However, all these considerations became somewhat academic, since the synthesis problems en-countered in trying to prepare the *N*-heterocyclic carboxamides of the 4-hydroxy-1,2-benzothiazine 1,1-dioxide series had been resolved. The synthe-tic route discussed above (Figure 7) permitted for the first time the preparation of a variety of *N*-heterocyclic amides from methyl 4-hydroxy-2-methyl-2*H*-1,2-benzothiazine-3-carboxylate 1,1-dioxide and heterocyclic amines of various types. So many of the initially prepared heterocyclic amide analogues clearly possessed both high potency and extended plasma half-life (Table 7) that exten-sive synthesis and testing efforts were focused on these compounds.[16,17]

The first few *N*-heterocyclic analogues were prepared from some readily ac-cessible heterocyclic amines. It quickly became apparent that almost any 2-amino-heterocycle, ranging from 2-aminothiazole, to 2-aminopyridine, to 2-aminopyrazine, to 2-aminopyridazine could be converted to an *N*-heterocyclic 3-carboxamide of 4-hydroxy-2*H*-1,2-benzothiazine 1,1-dioxide exhibiting anti-inflammatory activity.[16,17] This pioneering observation paved the way for additional work in our own laboratory and in other laboratories that continues today.[18,19]

Structure-activity relationships were determined on almost 30 analogues prepared in this series. Table 7 presents a sample of the compounds made; more complete compilations have been published.[17] Activity was widespread in the series, with several analogues (7-**1**, 7-**2**, 7-**7**, etc.) equaling or exceeding indomethacin in antiedema potency.

The *N*-heterocyclic carboxamides were generally more acidic than the *N*-aryl-carboxamides derived from the same 1,2-benzothiazine system, many analogues having pK_a values in the range of 4-6.[17] To explain such an enhanced

Table 7
N-Heterocyclic-3-Carboxamides of 4-Hydroxy-2-Methyl-2H-1,2-Benzothiazine 1,1-Dioxide

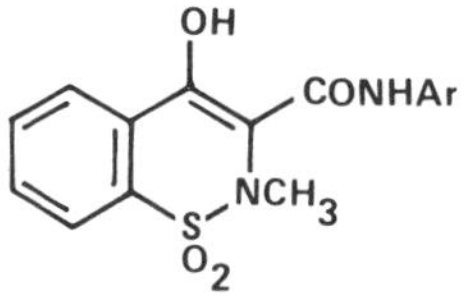

No.	Ar	Anti-inflammatory activity
7-1	2-Thiazolyl	+ + + + + +
7-2	4-Methyl-2-thiazolyl	+ + + + +
7-3	4,5-Dimethyl-2-thiazolyl	+ + + + +
7-4	2-Benzothiazolyl	+ + + + +
7-5	2-Pyrazinyl	+ + + +
7-6	6-Methoxy-3-pyridazinyl	+ + + +
7-7	2-Pyridyl	+ + + + +
7-8	5-Bromo-2-pyridyl	+ + + +
7-9	5-Chloro-2-pyridyl	+ + +
7-10	4-Methyl-2-pyridyl	+ + +
7-11	5-Methyl-2-pyridyl·HCl	+ + +
7-12	6-Methyl-2-pyridyl	+ + + + + +

acidity, a contribution from a structure such as A [illustrated for the N-(2-pyridyl)carboxamide in Table 8] to stabilization of the enolate anion was postulated. In addition to A, some contributions from the tautomeric structure B may further stabilize the enolate anion in the present series of N-heterocyclic carboxamides. Such stabilization of the enolate ion would result in an increased acidity for the conjugate acid. Table 8 presents additional pK_a' values, as well as other physical data on certain carboxamides of the 1,2-benzothiazine system. In animal tests, these compounds showed anti-inflammatory activity in the range of that of indomethacin. Within the series, acidities ranged from pK_a' 4.6 to 7.3, and partition coefficients were 0.5-5.0. Many of these compounds exhibit extended plasma half-lives in laboratory animals, and two, sudoxicam (7-1) and piroxicam (7-7), have been examined in man.

Table 8

Physiochemical Properties and Plasma Half-Lives of Selected N-Heterocyclic Carboxamides of 4-Hydroxy-2-Methyl-2H-1,2-Benzothiazine 1,1-Dioxide

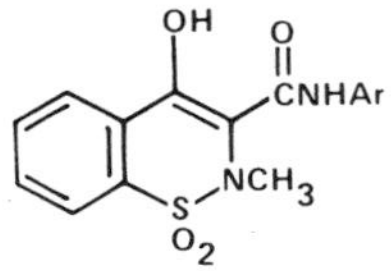

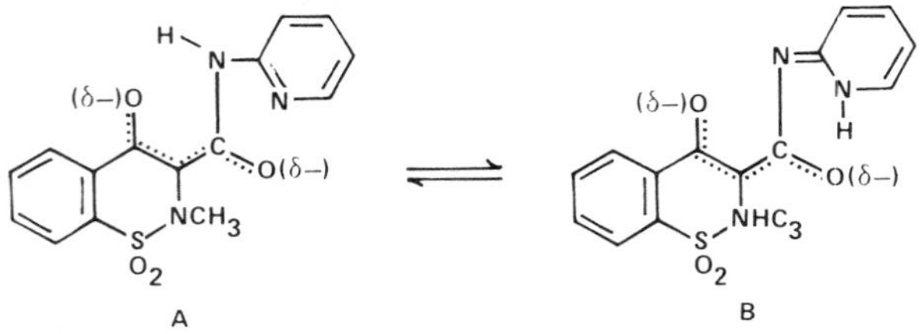

Ar	Partition coefficient	pK_a'	Plasma half-life (hours)				
			Rabbit	Dog	Rat	Monkey	Man
2-Thiazolyl (sudoxicam)	0.5	5.3	3.5	60.0	13.0	8.0	24-96
4-Methyl-2-thiazolyl	1.3	5.7	4.0	42.0	5.4		
4,5-Dimethyl-2-thiazolyl	4.8	5.8	2.8	53.0	3.7		
2-Pyridyl (piroxicam)	1.8	6.3	4.5	37.0	5.8		45
6-Methyl-2-pyridyl	4.0	6.6	1.3	12.0	3.6	6.0	

Sudoxicam

Piroxicam (Feldene)

In the RFE test sudoxicam significantly inhibited edema formation at doses as low as 0.1 mg/kg p.o.[20] In a comparative study with indomethacin, sudoxicam was 2.9 (1.5-5.9) times as effective as indomethacin (Figure 8) and was the most potent of 14 NSAID examined in the carrageenan-edema test.[21] Sudoxicam is a slightly water soluble, lipophilic, moderately strong acid that is extensively bound to plasma proteins. Absorption of sudoxicam occurs smoothly after oral administration and it is eliminated by extensive metabolism, less than 5% being recovered unchanged (Figure 9).[22] In man after an oral dose of 50 mg (approximately 0.7 mg/kg), peak plasma concentrations of 4 μg/ml were reached within 3 hours. The extended half-life of sudoxicam would lead to the expectation that, upon repeated administration, plasma concentrations would tend to plateau at a level above that seen upon acute administration. Indeed, in man, after an oral dose of 20 mg, plasma concentrations 24 hours after administration of the first dose were below 1 μg/ml, increasing to 3-7 μg/ml,

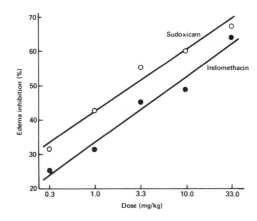

Figure 8. Anti-edema effects of sudoxicam and indomethacin in normal rats.

measured 24 hours after the fourteenth successive daily dose. Upon daily administration of 50 mg, human plasma concentrations reached 15-26 μg/ml, measured 24 hours after the eighth dose. After drug withdrawal from these subjects, the rate of disappearance of drug from plasma constantly changed, such that, depending on the initial plasma concentration, the apparent half-life ranged from as long as 12 days to a minimum of 24 hours (Figure 10).[20] Since such variable pharmacokinetic behavior was undesirable, a further representative of this series, piroxicam, with a potentially much simpler route of metabolism, was evaluated.

Piroxicam is an acid of pK_a' 6.3 (in dioxane H$_2$O) with a partition coefficient (octanol-pH 7.4 buffer) of 1.8. It has potent activity in a variety of anti-inflammatory tests in laboratory animals (Figure 11).[23,24] While potency in the RFE test is slightly less than that of indomethacin (Figure 12), piroxicam is outstandingly potent in the ultraviolet-light-induced erythema test in the guinea

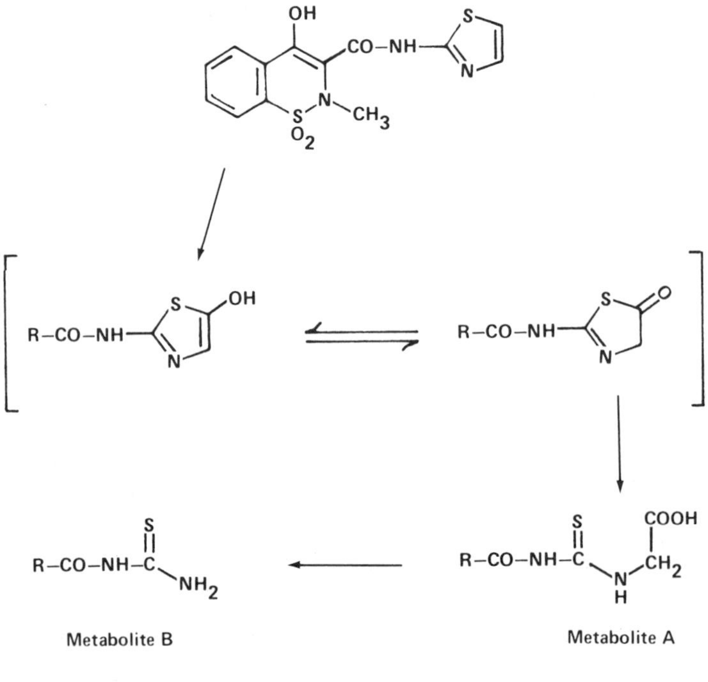

Figure 9. Proposed biotransformation pathway for sudoxicam.

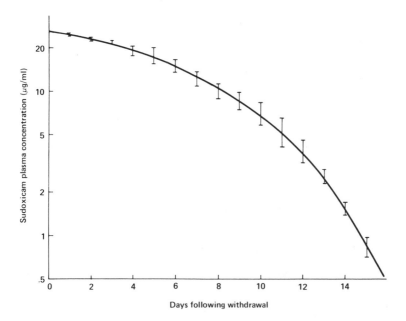

Figure 10. Decay of sudoxicam plasma concentrations after withdrawal of drug from subjects who received repeated oral doses of sudoxicam.

pig; in this test it is about 10 times as potent as indomethacin (Figure 13).[25] Piroxicam's anti-inflammatory activity is not dependent on stimulation of the adrenals, being as potent in adrenalectomized rats as in intact animals.[23] Piroxicam is a potent, competitive inhibitor of prostaglandin biosynthetase *in vitro*.[26] Piroxicam has an extended plasma half-life in animals and man (45 hours),[27] and this half-life does not vary with the plasma concentration, as is the case with sudoxicam. Biotransformation follows the steps shown in Figure 14.[28] Extensive preclinical studies demonstrated the safety of piroxicam in laboratory animals, and this safety has been corroborated in the broad clinical studies that have established the safety and efficacy of single daily doses of piroxicam in a wide variety of human inflammatory diseases.[29] Piroxicam represents the first clinically useful member of a growing class of anti-inflammatory benzothiazine carboxamides known as "oxicams".[32,31]

PHARMACOLOGIC PROFILE OF PIROXICAM

Antiedema activity
  Carrageenan-induced foot edema in rats
Antiinflammatory activity
  Ultraviolet-induced erythema in guinea pigs
Antiproliferative activity
  Cotton-string granuloma in rats
Antiarthritic activity
  Mycobacterium/adjuvant-induced arthritis in rats
Antigout activity
  Urate-crystal-induced synovitis in dogs
Analgesic activity
  Phenylbenzoquinone-induced writhing in mice
Antipyretic activity
  E. coli-induced fever in rats
Prostaglandin biosynthetase activity
  Synthesis of prostaglandins from arachidonic acid in vitro
Antithrombogenic activity
  Collagen-induced aggregation of human and animal platelets
  in vitro
Cardiovascular system
  No activity in dogs
Central nervous system activity
  No behavioral effects in rats or mice

Figure 11.   Pharmacological profile of piroxicam.

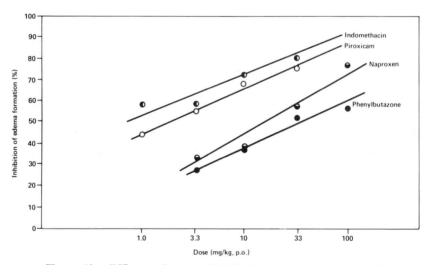

Figure 12.   Efficacy of some NSAIDs in carrageenan-induced foot edema in rats.

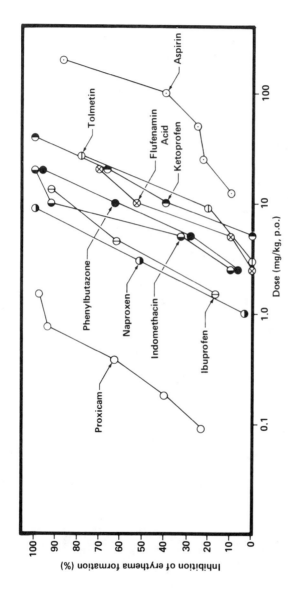

Figure 13. Inhibition of ultraviolet light-induced erythema in the guinea pig by administration of NSAIDs.

197

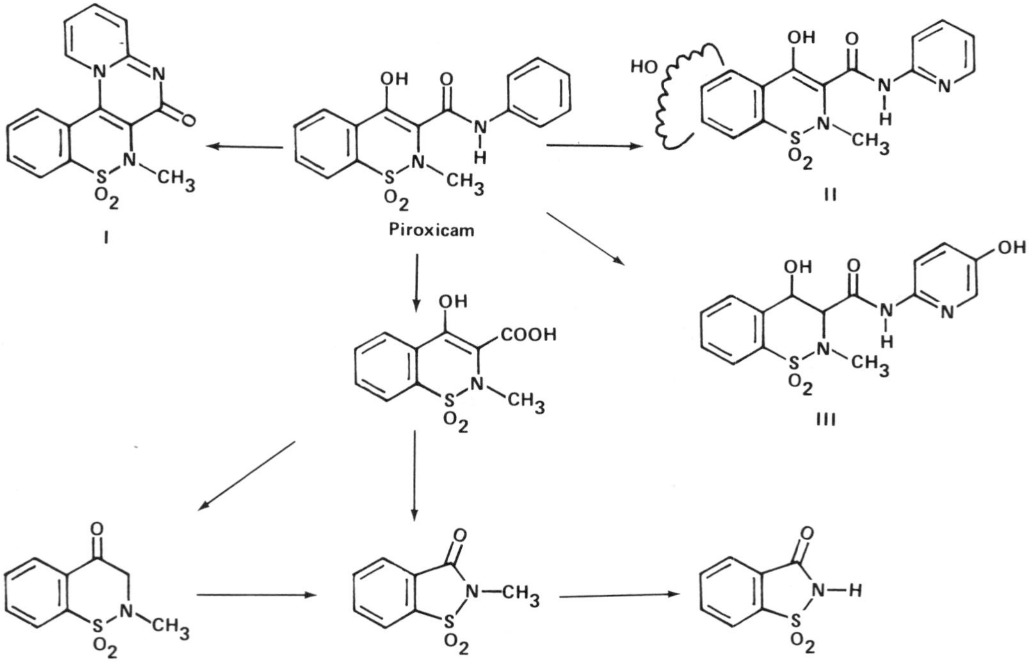

Figure 14. Biotransformation of piroxicam.

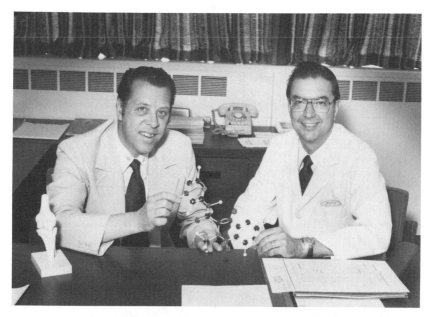

Figure 15. Dr. E. H. Wiseman (left), Executive Director of Research Administration, and Dr. J. G. Lombardino (right), Research Advisor, both of Pfizer Central Research, discussing a molecular model of piroxicam. Dr. Wiseman carried out the biological and pharmacokinetic studies on the compounds discussed in this review. Piroxicam and all the other β-dicarbonyl compounds, except for the dioxoisoquinolines, discussed herein were synthesized in Dr. Lombardino's laboratory.

CONCLUSION

The task took longer than anticipated. However, it is a source of considerable satisfaction to view piroxicam as an ordered progression, from an idea through chemical synthesis and structure-activity relationships developed in several chemical classes of compounds, and finally to a clinical candidate with the attributes (Figure 1) thought desirable at the inception of the program. The combination of high potency and long half-life, permitting maintenance of therapeutic plasma concentrations throughout the day from a single daily dose, gives piroxicam the attributes that contribute to, and are positively correlated with, excellent patient compliance.[32] As such, it is likely to be a significant contribution to the therapeutic armamentarium with which to treat human inflammatory diseases.

REFERENCES

1. J. G. Lombardino, "Enolic Acids with Antiinflammatory Activity" in *Antiinflammatory Agents, Chemistry and Pharmacology,* Vol. I, R. A. Scherrer and M. W. Whitehouse, Eds., Academic Press, 1974, pp. 129-157.
2. J. G. Lombardino, I. G. Otterness, and E. H. Wiseman, *Arzneim.-Forsch.,* **25,** 1629 (1975).
3. E. H. Wiseman, "Drug Kinetic Studies with Non-Steroidal Anti-Inflammatory Agents in Animals and Man," in *Antiinflammatory Agents, Chemistry and Pharmacology,* Vol. II, R. A. Scherrer and M. W. Whitehouse Eds., Academic Press, 1974, pp. 235-243.
4. J. G. Lombardino and E. H. Wiseman, *J. Med. Chem.,* **11,** 342 (1968).
5. L. Fontaine, M. Odievre, Y. Achet, and B. Drevon, *Therapie,* **16,** 34 (1961).
6. J. G. Lombardino and E. H. Wiseman, *J. Med. Chem.,* **13,** 206 (1968).
7. E. H. Wiseman and H. Reinert, *Agents Actions,* **5,** 322 (1975).
8. S. B. Kadin and E. H. Wiseman, *Nature,* **222,** 275-276 (1969).
9. E. H. Wiseman, E. J. Gralla, J. Chiaini, J. R. Migliardi, and Y.-H. Chang, *J. Pharmacol. Exp. Ther.,* **172,** 138 (1970).
10. A. Burger, "Relation of Chemical Structure and Biological Activity," in *Medicinal Chemistry,* A. Burger, Ed., 3d ed., Wiley-Interscience, New York, 1970, p. 77.
11. J. G. Lombardino and E. H. Wiseman, *J. Med. Chem.,* **14,** 973 (1971).
12. J. G. Lombardino, E. H. Wiseman, and W. M. McLamore, *J. Med. Chem.,* **14,** 1171 (1971).
13. K. Abe, S. Yamamoto, and K. Matsui, *J. Pharmacol. Soc. Jap.,* **76,** 1058 (1956); *Chem. Abstr.,* **51,** 3499d (1957).
14. H. Zinnes, R. A. Comes, and J. Shavel, Jr., *J. Org. Chem.,* **31,** 162 (1966).
15. J. Chiaini, E. H. Wiseman, and J. G. Lombardino, *J. Med. Chem.,* **14,** 1175 (1971).
16. J. G. Lombardino and E. H. Wiseman, *J. Med. Chem.,* **15,** 848 (1972).
17. J. G. Lombardino, E. H. Wiseman, and J. Chiaini, *J. Med. Chem.,* **16,** 493 (1973).
18. G. Steiner, Justis *Liebigs Ann. Chem.,* **1978,** 635.
19. H. Zinnes, N. A. Linds, J. C. Sircar, M. L. Schwartz, and J. Shavel, Jr., *J. Med. Chem.,* **16,** 44 (1973).
20. E. H. Wiseman and J. Chiaini, *Biochem. Pharmacol.,* **21,** 2323 (1972).
21. J. G. Lombardino, I. G. Otterness, and E. H. Wiseman, *Arzneim.-Forsch.,* **25,** 1629 (1975).
22. D. C. Hobbs and T. M. Twomey, *Drug Metab. Disposition,* **5,** 75 (1977).
23. E. H. Wiseman, Y-H. Chang, and J. G. Lombardino, *Arzneim.-Forsch.,* **26,** 1300 (1976).
24. E. H. Wiseman, *Roy Soc. Med., Int. Cong. Symp. Ser.,* **1,** 11 (1978).
25. I. G. Otterness, E. H. Wiseman, and D. J. Gans, *Agents Actions,* **9,** 177 (1979).
26. T. J. Carty, J. D. Eskra, J. G. Lombardino, and W. D. Hoffman, *Prostaglandins,* **19,** 51 (1980).
27. D. C. Hobbs and T. M. Twomey, *J. Clin. Pharmacol.,* **19,** 270 (1979).
28. D. C. Hobbs and T. M. Twomey, *Drug Metabol. Disposition,* **9,** 114 (1981).
29. E. H. Wiseman and J. A. Boyle, *Clinics in Rheum. Diseases,* **6,** 585 (1981).
30. J. G. Lombardino and E. H. Wiseman, *Trends in Pharmacol. Sciences,* **2,** 132 (1981).
31. E. H. Wiseman and J. G. Lombardino, *European J. Rheumatol. Inflamm.,* **4,** 280 (1981).
32. J. D. Fitzgerald, "The Influence of the Medication on Compliance with Therapeutic Regimens," in *Compliance with Therapeutic Regimens,* D. L. Sackett and R. B. Haynes, Eds., Johns Hopkins University Press, Baltimore, 1976.

Rifampicin

9

P. Sensi

1. INTRODUCTION

The starting point in the search for new antibiotics is a process consisting of an extensive systematic investigation of microorganisms as a potential source of secondary metabolites with antibacterial activity. Although there are many and sometimes significant differences in the details adopted by the various laboratories to improve its efficiency, the process was and still remains a blind screening of potential useful drugs, according to the terminology of medicinal chemistry. From this standpoint the discovery and development of a new natural antibiotic follow general schemes that are relatively traditional to the experts in the field. The modulation of the biological properties of a natural product through structural modifications, on the other hand, represents a very challenging research area, where the chemical approaches are continuously confronted with biological effects.

The history of the discovery of rifampicin presents some peculiarities, the most relevant one being, perhaps, the fact that all the chemical studies leading to very active derivatives were performed on a molecule (rifamycin B) practically inactive per se. It should be mentioned also that at the time (1959) when we started the program of chemical modifications of rifamycin B, the very many previous attempts to improve the biological properties of the natural antibiotics had been met with relatively little success and in fact some scientists believed that whatever was produced by a microorganism was already the product selected for its greatest activity. Instead of beginning with this belief, we started from the hypothesis that the production of a large series of structurally related antibiotics by a microorganism is a sign that it has biosynthesized a certain

number of variations on a basic structure and that these variations do not greatly affect the activity. In such a situation, chemical modifications in the
laboratory might well produce other variations with potential biological interest
that the producing microorganism "had not thought of." This was the case of
rifamycins.

The selection of rifamycin B as a lead for extensive chemical studies was due
to a series of fortuitous circumstances, especially its unusual ability to undergo
a spontaneous "activation." Also, the first chemical modifications led to the
discovery of rifamycin SV. In industry, research projects are continuously
challenged by management, whose opinion in respect to a specific project may
be different from that of the researchers. A research project can be quite
vulnerable in such a conflict situation. The early introduction into therapeutic
use of rifamycin SV, although resulting in a moderate commercial success,
made it possible for the researchers to overcome some recurrent criticisms inside the company on expense allocation to the antibiotic projects and to continue their activity in the field of chemical modifications of rifamycins with enthusiasm. This effort led eventually to the discovery of rifampicin.

2. THE PRODUCING STRAIN

In our laboratories the screening program for new antibiotics was initiated in
1952, some time after the company decision to build a plant for the production
of penicillin in Torre Annunziata near Naples. The first approach followed by
our research team, initially very small, was quite conventional if considered
retrospectively. The *Streptomyces* genus was considered the most promising
source of new microbial metabolites with antibacterial activity. The total
number of antibiotics described in the literature at that time was of the order of
a few dozen, although it was increasing very rapidly. During the course of a 4
year screening program (1953-1957), we examined approximately 2000 soil
samples, isolated about 18,000 streptomyces strains and, following obvious
selection criteria, identified some new antibiotics.

Most of the soil samples were collected by the laboratory workers directly involved in the screening program. It was in the summer of 1957 that one
member of our research team, H. Pagani, while on a holiday on the Cote
d'Azur, collected a soil sample at a pine arboretum near St. Raphael and
brought it to the laboratory. Among the microorganisms isolated from this soil
sample, the strain receiving our collection number ME/83 produced in
submerged culture a high activity against gram-positive bacteria and
Mycobacterium tuberculosis, and a moderate activity against gram-negative
organisms. The crude brown product extracted from the fermentation broths
showed high *in vitro* activity, protective effect against gram-positive infections
in mice, and low toxicity.

From these data and from the chemical and physical properties of the crude product, it was evident that we had in hand a new group of antibiotics.[1] Considerable effort was therefore spent to characterize the strain and its fermentation conditions and to isolate, identify, and evaluate the various active components formed. A comparative taxonomic study of the strain revealed that the strain ME/83 represented a new species, which was indicated as *Streptomyces mediterranei*.[2] Only some years later the strain was reclassified as belonging to the genus *Nocardii (Nocardia mediterranea)* mainly on the basis of the presence in its cell wall of *meso*-diaminopimelic acid.[3]

3. THE NAME

The thousands of microorganisms tested in a screening program are generally identified with number codes, often difficult to remember. We adopted the very informal rule of assigning, in addition to the code number, a nickname to the few antibacterial substances isolated during the screening and selected for more extensive evaluation. The laboratory books of my colleagues and myself in the late fifties report the experiments carried out on a number of new antibiotics, with nicknames such as Pecos Bill, Gengis Khan and Mickey Mouse. For publication the nicknames were replaced by common names acceptable by scientific journals [e.g., matamycin[4] was in fact, in our laboratory books, Mata Hari].

The crude antibiotic extracted from the strain ME/83 was named Rififi (an argot word meaning struggle among gangsters), which was the title of a French movie, directed by J. Dassin, rather popular at that time in Europe. The common name rifomycins given in the first publications to the "Rififi" antibiotics was later changed into rifamycins to avoid possible confusion with the trademark of another antibiotic. The various natural and semisynthetc members of the rifamycin family have been identified with suffixes or with names deriving from the common root "rifa" (e.g., rifamycin SV, rifamide, rifazine, rifampicin). The suffixes were often selected on the basis of some laboratory association. For example, when we encountered the problem of a chromatographic spot appearing now and then in unpredictable conditions among the degradation products of the 3-dialkylaminomethyl rifamycin SV, the name "rifamycin AF" (Araba Fenice) was given to the not yet isolated substance. In fact there is a popular saying, combining the Erodotus tradition with later centuries' skepticism, that states that the Phoenix exists, but nobody can tell where it is.

Rifamycin AF was later identified as 3-formylrifamycin SV. The hydrazone with *N*-amino-N′-methylpiperazine was coded rifamycin AF/AMP, which when introduced into therapy, received the INN (international nonproprietary name) of rifampicin and the USAN (United States adopted name) of rifampin.

4. FROM RIFAMYCIN-COMPLEX TO RIFAMYCIN SV

The active crude brown powder extracted from the fermentation broths of the strain ME/83 consisted of a mixture of at least five products, which was named rifamycin-complex. We encountered a great number of difficulties in the characterization and evaluation of the individual components of the complex, indicated as rifamycins A, B, C, D, E according to their mobility in paper chromatography. Their isolation was achievable using techniques, such as countercurrent distribution, by which only small amounts of material could be obtained.[5] Most of the individual components were quite unstable. Furthermore, although active *in vitro* and effective *in vivo,* the local tolerability of the complex on the site of injection was very poor.

The only product of the complex isolated in pure, crystalline form was rifamycin B, but it was a minor component (5-10%) of the mixture. Therefore, it was a very important step in the development of rifamycins when, in a study of various fermentation media, it was found that *N. mediterranea,* in a medium containing 0.2% sodium diethylbarbiturate, produced practically only rifamycin B,[6] together with small quantities of a new inactive rifamycin (rifamycin Y). Although rifamycin B was the less active component of the original complex, at least we had solved the problem of producing a single compound to submit for proper biological evaluation. Rifamycin B showed extremely low toxicity and a moderate therapeutic activity in animal infections by parenteral administration. Only later did we realize that rifamycin B has no effect per se against bacterial cells.[7]

Rifamycin B might well have been ignored and its description only added to the thousands of products of bacterial metabolism described in the scientific literature, were it not for the fact that it had an unusual property. In aqueous solution and in the presence of oxygen, rifamycin B was spontaneously transformed into other substances with great antibacterial activity. The idea of developing a pharmaceutical formulation that, instead of the usual expiration period, should indicate the "activation" period, increasing its therapeutic and commercial value with aging like champagne, was dwelt on as an encouraging joke in the lab. Therefore, we began studying the activation process of rifamycin B in oxidative conditions.[8] We found that rifamycin B is converted reversibly into rifamycin O, which is hydrolyzed to rifamycin S, losing one molecule of glycolic acid. Rifamycin S is the true "activation" product of rifamycin B.

Mild reduction of rifamycin S yielded rifamycin SV, whose sodium salt showed high *in vitro* activity against gram-positive bacteria and *Mycobacterium tuberculosis,* moderate activity against gram-negative bacteria, no cross resistance to the other antibiotics, good protective effect in various experimental animal infections, and low toxicity.[9,10] The therapeutic efficacy of rifamycin SV by parenteral administration against infections caused by gram-positive bacteria was confirmed by extensive clinical investigations.[11] Additional interest in the biological properties of rifamycin SV derived from the fact that it is excreted predominantly by the liver, reaching high concentrations in the bile. For this reason rifamycin SV is particularly useful in the therapy of the infections of the biliary tract, even those caused by gram-negative microorganisms. In spite of the high *in vitro* activity against *M. tuberculosis,* poor therapeutic results have been obtained in the treatment of tuberculosis, mainly because the blood levels of rifamycin SV have a relatively short half-life.

Rifamycin SV sodium salt was first introduced into therapeutic use in 1962 and is currently used in various countries for the parenteral and topical treatment of infections due to gram-positive bacteria and infections of the biliary tract also due to gram-negative bacteria.

5. THE STRUCTURE

After the isolation of the crystalline rifamycin B, various attempts were made in our laboratories to elucidate its structure. Although we had acquired information on various aspects of the rifamycin B chemistry and prepared a series of derivatives including the therapeutically used rifamycin SV, the structure elucidation appeared to be a very difficult problem. In the beginning of 1960, V. Prelog agreed to study the structure of rifamycin B in his laboratory at the Polytechnical School of Zurich, assigning the experimental work to W. Oppolzer as a Ph.D. thesis. After about 3 years of extensive chemical degradation studies and extensive use of NMR spectroscopy on the various fragments of the molecule, it was possible to assign to rifamycin B and its congeners the structures indicated in Figure 1. The structural problem of rifamycin B was also studied in the same period by M. Brufani, W. Fedeli, G. Giacomello, and A. Vaciago at the University of Rome through X-ray crystallographic analysis of rifamycin B *p*-iodoanilide, and they reached the same conclusion.

Being in continuous contact with the two groups, I remember having seen in Rome the molecular model of rifamycin B derived from X-ray analysis reproducing the same structure drawn in Zurich on the basis of chemical studies. But when Prelog received the picture of the model he stood quite perplexed and his confusion was erased only after a series of telephone calls between Zurich and Rome. Part of the rigid model structure had collapsed when in the hands of the photographer, who, relying on his memory, had just patched it up in what he thought was the correct way.

The papers describing the elucidation of the rifamycin structure by the two independent approaches appeared in the same issue of *Experientia.*[12-14]

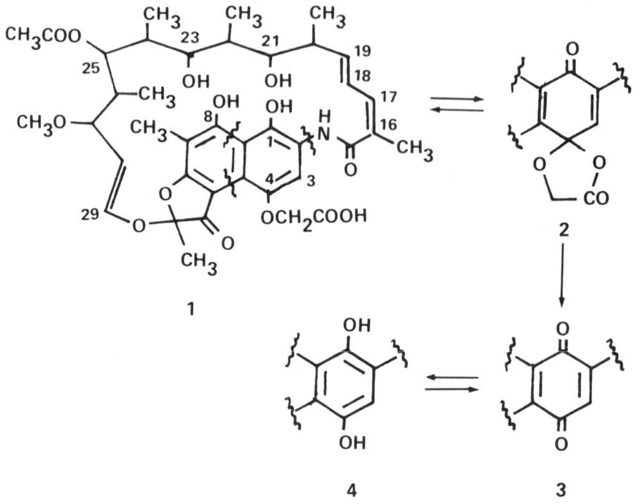

Figure 1.   Structure of rifamycin B (1), rifamycin O (2), rifamycin S (3), and rifamycin SV (4).

Rifamycins were the first natural compounds to be assigned an ansa structure with an aromatic moiety spanned by an aliphatic bridge. Now several natural products with ansa structures are known (Table 1). Some are metabolites of microorganisms of the order *Actinomycetales,* for which Prelog suggested the general name of "ansamycins." Others have been isolated from higher plants. It is noteworthy that all ansa compound so far described possess interesting biological properties, but only members of the rifamycin family have been introduced into therapeutic use.

6.   CHEMICAL MODIFICATIONS OF RIFAMYCINS LEADING TO RIFAMPICIN

The elucidation of the complete structure of rifamycin B in 1963 gave renewed impetus to the program of chemical modifications of the molecule that had been pursued until then only on the basis of a partial knowledge of the structure. Furthermore, a research agreement between Lepetit and Ciba in the same period opened a fruitful and challenging collaboration for a larger investigation of the many possibilities that the rifamycin field appeared to offer.

Table 1
Natural Ansa Products

Name	Origin	Biological Activities
Rifamycins	*Nocardia mediterranea*	Antibacterial (antiviral) (inhibitors of "reverse transcriptase")
Streptovaricins	*Streptomyces spectabilis*	Antibacterial (antiviral) (inhibitors of "reverse transcriptase")
Tolipomycin Y	*Streptomyces tolypophorus*	Antibacterial
Halomicin B	*Micromonospora halophytica*	Antibacterial
Naphtomycin	*Streptomyces collinus*	Antibacterial
Geldanamycin	*Streptomyces hygroscopicus*	Antiprotozoal
Maytansine	*Maytenus ovatus*	Antileukemic, antitumor
Maytanbutine	*Maytenus buchanii*	Antileukemic, antitumor
Maytanprine	*Maytenus buchanii*	Antileukemic, antitumor
Colubrinol	*Colubrina texensis*	Antileukemic, antitumor
Colubrinol acetate	*Colubrina texensis*	Antileukemic, antitumor
Ansamitocins	*Nocardia sp.* No. C-15003	Antitumor, antifungal
Macbecins	*Nocardia sp.* No. C-14919	Antitumor

Systematic studies of the chemical modifications of rifamycin were planned with the aim of obtaining a new rifamycin presenting the following advantages over rifamycin SV: oral absorption, more prolonged therapeutic blood levels, and higher activity in the treatment of mycobacterial and gram-negative bacterial infection.

As is mentioned earlier, rifamycin SV is partially (although very irregularly) absorbed from the gastrointestinal tract; oral treatment does not give rise to detectable blood levels because the drug is rapidly eliminated in the bile. The rate of biliary excretion of rifamycin SV is the main factor affecting the achievement of therapeutic blood levels after oral administration and the duration of effective blood levels after parenteral administration. The possibility of preparing a new oral rifamycin was thus linked to the probability that modifications of the natural antibiotic molecule, without affecting the *in vitro* activity, would lead to greater absorption in the gastrointestinal tract and to slower biliary elimination compared with rifamycin SV. The possibility of obtaining a new broad spectrum rifamycin was based on the fact that rifamycin SV itself possesses limited but not negligible activity also on gram-negative microorganisms.

Several hundred semisynthetic rifamycin derivatives have been prepared in the effort to obtain substances with improved biological properties over rifamycin SV.[15]

Chemical modifications have been made of the aliphatic ansa, on the glycolic chain and on the chromophoric nucleus of rifamycin B. Some of the most active derivatives are reported in Table 2.

Changes on the aliphatic ansa have generally led to rifamycins with much lower activity than rifamycin SV, with the exception of the 27-0-demethyl and 25-0-deacetyl derivatives, which show antibacterial activity only slightly inferior to that of the parent compounds.

Modifications on the glycolic chain were performed on the basis of the hypothesis that the low activity of rifamycin B could be due to the presence of a free carboxyl group in the molecule. This hypothesis was found to be correct, because most of the amides, hydrazides and esters prepared showed antibacterial activity of the same order as rifamycin SV. The negative influence of the free carboxyl group on the antimicrobial activity of rifamycin was later confirmed in other series of derivatives and is attributed to poor penetration through the bacterial cell wall.[16]

The series of rifamycinamides furnished interesting information relative to the possibility of varying the pharmacokinetic properties and the therapeutic efficacy on oral administration through suitable structural modifications. In fact in a series of homologous amides we observed that the rate of biliary excretion decreases with the length of the alkyl chains and that the oral ED_{50} approaches the subcutaneous dose.[16]

Among the active amides, the diethylamide was found to possess the highest *in vivo* activity and the lowest toxicity and was selected for more extensive studies.[17-19] Although similar to rifamycin SV in antibacterial spectrum, absorption, and elimination, the diethylamide demonstrated an improved therapeutic index, probably because of a better distribution in the tissues. Rifamycin B diethylamide was introduced into therapeutic use in some countries under the name of rifamide, practically with the same therapeutic indications and the same limitations of use as those of rifamycin SV.

Chemical modifications of the chromophoric nucleus of rifamycin S or SV, leaving the aliphatic chain intact, gave several series of derivatives, some of them with improved activity *in vitro* and *in vivo* in comparison to the parent compounds.

Rifamycin derivatives modified at position 4 included a large series of 4-amino rifamycins obtained by condensation of rifamycin 0 with aromatic amines, hydrazides, amidrazones, and aminoguanidines.[20] The *in vitro* activity of many of these derivatives was astonishingly high, for example, in the case of rifamycin AG (see Table 2) reaching MIC as low as 0.001 µg/ml against *S. aureus* and 0.005 µg/ml against *M. tuberculosis*. Unfortunately, their *in vivo* activity was negligible because of their insolubility in water.

Rifamycins substituted at both positions 3 and 4 include the products obtained by condensation of rifamycin S with *o*-phenylenediamines (phenazino{2,3-c}rifamycin SV derivatives)[21] and with *O*-aminophenols (phenoxazino{2,3-c}rifamycin SV derivatives.[22] Many of these derivatives showed very good *in vitro* and *in vivo* activity. Rifazine (Table 2) was studied more extensively because its *in vivo* activity in staphylococcal infections was greatly superior to that of rifamycin SV, in particular, it showed lower toxicity. Oral absorption was confirmed in man. However, studies on rifazine were discontinued for toxicological reasons.

The investigation of rifazine gave the first useful indications as to the possibility of obtaining an orally active rifamycin and confirmed that the blood levels obtained after oral administration were due to modification of the rate of biliary excretion, which in rifazine is much slower than in rifamycin SV and rifamide.

Rifamycin derivatives at position 3 include the 3-thioethers of rifamycin SV,[23] the 3-amino derivatives of rifamycin SV,[22] and the 3-dialkyl aminomethyl derivatives of rifamycin SV.[24] Most of these derivatives were very active both *in vitro* and *in vivo*. In particular, some derivatives of the last two classes showed, on oral administration, *in vivo* activity quite superior to that of rifamycin SV,

Table 2

Examples of the Most Active Semisynthetic Rifamycins in Various Groups of Derivatives Obtained in the Lepetit Laboratories from Rifamycin B

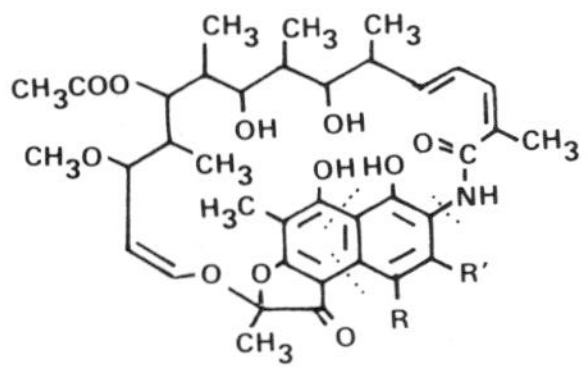

R	R'	Common name or laboratory code	MIC (µg/ml)			ED_{50} S. aureus in mice (mg/kg)	
			S. aureus	E. coli	M. tuberculosis $H_{37}Rv$	O.s.	S.c.
OCH_2COOH	H	Rifamycin B	0.025	1.000	0.005	>500	305
OH	H	Rifamycin SV	0.005	2.5	0.05	74	17
$OCH_2CON(C_2H_5)$	H	Rifamide	0.01	6.2	0.075	21	2.6
$NHNHCNH_2$ $\overset{\parallel}{NH}$	H	Rifamycin AG	0.001	0.75	0.005	>100	>100

	Compound					
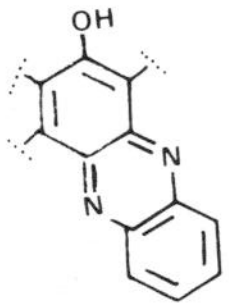 OH	Rifazine	0.005	5.0	0.5	2.7	1.7
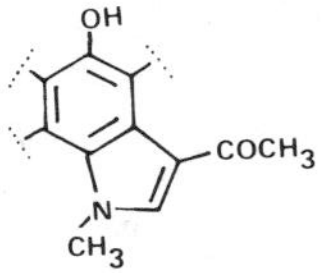 OH	Rifamycin PR/14	0.01	5.0	0.5	1.87	1.74
OH SCH$_2$CH$_2$NH$_2$	Rifamycin PF/48	0.005	5.0	0.5	32	5.7
OH CH$_2$N(CH$_3$)$_2$	Rifamycin PF/75	0.015	1.0	0.1	13.9	2.0
OH CHO	Rifamycin AF	0.002	2.0	0.1	4.6	2.46
OH CH=N—N(CH$_3$)$_2$	Rifamycin AF/DMI	0.001	5.0	0.05	0.30	0.26
OH CH=NOC$_2$H$_5$	Rifamycin AF/EO	0.005	5.0	0.1	0.87	0.76
OH CH=N—N[piperazine]NCH$_3$	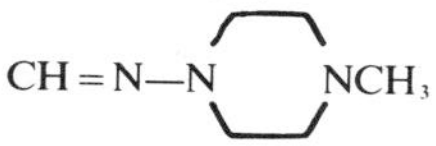 Rifamyin AF/AMP, Rifampicin, Rifampin, USAN	0.005	1.0	0.5	0.12	0.11

211

but experiments in man with 3-dimethylaminomethyl rifamycin SV (PF/75, Table 2) yielded results that were unsatisfactory with respect to the constancy of the blood levels.

The studies on the dialkylaminomethyl derivatives revealed their instability in the presence of oxidizing agents. One of the degradation products, rifamycin AF, separated from the others in minute amounts by thin layer chromatography, showed high antibacterial activity, but for some time the formation and isolation of the compound represented a very difficult problem. After various attempts, the proper oxidation conditions were found and the product turned out to be the 3-formylrifamycin SV. Rifamycin AF opened the way to the preparation of a large series of derivatives, including imines, hydrazones, oximes, and hydrazide-hydrazones.[25,26]

All these derivatives showed high antibacterial activity, and the majority of the N,N-disubstituted hydrazones and some oximes presented exceptionally high in vivo activity on staphylococcal infections in mice, with the oral and subcutaneous ED_{50} values almost equal (Table 2). The most active derivative was the hydrazone of 3-formylrifamycin SV with N-amino-N'-methylpiperazine, initially coded as rifamycin AF/AMP, and later rifampicin (rifampin USAN).

Considering that some other derivatives also exhibited good oral activity in experimental infections, although slightly inferior to that of rifampicin, experiments on oral absorption in man were performed on a selected group of compounds which had passed 2 week toxicity studies. It is worthy of mention that in Italy at that time there were no formal IND procedures and experiments for the selection of the product giving the highest blood levels in man after oral administration, which in fact turned out to be rifampicin, were performed in a period of a couple of months. Needless to say, the same experiments now, in the same country, with the present lengthy, time-consuming procedures for the approval of experiments in man, would require an unpredictable time, probably of the order of a couple of years. This comment is a criticism not of the control by the health authorities on experiments in man, but on the way it is sometimes exercised.

All the results obtained in the preliminary studies indicated that rifampicin possessed most of the properties sought in the program of chemical modification of rifamycins. In the course of the years since the synthesis of rifampicin, many other rifamycin derivatives have been prepared, for example, other oximes, hydrazones, semicarbazones and dimeric hydrazones of 3-formyl rifamycin SV, and pyrrolo(2,3-c)rifamycins. In some cases these were prepared in the search for a potential activity outside the antibacterial area (antiviral, antitumor).[27,33]

Until now no other rifamycin has shown an oral ED_{50} in the staphylococcal infection in mice lower than that of rifampicin. However, recently the hydrazone of 3-formylrifamycin SV with N-amino-N'-cyclopentylpiperazine (rifamycin AF/ACPP, DL 473) has been selected for clinical investigation in consideration of its activity on mycobacteria and its pharmacokinetic properties.[34,35]

Besides the studies on chemical modification of rifamycin B and congeners, extensive studies have been done for the isolation of other natural rifamycins from the original strain of *N. mediterranea* or from its mutants, yielding 37-demethylrifamycins, rifamycin W, rifamycins P, Q, and R.[36] Rifamycin P is the most active natural rifamycin so far isolated.

7. STRUCTURE-ANTIBACTERIAL ACTIVITY RELATIONSHIPS IN THE RIFAMYCINS

By making use of the large range of semisynthetic rifamycins available, it has been possible to identify clear relationships between structural features and antibacterial activity.[15,37-40]

With the exception of rifamycins possessing a free carboxy group, which do not enter the bacterial cell, the minimal requirements for antibacterial activity in the other rifamycins appear to be the presence of two free hydroxyls in positions 21 and 23 on the ansa chain and two polar groups (either free hydroxyl or carbonyl) at positions 1 and 8 of the aromatic nucleus, together with a conformation of the ansa chain that results in certain specific geometrical relationships among these four functional groups, as indicated in the molecular model of rifamycin S based on X-ray crystallographic analysis (Figure 2). The conformation of the rifamycin molecule in solution has been proved to be the same as that in the crystal state.[41]

The minimal requirements for antibacterial activity were determined from the following data:

1. Substitution or elimination of the 21- or 23-hydroxyls gives inactive products.
2. Modifications of the ansa chain that alter its conformation (e.g., 16-17 and 18-19-mono and diepoxy derivatives) give inactive or less active products. Also, the stepwise hydrogenation of the ansa chain double bonds results in a gradual decrease in activity as a consequence of the increase in flexibility of the ansa diverging from the most active conformation.
3. The oxygenated function at carbons 1 and 8 must be either free hydroxyl or carbonyl for maintaining the biological activity.
4. All modifications at the 3(4)-positions that do not interfere with the previous requirements do not affect the activity of the products.

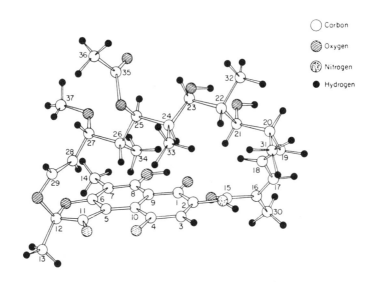

○ Carbon
◉ Oxygen
⊛ Nitrogen
● Hydrogen

Figure 2. Stereo model of rifamycin S according to X-rays (from Reference 41).

The nature of the substituents at the 3(4)-positions influences the physico-chemical properties of the derivatives, especially lipophilicity. The various derivatives show a minor degree of variation in antibacterial activity against intact cells, because transport through bacterial wall and membrane is the major factor affected by these substituents. Other biological characteristics influenced by the various modifications at the 3(4)-positions are absorption from the gastrointestinal tract and kinetics of biliary elimination.

8. MECHANISM OF ACTION

Just at the time when rifampicin was first introduced into clinical use, it was discovered that the rifamycins act on the sensitive bacteria by inhibiting specifically the enzyme DNA-directed RNA polymerase (DDRP).[42,43] Most rifamycins, including those in clinical use, are not effective on the mammalian RNA polymerase. Therefore, they possess the necessary requisite for ideal chemotherapeutic agents, that is, a selective toxicity against pathogens. Detailed studies on the mechanism of action of rifamycins revealed that they inhibit the initiation of RNA synthesis, inactivating the enzyme before the incorporation of the first purine nucleotide of the RNA chain. Rifamycins form a rather stable complex, with the bacterial DDRP, by binding with the β subunit of the enzyme, but no covalent linkages are involved. Probably the oxygens at positions 1, 8, 21, and 23 form hydrogen bonds with functional groups of the enzyme. Bacterial mutants resistant to rifamycins possess an altered RNA-polymerase that is not inhibited by rifamycins.

The discovery of the inhibitory effect of rifamycins on the bacterial DDRP gave rise to the hope that structural modifications of the rifamycin molecule could yield products with an inhibitory effect on other RNA or DNA polymerizing enzymes, such as the DDRP of resistant bacteria, the DDRP of cytoplasmic DNA viruses, and the RNA-directed DNA polymerase (RDDP, reverse transcriptase) of oncogenic RNA viruses. Preliminary results stimulated intensive chemical studies with the aim of obtaining rifamycin derivatives active as antiviral or antitumor agents.[44-46] Unfortunately, most of the rifamycins with some inhibitory effect on the indicated target enzymes also present a broad spectrum of activity against nucleotide polymerases and therefore poor selectivity. Several reviews on the mechanism of action and on the various effects of rifamycins at subcellular level have been published.[37,47-49]

9. RIFAMPICIN, TODAY
In the 12 years since the first introduction into therapeutic use of rifampicin, a large amount of information has been accumulated on the biological and clinical properties of this antibiotic. More than 5000 papers on this subject have been published. Two extensive reviews on the activity and the clinical applications of rifampicin are available.[50,51]

The data concerning its antibacterial activity shown in Table 3 represent a summary of the results obtained in many laboratories. Rifampicin has a very high activity against gram-positive bacteria, some gram-negative bacteria (*Neisseria, Haemophilus*), anaerobes (*Clostridia, Bacteroides fragilis*), *Mycobacteria,* and *Chlamidia.* The activity against other gram-negative bacteria is also of therapeutic interest. The effect of rifampicin is bactericidal. The mutation rate from sensitivity to resistance is of the order of 10^{-8} or lower for *S. aureus* and *E. coli*. The frequency of resistant mutants in sensitive bacterial populations is somewhat higher, of the order of 10^{-7}. No transferable resistance has been observed so far. There is no cross resistance with the other antibiotics or chemotherapeutic agents in clinical use, with the exception of rifamycin SV and rifamide.

The *in vivo* activity of rifampicin in various experimental infections with gram-positive, gram-negative, and mycobacteria is still the basis for the rational use in the therapy of human infections because of microorganisms sensitive to it.[52] In particular, the excellent antitubercular activity has been confirmed by many investigators, using various animal models, schedules of treatment, and criteria of evaluation. The overall results indicate that rifampicin has a high bactericidal effect and a therapeutic efficacy of the order of that of isoniazid

Table 3
In Vitro Antibacterial Activity of Rifampin

Microorganism	No. tested strains	MIC (g/ml)
Staphylococcus aureus	1744	0.001-0.1
Staphylococcus epidermidis	52	0.001-0.1
Streptococcus pneumoniae	175	0.001-1.0
Streptococcus pyogenes	383	0.001-0.1
Corynebacterium diphtheriae	114	0.001-0.1
Clostridium perfrigens	75	0.001-0.1
Pseudomonas aeruginosa	439	1-20
Escherichia coli	589	1-10
Klebsiella pneumoniae	43	5-50
Proteus vulgaris	50	1-10
Salmonella tiphi	54	1-10
Shigella spp.	218	5-10
Brucella melitensis	33	0.1-5
Haemophilus influenzae	230	0.1-1.0
Neisseria gonorrhoeae	531	0.001-0.1
Neisseria meningitidis	103	0.001-1.0
Bacteroides fragilis	515	0.1-1.0
Legionella pneumophila		0.3
Mycobacterium tuberculosis	1000	0.1-1.0
Mycobacterium leprae		0.1-0.5
Atypical mycobacteria: Group I	76	0.1-1.0 (90%)
Group II	32	0.1-1.0 (80%)
Group III	80	0.1-1.0 (40%)
Group IV	90	0.1-1.0 (30%)
Chlamidia trachomatis		0.007

and superior to all the other antitubercular drugs. The combination of rifampicin with isoniazid has been shown to produce a more rapid, complete, and durable sterilization of infected animals than any other combination.[53]

Rifampicin is excreted in bile and urine in a ratio related to the administered dose. The main metabolite is the 25-O-desacetylrifampicin, which shows antibacterial activity slightly inferior to that of rifampicin.[58]

The principal clinical application of rifampicin is the treatment of tuberculosis in combination with other antibacterial drugs. During the last years several combinations and different regimens have been investigated in carefully controlled clinical trials and evaluated in terms of length of treatment, efficacy at the end of treatment, and number of relapses after discontinuation of treatment. There is no doubt that the most successful regimens for a short-course treatment of tuberculosis include both rifampicin and isoniazid.[59-63] In fact, while the treatments based on the isoniazid-streptomycin combination, with the addition of a third drug, must be continued for 12-18 months to minimize or avoid failures during the treatment and relapses after its discontinuation, the combination of rifampicin plus isoniazid with the addition of a third drug in the first two months yields the same or better results in 6-9 months. In addition, the treatment with rifampicin-isoniazid combination leads to sputum conversion in a time shorter than any other combination.

Rifampicin has shown a very low incidence of adverse reactions when administered daily.[64] In addition, the risk of liver toxicity is very low in patients with no previous history of liver disease. A high incidence of severe untoward effects of immunological nature have been observed only in the intermittent therapy of tuberculosis; with proper adjustment of the sizes of each single dose, the interval between doses, and the length of treatment, it has been possible to reduce this incidence.

Rifampicin is also in clinical use for the treatment of leprosy with very good results because of its high and rapid bactericidal effect on *Mycobacterium leprae*.[65-68]

Beside the mycobacterial infections, rifampicin has been found effective in a variety of disease caused by sensitive bacteria (e.g., staphylococcal infections, respiratory tract infections, Legionnaires' disease, gonorrhoea, brucellosis, chlamidial infections). The increasing use of rifampicin in these diseases is often related to the results found in the bacteriological laboratories indicating the high activity of rifampicin on a variety of pathogenic bacteria.[69-72]

Because rifampicin is a drug of great value in the treatment of mycobacterial infections, its use for other infections has been questioned in view of the potential risk of development of widespread rifampicin-resistant *M. tuberculosis*. However, it has been recently demonstrated that this risk is virtually nonexistent. In fact a survey on primary resistance of *M. tuberculosis* to rifampicin comparing countries where the use of the antibiotic is restricted to tuberculosis to those where it is also freely available for the treatment of nontubercular infections indicates that *M. tuberculosis* has remained uniformly sensitive to rifampicin after several years of use in both groups of countries.[73]

One of the disadvantages of the use of rifampicin in severe infections sustained by a large population of pathogens is the selection of one-step mutants with a high level of resistance.[74] To exploit the high bactericidal effect of rifampicin and eliminate the resistant mutants, it has been used with success in combination with other chemotherapeutic agents.[75] In particular, the combination of rifampicin and trimethoprim is synergistic against a wide range of microorganisms and appears very promising for the treatment of severe urinary tract infections.[76-80]

10. PERSPECTIVES OF RESEARCH ON RIFAMYCINS

The chemotherapeutic efficacy of rifampicin in the tubercular infections, although extensively investigated and to a large extent defined, requires further studies for the optimal use of this antibiotic, especially in developing countries. Rifampicin is now and will remain in the near future one of the most expensive antitubercular drugs because of the complicated technology involved in its production (fermentation plus several chemical steps). The short course chemotherapy of tuberculosis, where rifampicin plays a primary role, appears a very good answer in terms of cost/benefit ratio for a rational treatment of the disease and should be used in developing countries with the necessary adjustments of the proposed regimens taking into account the socioeconomic, epidemiological and medical situation of each country.

The current interest in the use of rifampicin in the therapy of leprosy is due to the high and rapid bactericidal effect of rifampicin against *M. leprae*. In fact, it has been established that a single 1500 mg dose of rifampicin accomplishes as much bacterial killing as dapsone monotherapy for several months. Long-term studies are now under way to define the best treatment schedules and companion drugs that eliminate or minimize resistance and persistence problems.

Although there is already a large body of evidence for the efficacy of rifampicin, alone or in combination with other antimicrobial drugs, in the treatment of a variety of nonmycobacterial infections, the chemotherapeutic role of this antibiotic in the treatment of certain diseases due to sensitive microorganisms still requires further investigation. Also, for the use of the combination of rifampicin with trimethoprim in severe urinary tract infections, additional data are necessary to convince opponents of fixed combinations.

A new area of investigation concerns the effect of rifampicin in the treatment of cutaneous leishmaniasis. The first favorable clinical reports[81,82] need confirmation on laboratory models and controlled clinical trials. Also, the combination of amphotericin B and rifampicin that was found to be synergistic against *Histoplasma capsulatum* and *Blastomyces dermatitidis* infections in mice[83] should be critically tested in human systemic infections with the aim of using low, nontoxic doses of amphotericin B for the treatment of these severe infections.

In addition to these studies, which will provide more information on the proper use of rifampicin, further research is under way in our laboratories on new natural and semisynthetic rifamycins. The extensive knowledge of the structure-antibacterial activity relationships in the rifamycins is the basis for the design of new derivatives with potential therapeutic advantages over rifampicin in the treatment of bacterial infections. The hydrazone of 3-formylrifamycin SV with N-amino-N'-cyclopentylpiperazine (rifamycin AF/ACPP, DL 473) has been prepared in the frame of a research program on rifamycins with more lipophilic side chains and, as a potential consequence, with a half-life in the blood longer than that of rifampicin. The selected product could hopefully show some practical advantage in the intermittent therapeutic regimens of tuberculosis and leprosy and, in view of its improved distribution in the tissues, also in the treatment of some nonmycobacterial infections.

The mechanism of inhibitory effect of some rifamycins on viruses, on reverse transcriptase, on cell transformation, and on growth *in vitro* of tumor cells is far from understood. Although the rifamycins that show one or more of these effects have not yet found practical application, some recent data on rifamycin SV concerning its clinical efficacy in the treatment of *Herpes zoster*[84,85] and in the intra-articular treatment of rheumatoid sinovities[86] indicate that the potential usefulness of rifamycins in nonbacterial diseases should be reevaluated. Studies on the already known and on new semisynthetic or biosynthetic rifamycins are in progress to clarify the more intriguing aspects of the biological activity of thse compounds. This research field is still open to unpredictable developments.

REFERENCES

1. P. Sensi, P. Margalith, and M. T. Timbal, *Farmaco, Ed. Sci.,* **14**, 146 (1959).
2. P. Margalith and G. Beretta, *Mycopathol. Mycol. Appl.,* **8**, 321 (1960).
3. J. E. Thiemann, G. Zucco, and G. Pelizza, *Arch. Microbiol.,* **67**, 147 (1969).
4. P. Sensi, R. Ballotta, and G. G. Gallo, *Antibiot. Chemother.,* **9**, 76 (1959).
5. P. Sensi, A. M. Greco, and R. Ballotta, *Antibiot. Ann.,* 262 (1959).
6. P. Margalith and H. Pagani, *Appl. Microbiol.,* **9**, 325 (1961).
7. S. Furesz and M. T. Timbal, *Chemotherapia,* **7**, 200 (1963).
8. P. Sensi, R. Ballotta, A. M. Greco, and G. G. Gallo, *Farmaco, Ed. Sci.,* **16**, 165 (1961).
9. P. Sensi, M. T. Timbal, and G. Maffii, *Experientia,* **16**, 412 (1960).
10. M. T. Timbal, R. Pallanza, and G. Carniti, *Farmaco, Ed. Sci.,* **16**, 181 (1961).
11. M. Bergamini and G. Fowst, *Arzneim.-Forsch.,* **15**, 951 (1965).
12. W. Oppolzer, V. Prelog, and P. Sensi, *Experientia,* **20**, 336 (1964).
13. M. Brufani, W. Fedeli, G. Giacomello, and A. Vaciago, *Experientia,* **23**, 508 (1967).
14. J. Leitich, W. Oppolzer, and V. Prelog, *Experientia,* **20**, 343 (1964).
15. P. Sensi, N. Maggi, S. Furesz, and G. Maffii, *Antimicrob. Agents Chemother.,* **1966**, 699 (1967).

16. N. Maggi, S. Furesz, and P. Sensi, *J. Med. Chem.*, **11**, 368 (1968).
17. P. Sensi, N. Maggi, R. Ballotta, S. Furesz, R. Pallanza, and V. Arioli, *J. Med. Chem.*, **7**, 596 (1964).
18. R. Pallanza, S. Furesz, M. T. Timbal, and G. Carniti, *Arzneim.-Forsch.*, **15**, 800(1965).
19. S. Furesz, V. Arioli, and R. Scotti, *Arzneim.-Forsch.*, **15**, 802 (1965).
20. P. Sensi, M. T. Timbal, and A. M. Greco, *Antibiot. Chemother.*, **12**, 488 (1962).
21. G. G. Gallo, C. R. Pasqualucci, N. Maggi, R. Ballotta, and P. Sensi, *Farmaco, Ed. Sci.*, **21**, 68 (1966).
22. H. Bickel, F. Knusel, W. Kump and L. Neipp, *Antimicrob. Agents Chemother.*, **1966** 352.
23. N. Maggi and R. Pallanza, *Farmaco, Ed. Sci.*, **22**, 307 (1967).
24. N. Maggi, V. Arioli, and P. Sensi, *J. Med. Chem.*, **8**, 790 (1965).
25. N. Maggi, R. Pallanza, and P. Sensi, *Antimicrob. Agents Chemother. 1965*, **1966**, 756.
26. S. Furesz, V. Arioli, and R. Pallanza, *Antimicrob. Agents Chemother. 1965*, **1966**, 770.
27. R. Cricchio, G. C. Lancini, G. Tamborini, and P. Sensi, *J. Med. Chem.*, **17**, 396 (1974).
28. R. Cricchio, G. Cietto, E. Rossi, and V. Arioli, *Farmaco, Ed. Sci.*, **30**, 695 (1975).
29. R. Cricchio, G. Carniti, G. Cietto, G. Tamborini, and V. Arioli, *Farmaco, Ed. Sci.*, **30**, 704 (1975).
30. R. Cricchio, V. Arioli, and G. C. Lancini, *Farmaco, Ed. Sci.*, **30**, 605 (1975).
31. N. Maggi, V. Arioli, and G. Tamborini, *Farmaco, Ed. Sci.*, **24**, 263 (1969).
32. A. N. Tischlr, U. R. Joss, F. M. Thompson, and M. Calvin, *J. Med. Chem.*, **16**, 1071 (1973).
33. R. Cricchio, *Farmaco, Ed. Sci.*, **31**, 791 (1976).
34. S. R. Pattyn and E. J. Saerens, *Ann. Soc. Belge Med. Trop.*, **57**, 169 (1977).
35. A. T. Birmingham, A. J. Coleman, M. Le Orme, B. K. Park, A. H. Short, and P. J. Southgate, *Br. J. Clin. Pharmacol.*, **6**, 455 (1978).
36. R. J. White, G. C. Lancini, and P. Sensi, *Proc. Int. Congr. IAMS, 3*, 483 (1974).
37. P. Sensi, *Pure Appl. Chem.*, **35**, 383 (1973).
38. G. Lancini and W. Zanichelli, in Structure-Activity Relationship Among the Semisynthetic Antibiotics, D. Perlam, Ed., Academic Press, New York, 1977, p. 531.
39. W. Wehli and M. Staehelin, *Biochim. Biophys. Acta*, **182**, 24 (1969).
40. M. Brufani, S. Cerrini, W. Fedeli, and A. Vaciago, *J. Mol. Biol.*, **78**, 409 (1974).
41. G. G. Gallo, E. Martinelli, V. Pagani, and P. Sensi, *Tetrahedron*, **30**, 3093 (1974).
42. G. R. Hartmann, K. O. Honikel, F. Knusel, and J. Nuesch, *Biochim. Biophys. Acta*, **145**, 843 (1967).
43. H. Umezawa, S. Mizuno, H. Yamasaky, and K. Nitta, *J. Antibiot.*, **21**, 234 (1968).
44. E. Heller, M. Agrman, H. Levy, and M. Goldblum, *Nature*, **222**, 273 (1969).
45. J. H. Subak-Sharpe, M. C. Timbury, and J. F. Williams, *Nature*, **222**, 341 (1969).
46. C. Gurgo, R. K. Ray, L. Thiry, and M. Green, *Nature*, **229**, 111 (1971).
47. S. Riva and L. G. Silvestri, *Ann. Rev. Microbiol.*, **26**, 199 (1972).
48. W. Wehrli and M. Staehelin, *Bactiol. Rev.*, **35**, 290 (1971).
49. C. Gurgo, *Pharmacol. Ther.*, **2**, 139 (1977).
50. G. Binda, E. Domenichini, A. Gottardi, B. Orlandi, E. Ortelli, B. Pacini, and G. Fowst, *Arzneim.-Forsch.*, **21**, 1907 (1971).
51. A. Blasi, L. Donatelli, and C. Zanussi, Eds., *Rifampicina*, Minerva Medica, 1978.
52. R. Pallanza, V. Arioli, S. Furesz, and G. Bolzoni, *Arzneim.-Forsch.*, **17**, 529 (1967).
53. F. Grumbach, G. Canetti, and M. Le Lirzin, *Rev. Tuberc. Pneumol., (Paris)*, **34**, 312 (1970).
54. S. Furesz, *Antibiot. Chemoter. (Basel)*, **16**, 316 (1970).
55. G. L. Mandell, *J. Clin. Invest.*, **52**, 1673 (1973).
56. G. L. Mandell and T. K. Vest, *J. Infect. Dis.*, **125**, 486 (1972).

57. C. S. F. Easman, *Br. J. Exp. Pathol.,* **60,** 24 (1979).
58. N. Maggi, S. Furesz, R. Pallanza, and G. Pelizza, *Arzneim.-Forsch.,* **19,** 651 (1969).
59. G. Brouet, *Bull. Union Int. Tuberc.,* **49,** 1 (1974).
60. British Thoracic and Tuberculosis Association, *Lancet,* **2,** 1102 (1976).
61. W. Fox and D. A. Mitchison, *Am. Rev. Respir. Dis.,* **111,** 325 (1975).
62. W. Fox, *Proc. Roy. Soc. Med.,* **70,** 4 (1977).
63. A. K. Dutt, L. Jones, and W. W. Stead, *Chest,* **75,** 441 (1979).
64. D. J. Girling and K. L. Hitze, *Bull. W.H.O.,* **57 (1),** 45 (1979).
65. R. J. Rees, J. M. Pearson, and M. F. R. Waters, *Br. Med. J.,* **1,** 89 (1970).
66. C. C. Shepard, L. L. Walker, R. M. Van Landingham, and M. A. Redus, *Am. J. Trop. Med. Hyg.,* **20,** 616 (1971).
67. S. R. Pattyn, *Int. J. Lepr.,* **41,** 489 (1973).
68. W.H.O. Expert Committee on Leprosy, 5th Report, W.H.O. Technical Report Series, No. 607, 1977.
69. L. D. Sabath, C. Garner, C. Wilcox, and M. Finland, *Antimicrob. Agents Chemother.,* **9,** 962 (1976).
70. M. Finland, C. Gardner, C. Wilcox, and L. D. Sabath, *Antimicrob. Agents Chemother.,* **9,** 274 (1976).
71. M. Finland, C. Gardner, C. Wilcox, and L. D. Sabath, *J. Infect. Dis.,* **134,** S 75 (1976).
72. J. M. T. Hamilton-Miller, *J. Antimicrob. Chemother.,* **1,** 273 (1975).
73. G. Acocella, J. M. T. Hamilton-Miller, and M. Brumfitt, *Lancet,* **1,** 740 (1977).
74. W. R. McCabe and V. Lorian, *Am. J. Med. Sci.,* **256,** 255 (1968).
75. G. L. Archer, M. J. Tenenbaum, and H. B. Waywood, *J.A.M.A.,* **240,** 751 (1978).
76. D. W. Kerry, J. M. T. Hamilton-Miller, and W. Brumfitt, *J. Antimicrob. Chemother.,* **1,** 417 (1975).
77. G. Acocella and R. Scotti, *J. Antimicrob. Chemother.,* **2,** 271 (1976).
78. J. M. T. Hamilton-Miller and W. Brumfitt, *J. Antimicrob. Chemother.,* **2,** 181 (1976).
79. V. Arioli, M. Berti, G. Carniti, E. Rossi, and L. G. Silvestri, *J. Antimicrob. Chemother.,* **3,** 87 (1977).
80. R. N. Grüneberg and A. M. Emerson, *J. Antimicrob. Chemother.,* **3,** 453 (1977).
81. M. Selim and E. Kandil, *J. Kwt. Med. Assoc.,* **6,** 159 (1972).
82. O. Iskandar, *J. Int. Med. Res.,* **6,** 280 (1978).
83. M. Kitahara, G. S. Kobayashi, and G. Medoff, *J. Infect. Dis.,* **133,** 663 (1976).
84. P. Franceschini, *Gazette Med. Fr.,* **82,** 4051 (1975).
85. L. Bruni, A. Califano, G. DeAngelis, A. Montagnani, M. Pisani, G. Pezzarossa, G. Pozzo, D. Reali, A. Rebora, and A. Zanca, *J. Int. Med. Res.,* **1,** 1 (1980).
86. I. Caruso and F. Montrone, Abstracts, 9th European Congress on Pneumatology, Wiesbaden, Sept. 2-8, 1979, Abstr. No. 684.

Cefoxitin

10

B.G. Christensen

1. INTRODUCTION

The advent of antibacterial chemotherapy during the past several decades has spearheaded the successful use of modern drugs to treat disease. Many different classes of antibiotics, synthetics, and semisynthetic derivatives have been discovered or invented during this interval and several types of antiinfectives have found their way into clinical practice. Indeed, virtually all known pathogens are susceptible to at least one of these agents. However, not all infections can be cured because of a variety of physiological, pharmacokinetic, or other factors. More importantly, the emergence of drug-resistant organisms frequently is a major reason for the lack of effectiveness of these antibacterials.

Although several reasons, including alteration of permeability or binding characteristics of the agents, may be cited for the development of drug-resistant strains, microbial inactivation is the most studied, if not the most prevalent, cause. Because of this fundamental knowledge available to the medicinal chemist, the design[1] of drugs that resist microbial inactivation has been one of the most successful chapters in the history of modern medicinal chemistry.

At the inception of the work that led to the discovery of cefoxitin (1),[2] useful β-lactam antibiotics were, with few exceptions, semisynthetic derivatives of

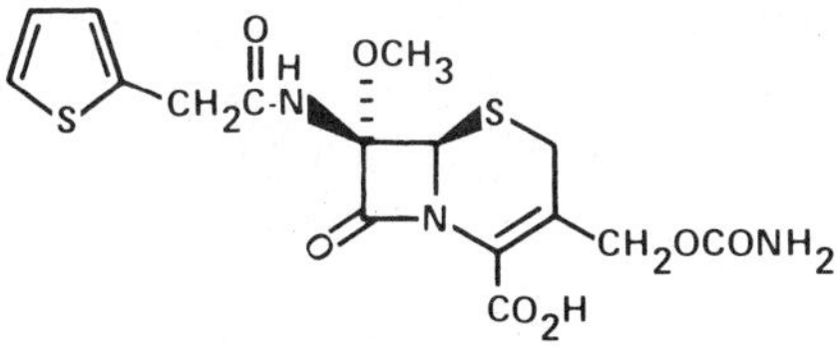

1

223

6-aminopenicillanic acid (6-APA) or 7-aminocephalosporanic acid (7-ACA). As such they could be classified as penicillins 2 or cephalosporins 3. Medicinal chemists throughout the world had made thousands of semisynthetic 6^7 amide derivatives in which the free amine had been functionalized with various acyl groups. Indeed, such acylation was the basis for the very successful modification[3] of the basic properties of these β-lactam nuclei.

A major reason for lack of susceptibility of organisms to existing β-lactam antibiotics is the existence of a group of enzymes called β-lactamases.[4] Although classified together, β-lactamases are a family of diverse enzymes of several basic types.[5] However, all inactivate the parent antibiotic by hydrolysis of the β-lactam functionality, generating biologically inactive products and thus protecting the organism that produces these enzymes from the bactericidal action of those agents. Although one strategy for the chemotherapy of β-lactamase producing organisms might be the concomitant administration of a β-lactamase inhibitor,[6] the diversity of these enzymes and the difficulties attendant on delivering two different drugs in optimal concentration to the same site and at the same time *in vivo*, as well as the difficulties in obtaining registration of fixed ratio drug systems, made a simpler alternative even more attractive. In principle, it should be possible to design a β-lactam antibiotic resistant to the various β-lactamases.

The commercial production of 6-APA[7] made possible the synthesis of 6-acylated penicillins. Of particular interest was the observation that penicillins with a sterically hindered side chain are resistant to hydrolysis by penicillinases. Methicillin,[8] oxacillin[9] and its halogenated derivatives, diphenicillin,[10] quinicillin,[11] and nafcillin[12] are examples of penicillins resistant to destruction by bacterial β-lactamases, especially staphylococcal penicillinase.

With the discovery of cephalosporin C,[13] its commercial conversion to 7-ACA,[14] and its subsequent acylation,[15] a family of cephalosporins of varying spectrum, oral absorption, and pharmacodynamic properties have been synthesized. However, one of the most important properties of the cephalosporins is their natural resistance to the staphylococcal enzymes. In addition to 7-acyl variations, displacement of the C-3' acetoxy function by nucleophiles, and

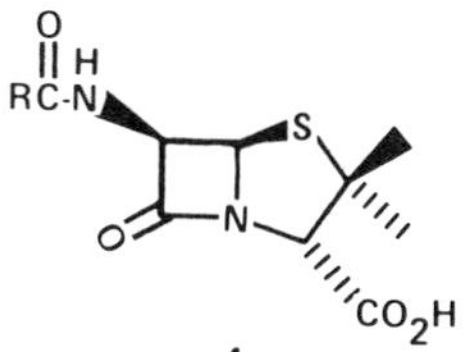

R =

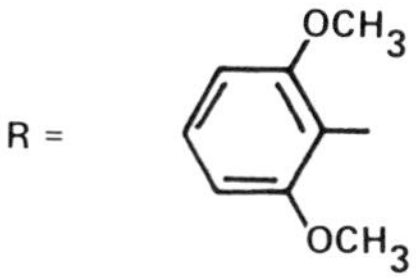

4a Methicillin

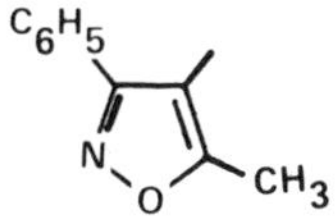

4b Oxacillin

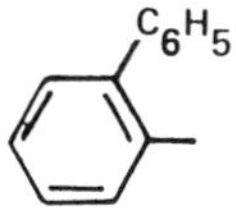

4c Diphenicillin

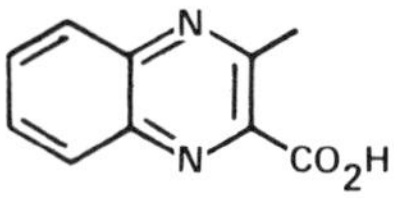

4d Quinicillin

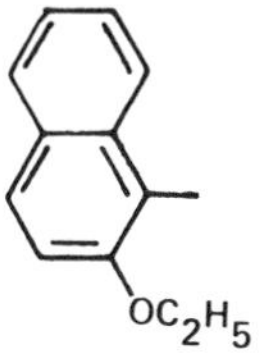

4e Nafcillin

4

particularly heterocyclic thiols, has led to additional semisynthetic variants of the cephalosporin family. However, until the very recent advent of cefuroxime[16] and cefotaxime,[17] none of these new cephalosporins had appreciably different stability to β-lactamases, especially those from gram-negative organisms.

2. THE CEPHAMYCINS

The cephamycins are a new family of β-lactam antibiotics, first reported in 1972.[18,19] All are structurally characterized as 7α-methoxycephems. All have the D-aminoadipoyl side chain at C_7, as does cephalosporin C, but the

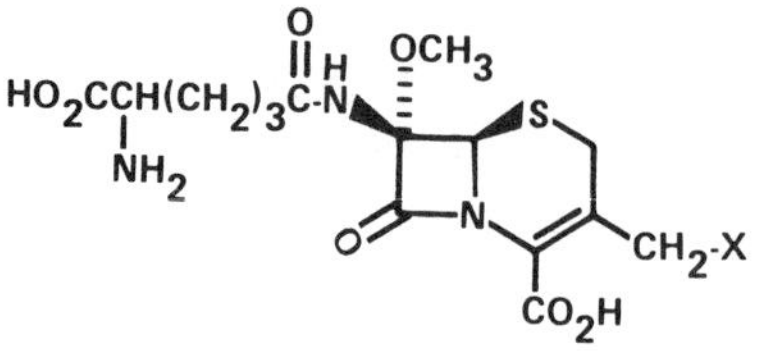

O
H
OCH3
HO2CCH(CH2)3C-N
S
NH2
N
O
CH2-X
CO2H

5

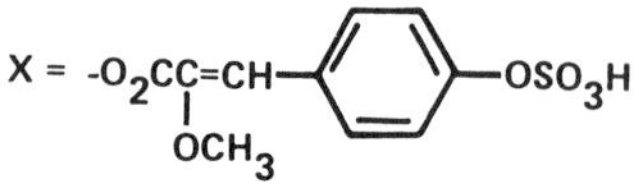

X = -O2CC=CH
OCH3
OSO3H

5a Cephamycin A

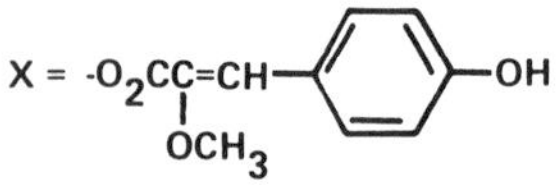

X = -O2CC=CH
OCH3
OH

5b Cephamycin B

X = $-O_2CNH_2$

5c Cephamycin C

X = -OAc

5d

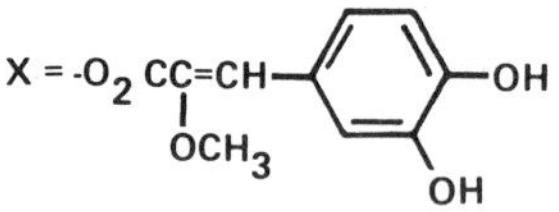

X = -O2 CC=CH
OCH3
OH
OH

5e C-2801X

cephamycins differ because of variations at C_3.[20] Because all are isolated from *Streptomyces,* this group has been called the cephamycins, recognizing their biological origin, as well as the common 3-cephem nucleus. Subsequently, **5e** has been isolated.[21]

Cephamycin C (**5c**) is the most important and best studied member of this series. Its *in vitro* spectrum[22] was qualitatively similar to cephalosporin C — poor gram-positive activity, but good gram-negative activity except for pseudomonal strains. However, cephamycin C showed activity against several gram-negative strains, especially *E. coli* and *proteus,* that were not susceptible to the cephalosporins. The reason for this activity was determined to be the stability to β-lactamases exhibited by cephamycin C as exemplified by the *E. cloacae* enzyme[23] (Table 1).

Table 1
Stability of Cephamycin C to *E. cloacae* β-Lactamase

Compound	V_{max} (x 10^{-3} μmol/min/mg protein)	K_m (x 10^{-2} μmol)
Cephamycin C (5c)	3.3	2.4
Cephalosporin C	200	14.3

It appeared reasonable to assume that enhanced gram-positive activity could be incorporated into a modification of cephamycin C by analogy to the increase in gram-positive activity in going from cephalosporin C to cephalothin.[24] If this could be achieved, a semisynthetic derivative of cephamycin C, with stability to clinically important β-lactamases, appeared to be a real possibility.

3. CHEMISTRY OF $C_{6(7)}$-SUBSTITUTED PENICILLINS AND CEPHALOSPORINS

Direct application of literature methods[25] to cleave the aminoadipoyl side chain of cephamycin C did not lead to the expected products. Presumably this is due to the instability of **6** under the acidic conditions employed, for example, nitrous acid/trifluoroacetic acid or phosphorous pentachloride. Because of the unsuitability of literature methods of cleavage, new chemical procedures for the synthesis of **6** were necessary.

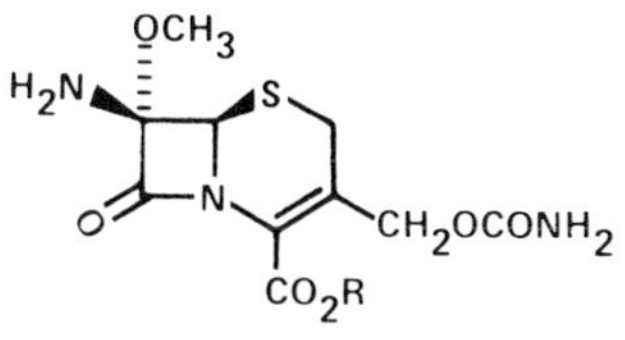

6

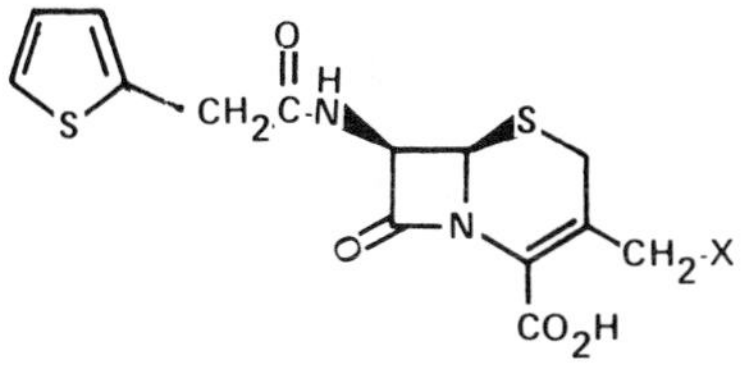

7a X = OCONH$_2$
7b X = OAc
7c X = OH

Second, it became necessary to determine which of the two novel functionalities in cephamycin C was responsible for the β-lactamase stability. Although the C_3 carbamoyloxymethyl seemed a less likely candidate on an intuitive basis, the chemistry seemed more amenable to solution. Accordingly, the synthesis of O-carbamoyldeacetylcephalothin (**7a**) was initiated. Deacetylcephalothin was a known entity and direct carbamoylation appeared to be the most direct route of synthesis. However, here again literature methods of carbamoylation were unsuccessful mainly because most involved acidic conditions resulting in lactonization. Finally, **7a** was prepared[26] using the method of Graf.[27] Clearly, the carbamoyl function was not responsible for the β-lactamase stability of cephamycin C, since **7a** was >99% destroyed by both *E. coli* and *E. cloacae* β-lactamases.[22] Then a new problem emerged. If, as deduced by elimination, the 7α-methoxyl group of cephamycin C is responsible for its β-lactamase stability, what other groups at this previously unexplored position might also confer β-lactamase stability? Indeed, the question of what effects a methoxy and other groups at the corresponding C_6 position of penicillin would have was also asked. Accordingly, a chemical program to introduce methoxy and other groups at the $C_{6(7)}$ position of penicillin and cephalosporin was launched.

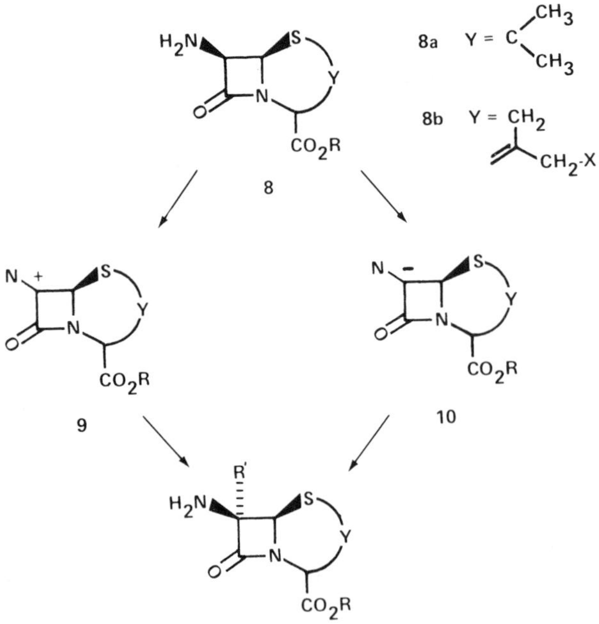

Since both 6-aminopenicillanic acid (**8a**, R = H) and 7-aminocephalosporanic acid (**8b**, R = H, X = OAc) are readily available, the general synthetic strategy for preparing a variety of 6(7)α-R's is shown. Stereocontrol should be attainable by virtue of the stereochemistry at $C_{5(6)}$. Approach from the least hindered side (α) would produce the desired stereochemistry in the product.

Generation of the incipient carbocation **9** was the first general solution to the generic problem of introduction of $C_{6(7)}$ substituents.[28] Diazotization of either **8a** or **8b** afforded the diazo intermediate **12**. Diazo esters have long been known to react with halogens to afford dihalo esters. However, reaction with pseudo-halogens was unknown. Treatment of **12** with bromine azide afforded **13** as a

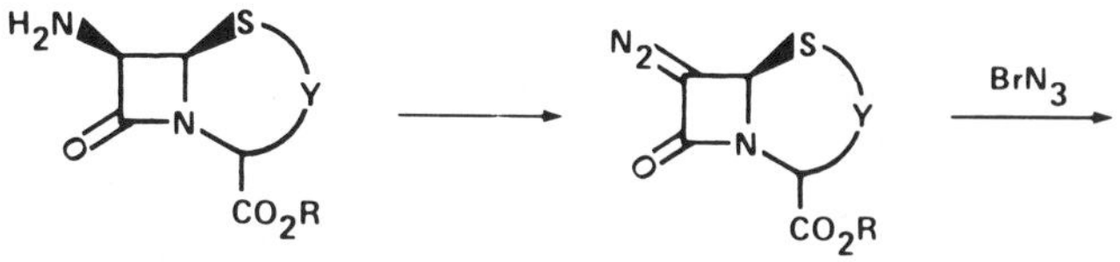

8

12

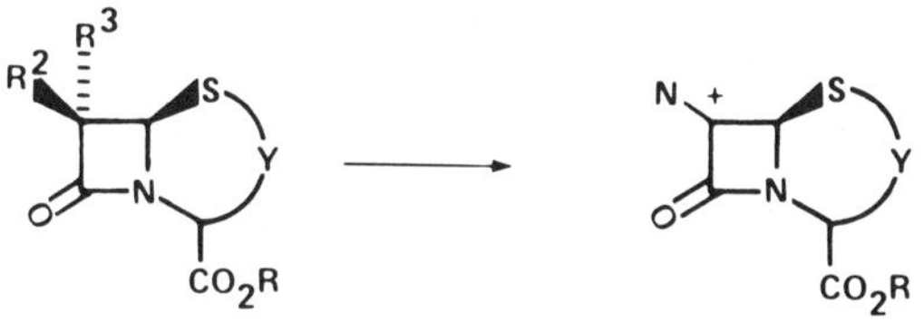

13

9

13a $R^2 = N_3$, $R^3 = Br$
13b $R^2 = Br$; $R^3 = N_3$

mixture of stereoisomers. However, either **13a** or **13b** or the mixture, upon treatment with methanolic silver perfluoroborate, afforded the methoxy azide **14** as a single stereoisomer. Presumably **9** is stable enough to have an appreciable half-life, so that all methanol adds from the least hindered α-face,

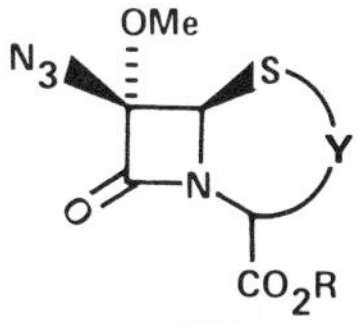

14

directed by the chiral center at $C_{5(6)}$. Reduction of **14** to the desired **6** in both the penicillin and cephalosporin series was readily effected. Other groups than methoxy could be added to the $C_{6(7)}$ position using this methodology.

Generation of the carbanion **10** was readily effected[29] by treatment with a non-nucleophilic base after activation by converting the amine to a Schiff base **15**. Reaction of **10** with a variety of electrophiles, for example, methyl iodide, gave **11** after hydrolysis of the Schiff base group. In this way, several new $C_{6(7)}$-substituted penicillins and cephalosporins were prepared.

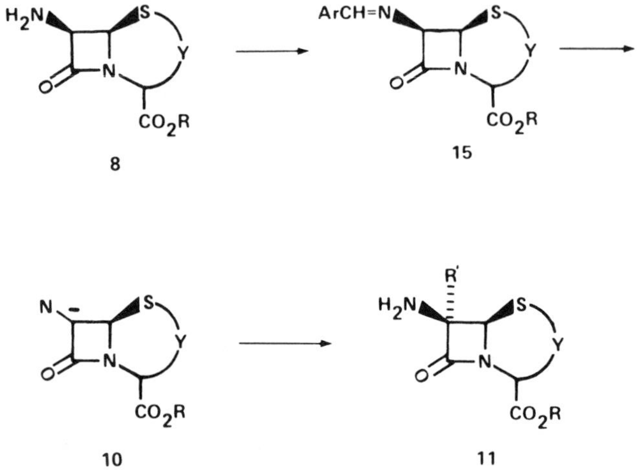

Of particular interest to the medicinal chemist was the synthesis of 6α-methylbenzyl penicillin.[29,30] Based on the structural similarity of D-Ala-D-Ala, the terminal amino acids of the pentapeptide strand involved in bacterial cell-wall synthesis, and penicillin, Strominger and Tipper[31] postulated that

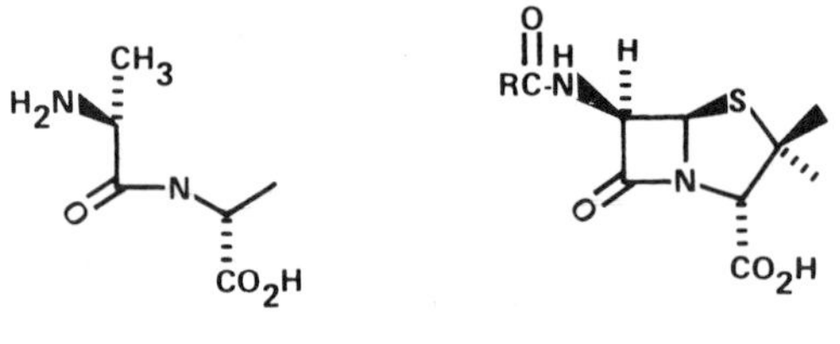

D-Ala-D-Ala   Penicillin

Figure 1.

penicillins acted by mimicking the terminal dipeptide and acylating the trans-peptidase responsible for cross-linking, thus preventing cell-wall synthesis. Because penicillins lack the methyl of D-Ala, these authors postulated that a 6α-methylpenicillin would be more potent. However, 6α-methylpenicillins are less potent than their natural counterparts.

At this point it was realized that where R ' of 11 was a good leaving group, extrusion of R ' occurred more rapidly than acylation to give medicinally useful products. Accordingly, a search for a method generally applicable to the synthesis of penicillins and cephalosporins bearing an electronegative $C_{6(7)}$ group was begun. Direct insertion of the group on a molecule bearing the preformed amide function appeared to be the most direct solution. Generation of the acylimine 17[32-34] was affected by halogenation of the amide, followed by base treatment. Acylimine 17 proved to be highly active and reacted with a variety of reagents, for example, methanol, to afford 18.

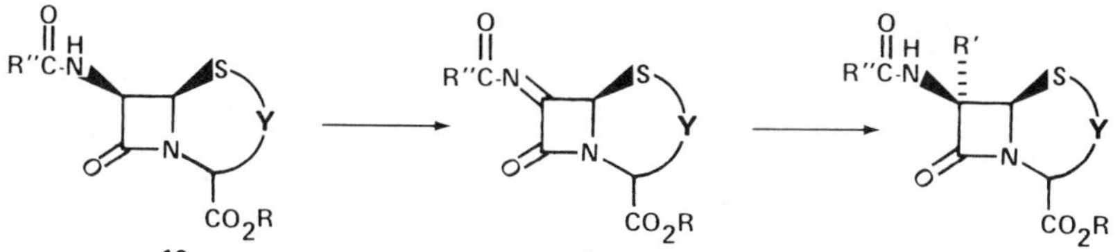

Using the above procedures, a large number of $C_{6(7)}$ groups have been intro-duced into the penicillin and cephalosporin molecules. Alkoxy,[28,32-36] alkyl,[29,30,37,38] acyl,[38,39] methylthio,[36,40] acetoxy,[41] hydroxy,[42] alkoxyform-amido,[43] and cyano[44] are some of those reported in the chemical literature.

In general, any group larger than hydrogen or methyl at C_7 of the cephalosporin nucleus imparts stability to β-lactamases.[22] 7α-Ethylcephalothin (19e) is also resistant to E. cloacae β-lactamase with a V_{max} of 3.9 x 10^3 μmol/min/mg protein and a K_m of 2.4 x 10^{-2} μmol. However, the lack of anti-

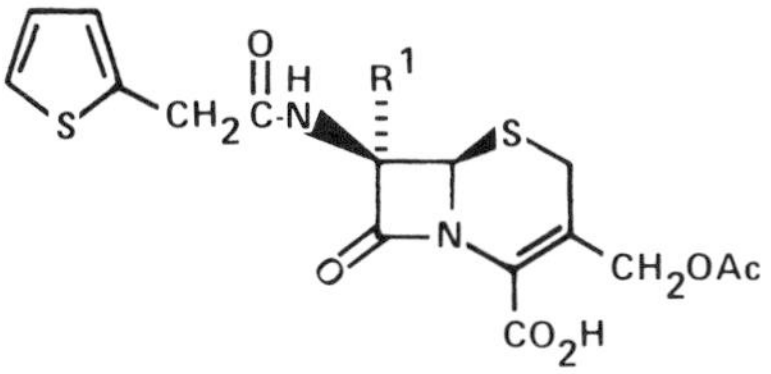

19a R^1 = -H
19b R^1 = -OC_2H_5
19c R^1 = -SCH_3
19d R^1 = -CH_2OH
19e R^1 = -C_2H_5

19

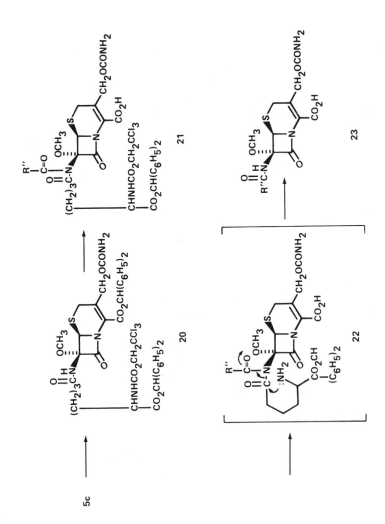

Table 2
β-Lactamase Stability Conferred by 7α-Substituent

Compound	% Destruction by β-lactamase	
	E. coli	E. cloacae
19a	> 96	76
19b	0	0
19c	20	0
19d	0	28

bacterial activity of all groups, with the exception of the 7α-methoxy group, makes their stability to β-lactamase of academic interest only. Finally, it should be noted that resistance to the action of the β-lactamase enzymes appears to be a function of steric bulk, any group containing at least two atoms other than hydrogen at the 7α-position protecting the β-face of the azetidinone from attack by the enzyme. While results in the penicillin series have not received as much attention, 6α-methoxybenzyl penicillin is about as active as methicillin and is stable to gram-positive pencillinases and 6α-methoxycarbenicillin is more potent than carbenicillin against many gram-negative organisms.[45]

With the solution of the general synthetic problem, namely, the introduction of a large variety of substituents at $C_{6(7)}$ of the penicillin and cephalosporin nuclei in hand, and with the demonstration of the unique biological reaction of the $C_7\alpha$-methoxy group in the cephalosporin nucleus, the problem of a specific side-chain interchange of the naturally occurring cephamycins could be addressed. Concomitant with the general solutions mentioned above, a specific side-chain interchange of cephamycin C was being developed.[46] The specific problem to be overcome in any side-chain interchange process is the instability of **6** when known literature procedures are applied. The obvious way to avoid this instability was to avoid the formation of **6**. Specifically, if the new acyl function could be added prior to cleavage of the aminoadipoyl side chain, the new cephamycin derivative could be generated without the intermediacy of **6**. The other salient feature of this scheme was to use the amino group of the aminoadipoyl side chain to promote its own cleavage. Thus, when cephamycin C (**5c**) was converted to its N-trichloroethoxycarbonyl-dibenzhydryl ester (**20**) by conventional means, it could be converted to the imide (**21**) by reaction with the appropriate acid chloride in the presence of $CF_3CONHSiMe_3$. Deblocking of the trichloroethoxycarbonyl protecting group afforded **23** directly,

Table 3

MICs (μg/ml)

Organism	Cephamycin C (5c)	Cefoxitin (1)	Cephalothin (7b)
Staphylococcus aureus (8)	>100	6.25-12.5	0.19-0.78
Streptococcus pyrogenes	>100	0.78	0.09
Streptococcus agalactiae	>100	0.78	0.05
Corynebacterium diphtheriae	>100	6.25	0.39
Erysipelothrix rhusiopathiae	>100	1.56	1.56
Diplococcus pneumoniae	>100	3.12	0.19
Pasteurella multocida (2)	3.12	0.78	0.09
Shigella sp. (2)	12.5-25	6.25-12.5	6.25
Klebsiella pneumoniae (3)	12.5-25	3.12-12.5	1.56-12.5
Escherichia coli (3)	25	6.25-12.5	6.25-50
Proteus vulgaris	1.56	1.56	100
Proteus mirabilis (3)	0.39-3.12	1.56-12.5	6.25-12.5
Proteus morganii (2)	25	6.25	>100
Salmonella schottmuelleri	25	3.12	1.56
Salmonella pullorum	6.25	1.56	0.78
Paracolobacterium arizonae	12.5	1.56	1.56

234

presumably by way of **22**. This route afforded a specific conversion of cephamycins to semisynthetic derivatives with a variety of side chains. Subsequent publications[47] have modified both reaction conditions and concept of mechanism, but the method remains the most practical route to cephamycin derivatives with different side chains.

3. CEFOXITIN

During the course of an extensive analogue program, over 300 7α-methoxycephalosporin derivatives were prepared utilizing all of the chemistry previously described. Of these, cefoxitin (**1**) appeared from the outset to have a desirable blend of features that makes it unique among the β-lactam antibiotics. The interchange of the thienylacetyl for the D-aminoacipoyl side chain of cephamycin C (**5c**) brought about a dramatic increase in gram-positive activity (Table 3) while retaining the excellent gram-negative potency of **5c**.[22] Indeed, the *in vitro* susceptibility of 5096 gram-positive isolates from five hospitals showed cefoxitin (**1**) to be nearly as effective as cephalothin (**7b**) (95% versus 98%).[23] *Enterococcus* is not susceptible to cefoxitin. Cefoxitin (**1**), however, is appreciably better than the cephalosporins, as exemplified by cephalothin (**7b**) against gram-negative isolates *in vitro*. Of 14,528 isolates from five hospitals, 88% were susceptible to cefoxitin while only 67% were susceptible to cephalothin (excluding *Enterobacter* and *Pseudomonas*). Especially important is the susceptibility of *Bacteroides fragilis* to cefoxitin. 74-95% are susceptible to 16 μmg/ml or less of **1**, while only 4-13% are susceptible to **7b**. These results are best rationalized by the β-lactamase stability conferred by the 7α-methoxy group, since cefoxitin is more stable than cephalotin to β-lactamases derived from both *E. cloacae* and *B. fragilis*.

Finally, the importance of the 3-carbamoyloxymethyl function of cefoxitin (**1**) should be mentioned. The *in vivo* deacetylation of cephalothin is well known[48] to result in conversion to a less active metabolite. The carbamoyl function of cefoxitin (**1**) is metabolically stable; 93% of **1** is recovered from the urine of monkeys after a parenteral dose.

Thus it can be seen that cefoxitin (**1**) differs from the related cephalosporin antibiotics in three important respects, each difference contributing to its unique biological profile (Figure 2).

Other 7α-methoxycephalosporin derivatives (Table 4) have now been reported in the literature. Cefoxitin is the first of the cephamycin derivatives to be marketed throughout the world. The newer analogues are either at an earlier stage of development or are not being developed at all. These new derivatives are reported to be two to eight times as active as cefoxitin, but none is active

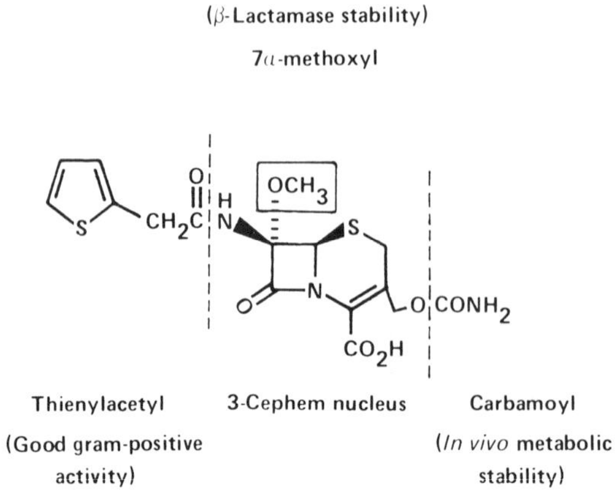

(β-Lactamase stability)

7α-methoxyl

Thienylacetyl	3-Cephem nucleus	Carbamoyl
(Good gram-positive		(*In vivo* metabolic
activity)		stability)

Cefoxitin (1)

Figure 2.

Table 4

Other 7α-Methoxycephalosporins

Name or code no.	R 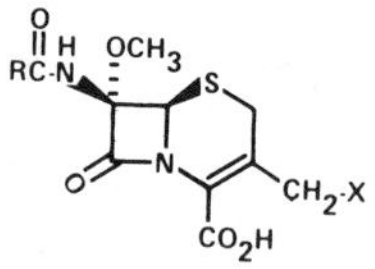	X
Cefmetazole (CS-1170)	$NCCH_2SCH_2-$	$-OCONH_2$
SKF-73678	CF_3SCH_2-	$-STet$
SQ-14359	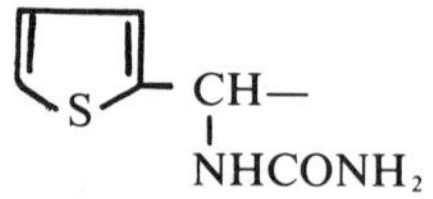 [thienyl]$-CH-$ $\quad$ $NHCONH_2$	$-STet$
YM-09330	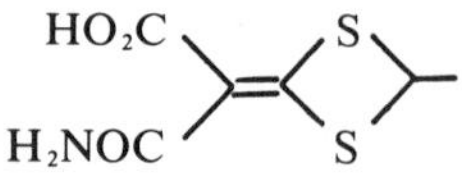 HO_2C / H_2NOC >=< S / S	$-STet$

against pseudomonas.[49] All have activity similar to that of cefoxitin (1) against anaerobes such as *B. fragilis.*

In conclusion, the structure of cefoxitin and the studies leading to its discovery have provided new insight into the synthesis of β-lactam antibiotics stable to the bacterial inactivating enzymes, the β-lactamases. It also provides the cephalosporin chemist with a new metabolically stable group at C_3. But most importantly, cefoxitin (1) is a new β-lactam antibiotic with a broad and extended spectrum when compared to existing cephalosporins by virtue of the β-lactamase stability conferred by the 7α-methoxy functionality.

REFERENCES

1. B. G. Christensen, L. J. Ruswinkle, and L. D. Cama, *Rev. Infect. Dis.,* 1, 64 (1979).
2. B. G. Christensen, M. Sletzinger, S. Karady, and L. D. Cama, Ger. Offen. 2,129,675, Dec. 23, 1971.
3. M. Gorman and C. W. Ryan, *Cephalosporins and Penicillins,* E. H. Flynn, Ed., Academic Press, New York, 1972, p. 533.
4. K. E. Price, *Structure-Activity Relationships among the Semisynthetic Antibiotics,* D. Perlman, Ed., Academic Press, New York, 1977, p. 1.
5. R. B. Sykes and M. Matthew, *J. Antimicrob. Chemother.,* 2, 115 (1976).
6. C. Reading and M. Cole, *Antimicrob. Agents Chemother.,* 11, 852 (1977).
7. F. R. Batchelor, F. P. Doyle, J. H. C. Nayler, and G. N. Rolinson, *Nature,* 183, 257 (1959).
8. G. N. Rolinson, S. Stevens, F. R. Batchelor, J. Cameron-Wood, and E. B. Chain, *Lancet,* 564 (1960).
9. F. P. Doyle, A. A. W. Long, J. H. C. Nayler, and E. R. Stone, *Nature,* 192, 1183 (1961).
10. M. M. Dolan, A. Bondi, J. R. E. Hoover, R. C. Stewart, and R. J. Ferlauto, *Antimicrob. Agents Chemother.,* 1962, 648.
11. H. C. Richards, J. R. Housley, and D. F. Spooner, *Nature,* 199, 354 (1963).
12. S. B. Rosenman and G. H. Warren, *Antimicrob. Agents Chemother.,* 1962 611.
13. E. P. Abraham and G. G. F. Newton, *Biochem. J.,* 58, 266 (1954).
14. R. B. Morin, B. G. Jackson, E. H. Flynn, and R. W. Roeske, *J. Am. Chem. Soc.,* 84, 3400 (1962).
15. R. R. Chauvette, E. H. Flynn, B. G. Jackson, E. F. Lavagnino, R. B. Morin, R. A. Mueller, R. P. Pioch, R. W. Roeske, C. W. Ryan, J. L. Spencer, and E. Van Heyningen, *J. Am. Chem. Soc.,* 84, 3401 (1962).
16. C. H. O'Callaghan, R. B. Sykes, D. M. Ryan, R. D. Foord, and P. W. Muggleton, *J. Antibiotics,* 29, 29 (1976).
17. R. Heymes, A. Lutz, and E. Schrinner, *Infection,* 5, 259 (1977).
18. R. Nagarajan, L. D. Boeck, M. Gorman, R. L. Hamill, C. E. Higgens, M. M. Hoehn, W. M. Stork, and J. G. Whitney, *J. Am. Chem. Soc.,* 93, 2308 (1971).
19. E. O. Stapley, J. Jackson, S. Hernandez, B. S. Zimmerman, S. A. Currie, S. Mochales, J. M. Mata, H. B. Woodruff, and D. Hendlin, *Antimicrob. Agents Chemother.,* 2, 122 (1972).
20. G. Albers-Schonberg, B. H. Arison, and J. L. Smith, *Tetrahedron Lett.,* 1972, 2911.
21. H. Fukase, T. Hasegawa, K. Hatano, H. Hidesuke, and M. Yoneda, *J. Antibiot.,* 29, 113 (1976).
22. E. O. Stapley, D. R. Daoust, D. Hendlin, A. K. Miller, S. B. Zimmerman, J. Birnbaum, L. D. Cama, and B. G. Christensen, *Microbial Drug Resistance,* Vol. II, S. Mitsuhashi, Ed., Japan Scientific Society Press, Tokyo, 1971, p. 405.

23. J. Birnbaum, E. O. Stapley, A. K. Miller, E. Celozzi, H. Wallick, B. A. Pelak, S. B. Zimmerman, D. Hendlin, and H. B. Woodruff, *Infection*, 7, S13 (1979).
24. J. R. E. Hoover and G. L. Dunn, *Burger's Medicinal Chemistry*, Part II, M. E. Wolff, Ed., Wiley, New York, 1971, p. 105.
25. F. H. Huber, R. R. Chauvette, and B. G. Jackson, *Cephalosporins and Penicillins*, E. H. Flynn, Ed., Academic Press, New York, 1972, p. 27.
26. B. G. Christensen, Abstracts, 13th National Medicinal Chemistry Symposium, Iowa City, Iowa, 1972, p. 107.
27. R. Graf, *Chem. Ber.*, **96**, 56 (1963).
28. L. D. Cama, W. J. Leanza, T. R. Beattie, and B. G. Christensen, *J. Am. Chem. Soc.*, **94**, 1408 (1972).
29. R. A. Firestone, N. Schelechow, D. B. R. Johnston, and B. G. Christensen, *Tetrahedron Lett.*, **1972**, 375.
30. E. H. W. Bohme, H. E. Applegate, B. Toeplitz, J. E. Dolfini, and J. Gougoutas, *J. Am. Chem. Soc.*, **93**, 4324 (1971).
31. J. L. Strominger and D. J. Tipper, *Am. J. Med.*, **39**, 708 (1965).
32. R. A. Firestone and B. G. Christensen, *J. Org. Chem.*, **38**, 1436 (1973).
33. J. E. Baldwin, F. J. Urban, R. D. G. Cooper, and F. L. Jose, *J. Am. Chem. Soc.*, **95**, 2401 (1973).
34. G. A. Koppel and R. E. Koehler, *J. Am. Chem. Soc.*, **95**, 2403 (1973).
35. G. A. Koppel and R. E. Koehler, *Tetrahedron Lett.*, **1973**, 1943.
36. W. A. Spitzer and T. Goodson, *Tetrahedron Lett.*, **1973**, 273.
37. D. B. R. Johnston, S. M. Schmitt, R. A. Firestone, and B. G. Christensen, *Tetrahedron Lett.*, **1972**, 4917.
38. G. H. Rasmusson, G. F. Reynolds, and G. E. Arth, *Tetrahedron Lett.*, **1973**, 145.
39. E. H. W. Bohme, H. E. Applegate, J. B. Ewing, P. T. Funcke, M. S. Puar, and J. E. Dolfini, *J. Org. Chem.*, **38**, 230 (1973).
40. T. Jen, J. Frazee, and J. R. E. Hoover, *J. Org. Chem.*, **38**, 2857 (1973).
41. W. A. Slusarchyk, H. E. Applegate, P. Funcke, W. Koster, M. S. Puar, M. Young, and J. E. Dolfini, *J. Org. Chem.*, **38**, 943 (1973).
42. W. A. Spitzer, J. Goodson, Jr., M. O. Chaney, and N. D. Jones, *Tetrahedron Lett.*, **1974** 4311.
43. M. M. Campbell and G. Johnson, *J. Chem. Soc. Chem. Commun.*, **1974**, 479.
44. H. Yanagisawa, M. Fukushima, A. Ando, and H. Nokao, *Tetrahedron Lett.*, **1976**, 259.
45. Unpublished results from these laboratories.
46. S. Karady, S. H. Pines, L. M. Weinstock, F. E. Roberts, G. S. Brenner, A. M. Hoinowski, T. Y. Cheng, and M. Sletzinger, *J. Am. Chem. Soc.*, **94**, 1410 (1972).
47. L. M. Weinstock, S. Karady, F. E. Roberts, A. M. Hoinowski, G. S. Brenner, T. B. K. Lee, W. C. Lumma, and M. Sletzinger, *Tetrahedron Lett.*, **1975**, 3979.
48. C. H. O'Callaghan and P. W. Muggleton, *Biochem J.*, **89**, 304 (1963).
49. L. D. Cama and B. G. Christensen, *β-Lactam Antibiotics*, S. Mitsuhashi, Ed., Japan Science Society Press, Tokyo, in press.

Cambendazole

11

D. R. Hoff

1. INTRODUCTION

Cambendazole (**1**), a potent broad-spectrum anthelmintic active principally against nematode parasites, was introduced in 1970.[1] It is widely used for control of gastrointestinal parasitism in cattle, horses, sheep, and swine.[2] Cambendazole is a direct descendent of thiabendazole (**2**) and was developed following an extensive study of the structure-activity relationships among thiabendazole analogues and, in particular, of the metabolic inactivation of thiabendazole. Discovery of thiabendazole by Brown, Sarett, Cuckler, and co-workers[3] followed recognition of the critical need for a livestock anthelmintic more effective than phenothiazine and from availability of a newly developed anthelmintic test (a modified *Nematospiroides dubius* assay in mice). An additional contribution to the success of the early anthelmintic research at Merck was the availability of a group of benzimidazoles, indoles, benzothiazoles, and benzoxazoles, many of which had anthelmintic activity and had been synthesized as part of an earlier antiviral project.

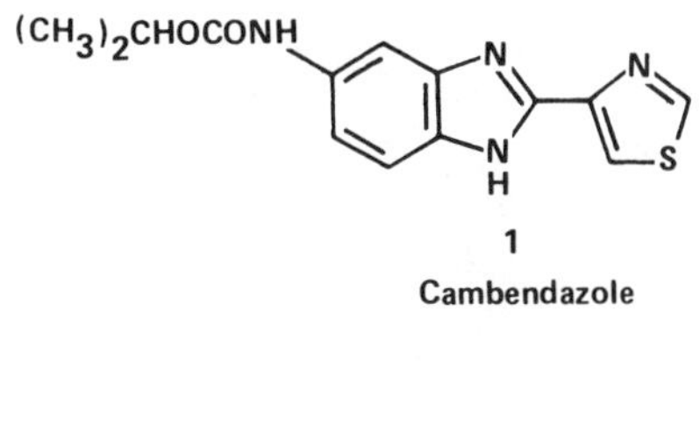

1	2
Cambendazole	Thiabendazole

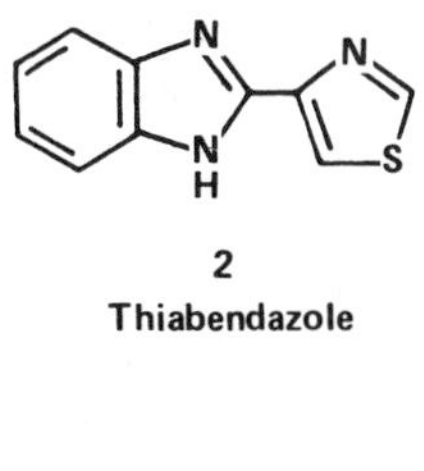

239

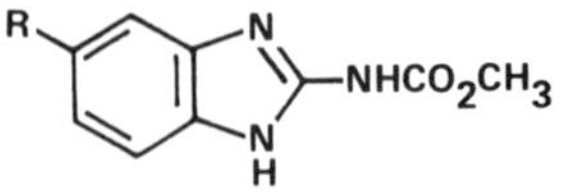

$$R-\text{(benzimidazole)}-\text{NHCO}_2\text{CH}_3$$

3

	Generic name	R	Reference
3a	Parbendazole (SKF)	$n\text{-}C_4H_9-$	9
3b	Mebendazole (Janssen)	C_6H_5CO-	8
3c	Albendazole (Janssen)	$CH_3CH_2CH_2S-$	6
3d	Oxibendazole (SKF)	$CH_3CH_2CH_2S-$	4
3e	Fenbendazole (Hoechst)	C_6H_5S-	7
3f	Oxfendazole (Syntex)	$C_6H_5S(O)-$	5

Figure 1

Appearance of thiabendazole was followed in time by discovery of a series of carbamate derivatives of 2-aminobenzimidazoles (**3**), starting with parbendazole (**3a**, SKF). Many of these proved to be potent and broad-spectrum anthelmintics.

Despite the stark dissimilarity of the substituents in the 2-position, both subclasses of benzimidazole anthelmintics (**1** and **2** versus **3**) are doubtless disparate examples of the same therapeutic lead. The evidence derives from cross-resistance studies[10] and related mode of action studies.[11,12] The benzimidazole anthelmintics are now thought to act by binding to tubulin and hence by interference with microtubule assembly.[10]

Some 1200 benzimidazoles were synthesized and evaluated as benzimidazoles during the course of the Merck project, but the search was not nearly as arduous as might be suggested by the scale of the effort. Benzimidazoles were included in the early rounds of screening, and only a limited number of analogues of the definitive lead were synthesized prior to the selection of thiabendazole as the preferred candidate for field trials.[13] The properties of thiabendazole and the perception of its potential importance stimulated a large follow-up effort. Perhaps 300 relatives had been made before the end of this phase. Somewhat later, analysis of the data then in hand pointed to the modification strategy that led to cambendazole. CBZ was one of the first dozen candidates synthesized in the second phase and a sizable effort was launched to exploit the new information. The goals were increased potency and altered activity spectrum.

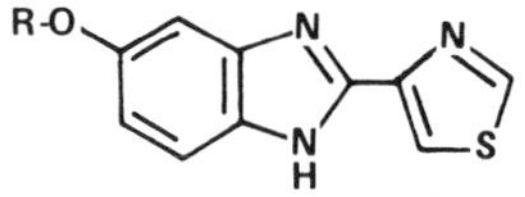

4a R = H
4b R = OSO$_3^-$
4c R = glucuronate

Figure 2. Metabolites of thiabendazole.[16]

The main body of the present discussion is dedicated to a summary of the information that was available concerning thiabendazole pharmacology and structure-activity relationships among the various analogues and data used to formulate the strategy that led to cambendazole.

2. ABSORPTION, METABOLISM, AND EXCRETION OF THIABENDAZOLE

Thiabendazole is rapidly absorbed, metabolized, and excreted in man, experimental animals, and farm animals.[14,15] In cattle, for example, following oral administration, peak plasma level of total drug-related materials was observed at 1-3 hours and consisted almost entirely of the metabolites 5-hydroxy-cambendazole **4a**, its sulfate **4b**, and glucuronide **4c**, all of which are essentially inactive as anthelmintics.[15] The half-life of unchanged thiabendazole in rat serum following i.v. administration is typically 10-20 min.

The recommended dose of thiabendazole in sheep is 44 mg/kg.[2] In view of the speedy absorption and bioconversion of thiabendazole to inactive products and the intestinal location of the target parasites, the effectiveness of the drug has to be attributed to extraordinary intrinsic activity or special physiologic mechanism(s) for delivery to the target organisms. In fact, Brown[3] pointed out the spectacular intrinsic activity (larvicidal and ovacidal) activity *in vitro* of certain benzimidazoles at concentrations as low as 10^{-5} mg/ml, or 5×10^{-11} M! Furthermore, McManus et al.[17] commented on an efficient reexcretion of thiabendazole and metabolites into the acidic abomasum. There must exist an effective absorption/re-excretion loop that magnifies the amount of drug reducing the intestinal parasites before inactivation during passage through the liver. A combination of such a delivery system, high intrinsic activity, and rapid metabolism must account for the favorable blend of therapeutic efficiency and high safety observed with thiabendazole.[18]

3. STRUCTURE-ACTIVITY RELATIONSHIPS: THIABENDAZOLE ANALOGUES

Some degree of anthelmintic activity was observed over a wide range of bicyclic aromatic heterocycles, including benzimidazoles, benzothiazoles, benzoxazoles, indoles, imidazo[1,2-a]pyridines, and pyrrolo[2,3-b]pyridines. The general formulation 5 summarizes the *essential* features of the best of these. Q

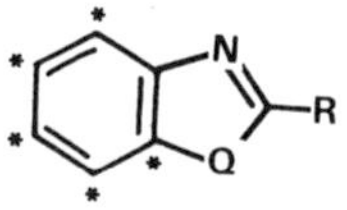

5

is C, NH, or S. The asterisked atoms are usually carbon, but one or two can be nitrogen. Of particular interest chemically was the thieno[2,3-d]imidazole 9, the first example of that novel ring system.[19] Its synthesis proceeded by way of the diaminothiophene derivative 8, which, despite the reputed instability of aminothiophenes, could be readily isolated and handled either as the free base or hydrochloride. Nitration of the amidothiophene 6 in acetic anhydride afforded the desired β-nitrothiophene 7, rather than the alternative α-nitrothiophene. Nitration *ortho* to an acylamido group is typical of nitrations employing acetyl nitrate. Thienoimidazole 9 was about as potent as thiabendazole itself when evaluated against rodent nematodes.

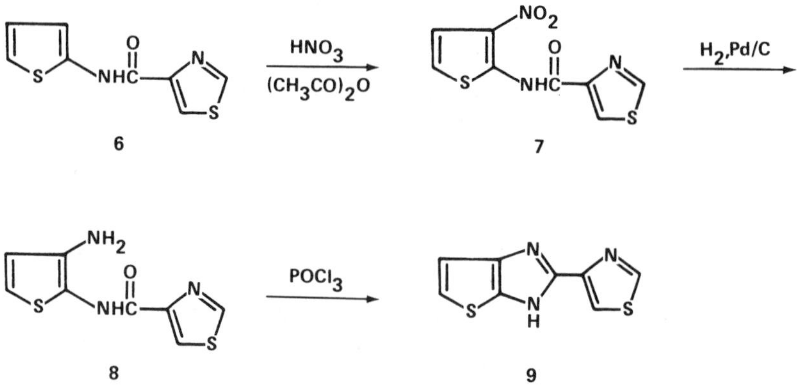

6   7

8   9

4. SEARCH FOR A MODIFIED THIABENDAZOLE

Despite, or perhaps because of, the wide acceptance of thiabendazole, several considerations dictated a continued search for new variants. Thorough patent coverage was of course one of these. Increased potency and altered spectrum were others. Many genera and species of worms can infest man and other animals. The parasites may be found in the stomach, upper or lower intestine, esophagus, lungs, liver, heart, bile ducts, blood vessels, or other somatic locations. The lungworm of cattle and sheep and the migrating ascarid of swine are examples of economically important parasites that spend a part of their life cycles in tissue rather than in the intestinal tract. It may not be realistic to expect a single drug to eradicate all of such a variety of pests. It did seem logical that the broadest spectrum of action would be achieved with a compound that would be broadly dispersed in all tissues and that would be more slowly metabolized and excreted than is thiabendazole. Metabolic blocking, that is, prevention of the rapid 5-hydroxylation of thiabendazole was a reasonable strategy for development of a more potent thiabendazole congener with a broader or altered anthelmintic spectrum. Still another objective was considered. Thiabendazole had been found active *in vitro* against saprophytic fungi and pathogenic fungi affecting man.[20] A more persistent antimycotic benzimidazole might prove of value for control of deep mycoses in man.

Two entirely different approaches were employed to overcome the problem of fast metabolic inactivation of thiabendazole. The first involved the use of specific additive agents capable of inhibiting enzymatic hydroxylation. The experimental method was straightforward. ^{14}C-Labeled thiabendazole (5×10^{-5} M) was incubated with a sheep liver homogenate. A series of test agents were added in turn to the test system and the effect of such additives on the extent of hydroxylation of thiabendazole relative to the controls was determined using a combination of thin-layer chromatography and scintillation counting.

This experimental assay revealed that a variety of classes of chemical substances were capable of inhibiting hydroxylation of thiabendazole by sheep liver enzymes. Most of these were regarded as competitive substrates for the hydroxylation reaction.

Compounds that were found to function as hydroxylation inhibitors were studied further for their effects on thiabendazole metabolism *in vivo* using rats, and, in some cases, sheep. It may be sufficient to describe in more detail two of the more interesting inhibitors uncovered in this study.

Phenothiazine (**10**), itself an anthelmintic, is capable of inhibiting hydroxylation of thiabendazole. This inhibition was first observed in the simple *in vitro* liver homogenate system described above. The plasma half-life of intravenously administered thiabendazole (sheep) was extended from 18 to 28 min

Table 1
Effect of Khellin on the Concentration (mg/ml) of Thiabendazole in Sheep Blood Serum

Animal no.	Khellin[a] dose (mg/kg)	TBZ dose (mg/kg)	15 min	30 min	1 hour	2 hours	4 hours	7 hours
195	None	50	0.0	0.0	0.0	0.26	0.32	0.10
217	None	50	0.0	0.0	0.34	0.50	0.16	0.0
201	40	50	0.30	1.3	3.2	3.6	5.4	7.6
223	40	50	0.28	1.6	2.8	3.6	4.6	5.6
153	20[b]	None	0.0	0.0	0.0	0.0	0.0	0.0

[a] Khellin (20 mg/kg) was administered orally 30 min before a second dose of khellin (20 mg/kg) and thiabendazole (50 mg/kg).

[b] Only one dose given 15 min before the first blood sample.

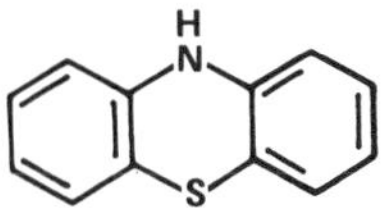

Phenothiazine
10

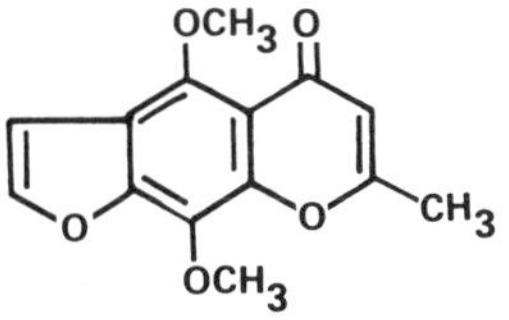

Khellin
11

after predosing with 300 mg/kg of phenothiazine. This small degree of thiabendazole-sparing activity may account for the modest synergism that can be demonstrated between thiabendazole and phenothiazine.

A systematic search for more effective hydroxylation inhibitors led ultimately to the finding that khellin (11), is highly potent in this respect. Oral administration of khellin (two 20 mg/kg doses 30 min apart) to sheep followed by intravenous treatment with thiabendazole (50 mg/kg, immediately after second khellin dose) gave not only increased plasma concentration of thiabendazole, but a greatly increased duration of thiabendazole residence in the blood. The data are given in Table 1.

As a practical demonstration of the anthelmintic efficacy of khellin/thiabendazole combinations, an experiment using swine with pulmonary infections of migrating ascaris larvae was employed. Thiabendazole alone or a combination of thiabendazole plus khellin was fed continuously in the diet. A five- to six-fold enhancement of the anthelmintic efficacy of thiabendazole in this infection was achieved by coadministration of khellin.

Although the experiments employing external hydroxylation inhibitors amply demonstrated the possibilities for improving the clinical potency of thiabendazole, the practical advantages of achieving the same result by way of alternative structural modification of the drug itself needs no elaboration. Efforts along this line succeeded and are the subject of the remainder of the discussion.

5. DIRECT BLOCKING OF THIABENDAZOLE METABOLISM

The traditional approach, direct blocking of the hydroxylation site, was complicated by the apparent symmetry of the benzimidazole ring structure, since the 5- and 6-positions are equivalent. One might imagine that blocking of both the 5- and 6-positions would be necessary. On the other hand, introduction of a substituent in either position might shield the other and redirect metabolic attack to another part of the molecule.

Table 2

	R	*in vivo* (thiabendazole = 1.0)	*in vitro* (μg/ml)	Relative stability in sheep liver homogenate (percent recovery)
1	H (thiabendazole)	1.0	10^{-5}	40
2	5-F	1	10^{-5}	
3	5,6-F$_2$	0.5	10^{-4}	57
4	5-Cl	0.5	100	
5	5,6-Cl$_2$	0.1	10^{-4}	
6	5-Br	0.1	10^{-3}	
7	5-CN	.05	—	
8	5-NO$_2$	.05	—	
9	5-CF$_3$	< 0.1	10^{-2}	20
10	5-CON(CH$_3$)$_2$	< 0.1	10	
11	5-CH$_3$	0.25	10^{-3}	
12	5-C$_6$H$_5$	1	10^{-5}	65
13	5-(*p*-F)-C$_6$H$_4$	1	10^{-4}	
14	5-(*p*-Cl)-C$_6$H$_4$	0.2	10^{-2}	
15	5-(α-thienyl)	0.5	10^{-3}	
16	5-OH	< 0.1	10	
17	5-OCH$_3$	0.2	10^{-2}	
18	5-OC$_6$H$_5$	1	10^{-6}	
19	5-SCH$_3$	0.25	10^{-1}	
20	5-SC$_6$H$_5$	0.5	10^{-3}	
21	5-NH$_2$	0.5	Inactive	
22	5-BrCH$_2$CONH	< 0.1	10	66

In fact, a variety of thiabendazole analogues, modified by substitution of any one or two places on the carbocycle, were synthesized for anthelmintic evaluation. Selected examples of these are shown in Table 2. In the second column is shown the *in vivo* anthelmintic activity of each compound relative to thiabendazole. The concentrations (in ppm) sufficient to inhibit helminth ova development *in vivo* are tabulated in the third column. The last column in the table supplies a rough indication of the relative metabolic stabilities of certain

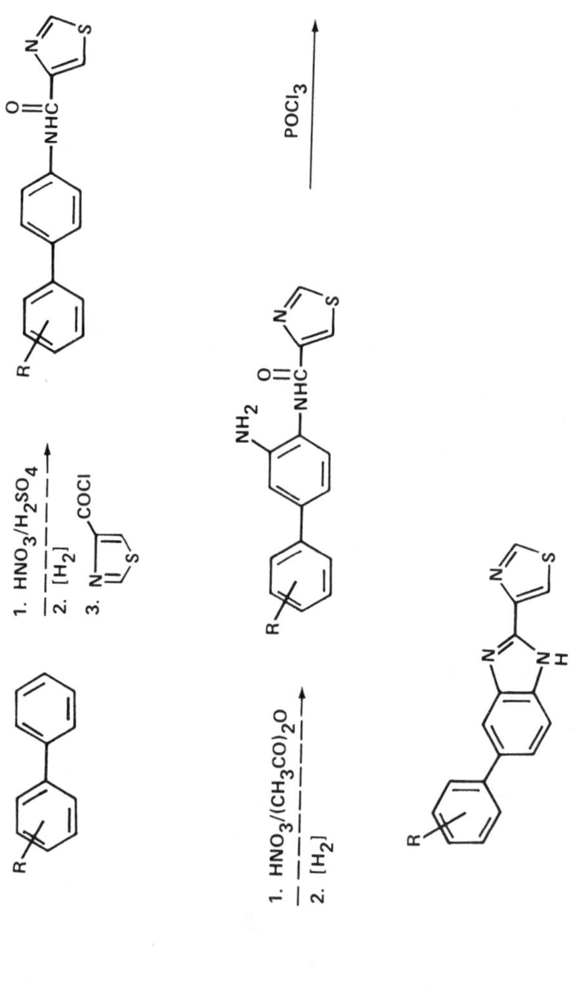

Scheme 1.

247

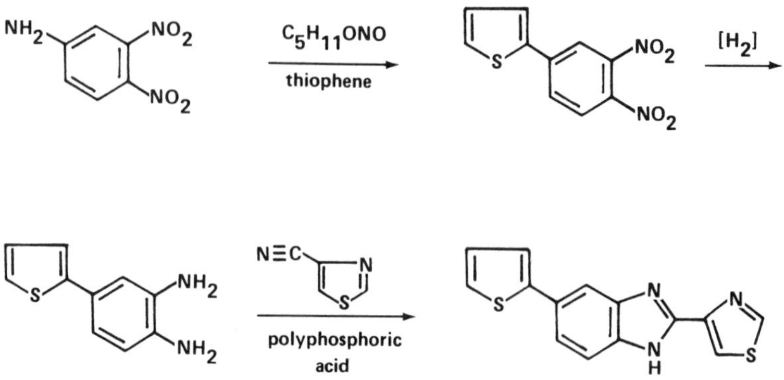

Scheme 2.

of the entries. These stabilities were determined in the presence of sheep liver homogenate, employing conditions under which thiabendazole is hydroxylated to the extent of about 50-60%. The numbers indicate percent recovery of unchanged benzimidazole under the fixed experimental conditions. Thus larger numbers indicate metabolically more stable compounds.

Many of the benzimidazoles in the table were accessible using standard benzimidazole syntheses.[20a] The 5-aryl-benzimidazoles (e.g., 12-14 Table 2) required manipulation of biphenyl derivatives (Scheme 1) prior to construction of the benzimidazole ring.

Entry 15, containing a thiophene ring, presented tactical problems, solved by using a modified Gomberg reaction (Scheme 2). A number of other novel thiabendazole congeners bearing heteroaromatic substituents in the 5-position required unique syntheses, but they are not central to the discussion.

The major conclusion was that none of these materials was demonstrably superior in potency to thiabendazole. Nonetheless, there are sufficient significant clues in this tabulation to point to a solution to the medicinal chemical problem.

The first entries in the table are some halogenated thiabendazole analogues. Note that but for the single exception of 5-fluorothiabendazole, halogenation led to a significant reduction in both *in vivo* and *in vitro* anthelmintic potency. These results should not be surprising, if blocking of hydroxylation is the sole mechanism for potency improvement. Extensive work at the NIH has shown that enzymatic hydroxylation can proceed unchecked by the presence of fluorine, chlorine, or bromine at the hydroxylation site. Seymour Kaufman[21] found that p-fluorophenylalanine is hydroxylated in the presence of rat-liver and sheep-liver hydroxylases with tetrahydropteridines as cofactors. The products were tyrosine and fluoride. Guroff et al.[22] showed that p-chlorophenylalanine and p-bromophenylalanine were transformed chiefly into m-chlorotyrosine and m-bromotyrosine, respectively (the NIH shift).

The second group of compounds shows the effect of typical electronegative substituents, namely, nearly total loss of significant anthelmintic effect. It is of interest to note that 5-trifluoromethyl-thiabendazole was quite unstable in the presence of liver homogenate, though the nature of the metabolism is not known.

The most prominent member of the third group is 5-phenylthiabendazole, which retained the full activity of the parent compound. The high metabolic stability of the material is noteworthy. Further substitution on the phenyl ring (fluorine, chlorine, nitro, amino, methoxyl) failed to improve the potency of this series.

The remainder of the table is made up of derivatives in which a heteroatom is bonded directly to the 5-position. 5-Phenoxy-thiabendazole is the outstanding member of this group. Unfortunately, its metabolic stability was not measured.

Several features of the 5-amino substitution are arresting. Anthelmintic activity was substantial, though inferior to that of thiabendazole. The bromoacetyl derivative, while showing poor activity, was the most stable of the thiabendazole analogues in the presence of sheep liver homogenate. The lack of *in vitro* activity of 5-aminothiabendazole, when contrasted with the extraordinary intrinsic efficacy of thiabendazole under the same conditions, was significant. It seemed likely that the amino group was metabolically altered; perhaps by acetylation, accounting for generation of *in vivo* activity.

It appeared reasonable to assume that 5-amino substitution should have led to a fundamental alteration in the mode of metabolism; and the demonstrated metabolic stability of an acylated derivative thereof raised the possibility that a useful strategy for the design of new thiabendazole analogues with substantially enhanced biological half-life in animals was then in hand.

Nitration of thiabendazole, followed by chemical or catalytic reduction, afforded 5-amino-thiabendazole, which was protected against oxidation by conversion to the hydrochloride **12**. General formula **13** represents a series of derivatives (amides, urethanes, ureas, etc.) synthesized for the purpose of optimizing the distribution and stability properties of the series. The first candidate chosen for synthesis was **13a**, the methyl carbamate derivative. Though the structure of parbendazole (**3a**), a methyl carbamate of 2-aminobenzimidazole, was familiar at the time, the choice of a carbamate as the first trial compound was influenced largely by our experience with ronidazole (**14**),[23]

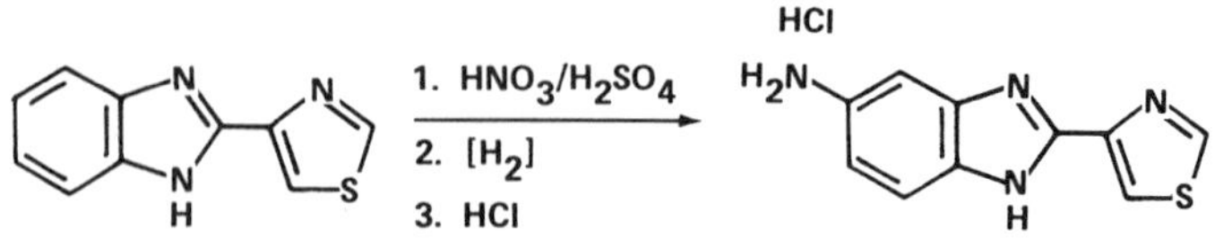

Thiabendazole   12

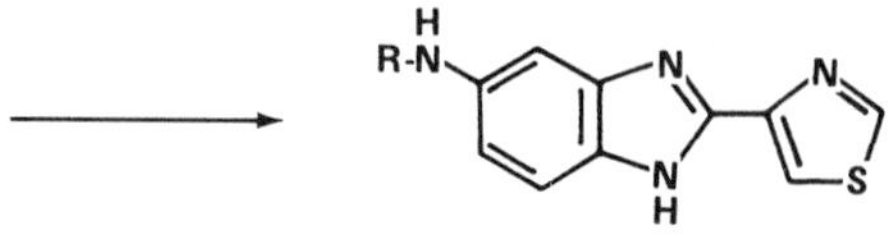

13

13a R = CH$_3$OCO-

13b R = (CH$_3$)$_2$CHOCO-

an antimicrobial nitroimidazole in which the mode of metabolism is strongly influenced by the presence of a carbamate group in the side chain. Carbamate

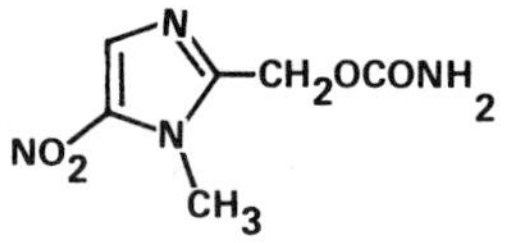

14

13a proved to be four to six times as potent as thiabendazole in the rodent anthelmintic trial, a result that echoed the potency enhancement achieved with khellin in the additive experiments described earlier. A large and varied group of 5-amino-thiabendazole derivatives was synthesized and evaluated. The carbamates proved best in overall activity and the isopropyl carbamate **13b**, cambendazole, was selected for field trials and eventual marketing.

Not all the objectives were achieved, however. Anthelmintic potency was enhanced, but the antifungal activity was diminished. Thus the hope for a systemic fungicide was dashed.

Cambendazole metabolism was studied in cattle, swine, and sheep.[24] The result had been anticipated in part. The benzimidazole ring was largely spared

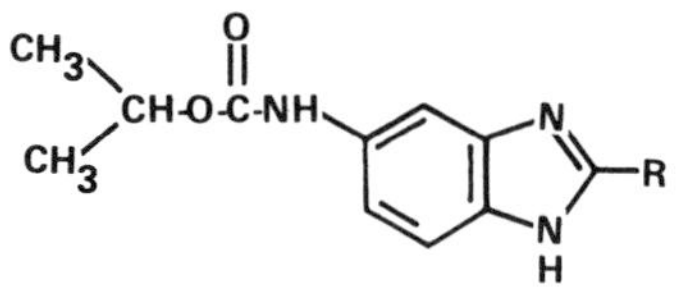

15a R = -CH$_2$CH(OH)SO$_2$CH$_3$

15b R = -CH(CH$_2$OH)NHCHO

15c R = -CH$_2$NHCHO

15d R = -CONH$_2$

15e R = -CO$_2$H

15f R = -CH(OH)CH$_2$OH

15g R = -CH(OH)CH$_3$

15h R = -COCH$_3$

15i R = -CH$_2$OH

15j R = -H

attack and metabolism was redirected against the thiazole ring. Ten of the identified urinary metabolites (15a-15j) were metabolized at the thiazole site. The remaining four metabolites isolated were 5-aminobenzimidazole, 5-acetylamino thiabendazole, and the hydroxylated products 16 and 17.

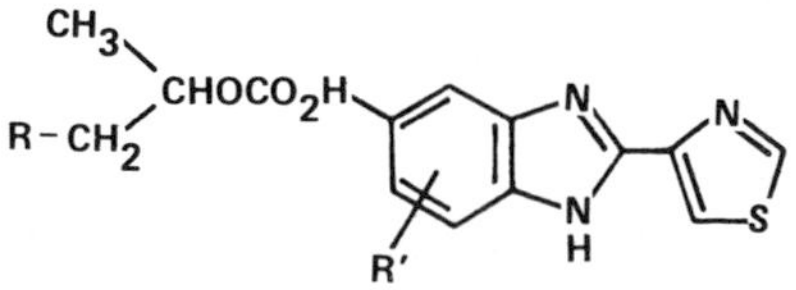

16 R = OH, R' = OH

17 R = H, R' = OH

6.   ATTEMPTS TO EXTEND THE METABOLIC BLOCKING STRATEGY

Systematic probing of the thiabendazole lead had generated a series of 2-heteroaryl benzimidazoles with good anthelmintic activity. Nothing was known about their metabolism, but would blind application of a parallel blocking strategy generate a new family of more highly active congeners? In fact, no. Attaching a CH$_3$OCONH— group at the 5-position of each of these generally destroyed or reduced the activity. As an example, MK340 (18), an isomer of thiabendazole, which was scarcely distinguishable from it with respect to anthelmintic efficacy, gave rise to the inactive carbamate 19.

Apparently thiabendazole metabolism is unique in the series, or, more likely, the dynamics of thiabendazole metabolism render it more susceptible to a blocking strategy.

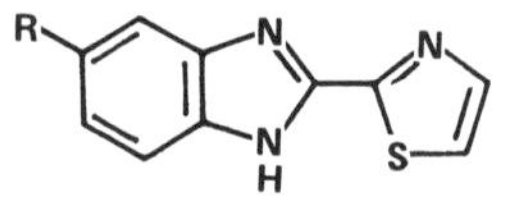

18 R = H
19 R = CH$_3$OCONH-

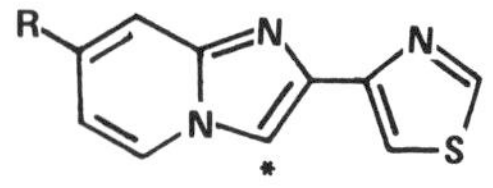

20 R = H
21 R = C$_2$H$_5$OCONH-

The second selected example had a more satisfying ending. The imidazo-[1,2-a]pyridine **20**, still another thiabendazole isomer, had at best borderline anthelmintic activity in rodents, but very high *in vitro* potency — readily diagnosed as speedy metabolic inactivation of some variety. The carbamate derivative **21** had excellent *in vivo* activity in both rodents and sheep, surpassing thiabendazole in potency.[25] Nonetheless, an initial misstep followed from a faulty assumption.

Imidazo[1,2-a]pyridines are usually substituted at C$_3$ (* in **20**) by electrophilic reagents. Since the enzymatic hydroxylation system was regarded as electrophilic, the block was first inserted at C$_3$, affording an inactive compound. Apparently the hydroxylating system was governed by steric rather than electronic factors in this instance.

As we conclude the cambendazole narration, a total silence on the subject of QSAR, statistical methods for unravelling substituent effects of compound series, may have been noted. This was not from lack of application or interest. Physical properties of the entire series of active benzimidazole anthelmintics were tabulated and thoroughly analyzed. Conclusions were drawn, but were largely invalidated by the discontinuous nature of the data. It appears that the compounds were broken into unrelated sets by differing modes of physiological disposition by the mammalian hosts.

7. APPLICATION OF BIOTRANSFORMATION FOR THE CONSTRUCTION OF SOLUBLE "PRE-CAMBENDAZOLES"

Cambendazole, like many benzimidazoles, has very low solubility in water and in most organic solvents. While this is not a serious drawback, there are applications wherein a more soluble cambendazole formulation would find use. The ultimate would be a water-soluble cambendazole for use by injection. The first hint that soluble benzimidazole anthelmintics might prove feasible was found in the new chemistry outlined in Scheme 3.[26] Incomplete reduction of the O-nitroanilide **22** afforded the benzimidazole-N-oxide or 1-hydroxy benzimidazole **23**, which arose by way of trapping of a hydroxylamine intermediate. Compound **23** was not active as an anthelmintic, but its alkylated derivatives **24**

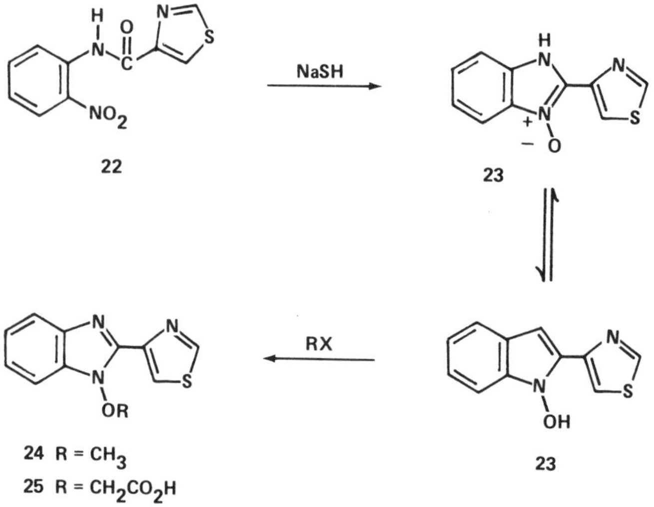

Scheme 3.

and **25** were nearly as active (orally, mice) as the parent thiabendazole. Bioactivation by enzymatic N-O cleavage seemed very efficient. This was an interesting result, because, by varying the R group, a nearly unlimited range of physical properties could be introduced without altering the desired biological activity. The concept was tested by synthesis of the cambendazole derivatives **26-28** (selected from a much larger series). Quite respectable water solubility (up to 25%) was achieved without sacrificing *oral* activity, but the anthelmintic effect proved variable and unsatisfactory when the compounds were administered i.v., or i.m. into mice or sheep.

The drugs were probably being excreted too rapidly by facile processes in the kidney. Oral dosing gave the compounds a chance to lose the polar groups, which were aiding renal clearance. N—O clearance may have been facilitated by intestinal bacteria, too. In one instance, activity was improved by coad-

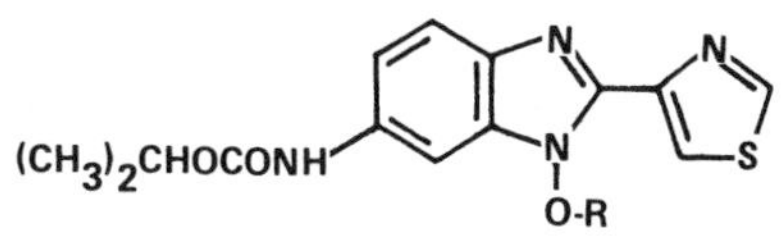

26 R = -OCH₂CO₂H
27 R = -OCH₂CH₂N(CH₃)₂
28 R = -OCH₂CH₂CH₂N⁺(CH₃)₃

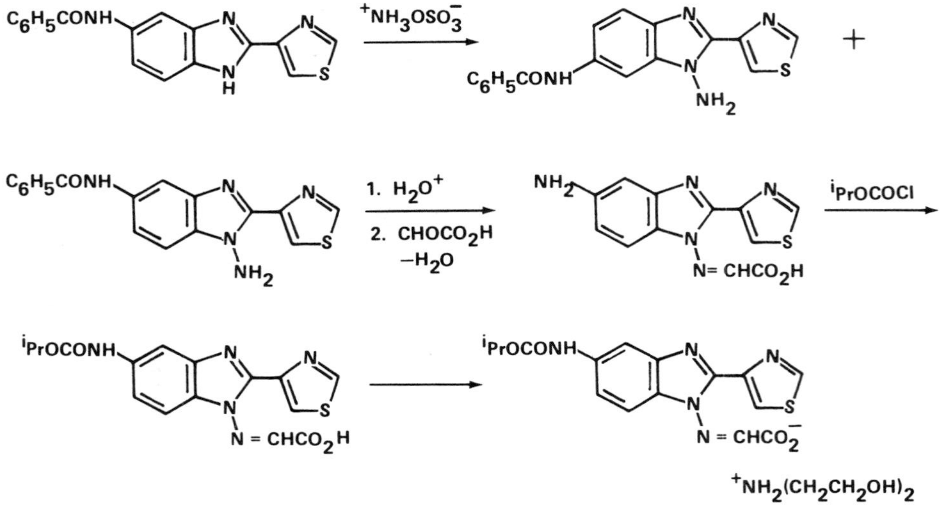

Scheme 5.

254

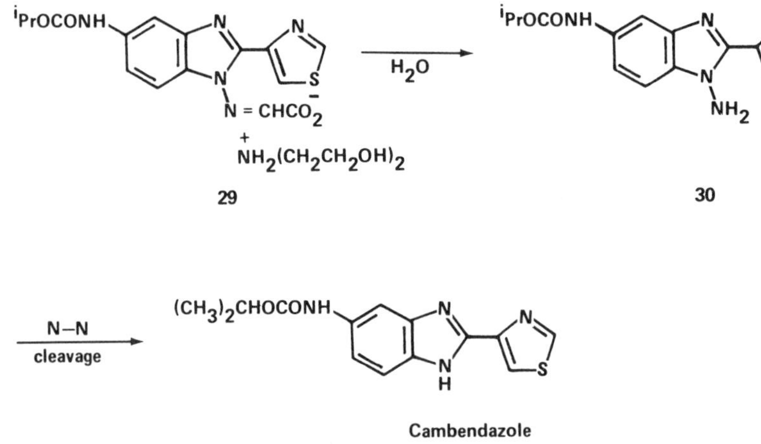

Scheme 4.

ministration of benenid, impairing clearance and supporting our explanation of the poor results.

The idea was salvaged through "fine-tuning", leading to the ultimate variant **29** in Scheme 4. Soluble cambendazole derivative **29** was highly water soluble (80%) and effective orally or by injection against parasites of cattle or sheep. It may be assumed that **29** is rapidly solvolized in plasma to N-amino-cambendazole **30**, which is resistant to renal elimination and which is cleaved to cambendazole, the active product of biotransformation. The scheme is supported by the lack of *in vitro* activity of **29** and **30**.

The N-amino group in **29** was introduced by the use of hydroxylamine-O-sulfate (Scheme 5). The soluble cambendazole **29** was not subjected to field trials, largely because of economic and other practical considerations. The questions of actual performance under rigorous field conditions and long-term stability of water solutions were not assessed.

8. ACKNOWLEDGMENTS

The foregoing discussion utilized illustrative examples from some 1200 benzimidazoles that were synthesized and evaluated as part of the thiabendazole and cambendazole development. The work described is thus the result of the efforts of a large group of individuals. The earlier thiabendazole discovery resulted from the collaborative efforts of Drs. H. D. Brown, L. H. Sarett, and A. C. Cuckler and numerous associates. Particular acknowledgment is due to Drs. W. C. Campbell and J. R. Egerton for biological evaluation of the cambendazole analogues and to Drs. M. H. Fisher and C. S. Rooney, who guided much of the chemical synthesis of the latter group of compounds. *In vitro* metabolism studies were executed by Drs. F. A. Kuehl and R. E. Harman, and the animal evaluation of thiabendazole/khellin combinations were the work of Dr. D. J. Tocco.

9. REFERENCES

1. D. R. Hoff, M. H. Fisher, R. J. Bochis, A. Lusi, F. Waksmunski, J. R. Egerton, J. J. Yakstis, A. C. Cuckler, and W. C. Campbell, *Experientia,* **26,** 550 (1970).
2. *The Merck Veterinary Manual,* 5th ed., Merck & Co., Inc., Rahway, NJ, 1979, pp. 673 – 698, 1554.
3. H. D. Brown, A. R. Matzuk, I. R. Ilves, L. H. Peterson, S. A. Harris, L. H. Sarett, J. R. Egerton, J. J. Yakstis, W. C. Campbell, and A. C. Cuckler, *J. Am. Chem. Soc.,* **83,** 1764 (1961).
4. V. J. Theodorides, J. Chang, C. J. Dicuello, G. M. Grass, R. C. Parish, and G. C. Scott, *Br. Vet. J.,* **129,** xcvii (1973).
5. E. A. Averkin, C. C. Beard, C. A. Dvorak, J. A. Edwards, J. H. Fried, J. G. Kilian, and R. A. Schiltz, *J. Med. Chem.,* **18,** 1164 (1975).
6. V. J. Theodorides, R. J. Gyurik, W. D. Kingsbury, and R. C. Parish, *Experientia,* **32,** 702 (1976).
7. C. Baeder, H. Bahr, O. Christ, D. Duwel, H.-M. Kellner, R. Kirsch, H. Loewe, E. Schultes, E. Schutz, and H. Weston, *Experientia,* **30,** 753 (1974).
8. G. Chaia, L. Chiari, S. deArdujo, and I. B. deAbreu, *Folia Med.,* **64,** 139 (1972).
9. P. Actor, E. L. Anderson, C. J. DiCuollo, R. J. Ferlauto, J. R. E. Hoover, J. F. Pagano, L. R. Ravin, S. F. Scheidy, R. J. Stedman, and V. J. Theodorides, *Nature,* **215,** 321 (1967).
10. J. D. Kelly, C. A. Hall, H. V. Whitlak, H. G. Thompson, N. J. Campbell, and I. C. A. Martin, *Res. Vet. Sci.,* **22,** 161 (1977).
11. L. C. Davidse and W. Flach, *Biochim. Biophys. Acta,* **543,** 82 (1978).
12. M. Borgers, S. DeNollin, M. DeBrabander, and D. Thienpont, *Am. J. Vet. Res.,* **36,** 1153 (1975).
13. H. D. Brown, private communication, Jan. 7, 1960.
14. D. J. Tocco, C. Rosenblum, C. M. Martin, and H. J. Robinson, *Toxicol. Appl. Pharmacol.,* **9,** 31 (1966).
15. D. J. Tocco, J. R. Egerton, W. Bowers, V. W. Christensen, and C. Rosenblum, *J. Pharm. Exp. Ther.,* **149,** 263 (1965).
16. D. J. Tocco, R. P. Buhs, H. D. Brown, A. R. Matzuk, H. E. Mertel, R. E. Harman, and N. R. Trenner, *J. Med. Chem.,* **7,** 399 (1964).
17. E. C. McManus, F. V. Washko, and D. J. Tocco, *Am. J. Vet. Res.,* **27,** 849 (1966).
18. H. J. Robinson, H. C. Stoerk, and O. E. Graessle, *Toxicol. Appl. Pharmacol.,* **7,** 53 (1965).
19. D. R. Hoff and L. H. Peterson, South African Patent 68,100,904 (Aug. 12, 1969), *Chem. Abst.,* **72,** P100702K (1970).
20. H. J. Robinson, H. F. Phares, and O. E. Graessle, *J. Invest. Dermatol.,* **42,** 479 (1965).
21. S. Kaufman, *Biochim. Biophys. Acta,* **51,** 619 (1961).
22. G. Guroff, K. Kondo, and J. Daly, *Biochim. Biophys. Res. Commun.,* **25,** 622 (1966).
23. J. A. Carlson, D. R. Hoff, and Clarence S. Rooney, U.S. Patent 3,646,027 (Feb. 29, 1972).
24. W. J. A. VandenHeuvel, D. E. Wolf, B. H. Arison, R. P. Buhs, J. R. Carlin, R. L. Ellsworth, T. A. Jacob, F. R. Koniuszy, J. L. Smith, N. R. Trenner, R. W. Walker, and F. J. Wolf, *J. Agric. Food Chem.,* **26,** 1357 (1978).
25. M. H. Fisher and A. Lusi, *J. Med. Chem.,* **15,** 982 (1972).
26. M. Sletzinger and D. R. Hoff, U.S. Patent 3,429,890 (Feb. 25, 1969).

Oxamniquine **12**

H. C. Richards

1. INTRODUCTION

What human diseases do you associate with the tropics?

If this question is put to people living in the temperate zones, only a minority would include schistosomiasis or give one of its alternative names, bilharzia, bilharziasis or "snail fever." The possible reason for this lack of awareness is that schistosomiasis is essentially a debilitating rather than a killing disease and, although it causes a great deal of suffering and hardship and can lead to death, it is less obviously dramatic in its effect than, say, malaria or sleeping sickness. Nevertheless, schistosomiasis certainly ranks as one of the major medical problems throughout tropical and subtropical regions. The number of people afflicted with the disease is estimated at 200 million — a figure comparable to the entire population of the United States or the USSR, or roughly 1 in 20 of the world's inhabitants — and the prevalence is increasing.[1]

The disease is caused by the schistosome parasite, a small flatworm (trematode or fluke) that inhabits certain blood vessels in the human host. Each female schistosome, permanently paired with her male counterpart, continually discharges eggs, a proportion of which are eventually excreted in the urine or feces of the infected person. Excreted eggs hatch to release larvae (miracidia) that seek certain species of water snail that act as intermediate host. Infected snails liberate large numbers of second-stage larvae (cercariae) and the schistosome life cycle is completed when these free-swimming larvae penetrate the skin of the (often unsuspecting) primary host. The increasing prevalence of the disease is linked to the introduction of new irrigation schemes and consequent enlargement of breeding grounds for the snails.

Three species of the parasite affect man. *Schistosoma haematobium* is widely distributed throughout Africa and the Middle East; *Schistosoma mansoni* occurs extensively in Africa, South America, and Central America; and *Schistosoma japonicum* is prevalent in Asia. Each of these species of schistosome gives rise to a typical clinical picture — arising from inflammatory reactions produced by schistosome eggs trapped in various tissues and organs of the body — *S. mansoni* and *S. japonicum* affecting primarily the intestine, liver, and spleen and *S. haematobium* affecting the bladder and urogenital tract.

Descriptions of the parasite and its life-cycle together with the epidemiology of the disease and its clinical manifestations appear in an informative monograph by Jordan and Webbe.[2] There have been good reviews by Standen,[3] Werbel,[4] Islep,[5] and Katz[6] on the chemotherapy of schistosomiasis and other (less successful) methods of control, for example, immunization and snail eradication. A recent publication,[7] presenting the proceedings of an Anglo-American Symposium on Tropical Medicine, explores recent advances and suggests avenues for future research.

2. BACKGROUND — THE STATE OF THE ART IN 1964

The search for a novel schistosomicidal agent was initiated at the Pfizer United Kingdom laboratories in 1964. At that time only two types of drugs were in general use, namely, the trivalent antimonials typified by stibocaptate (Astiban, sodium antimony-2,3-dimercaptosuccinate, **1**) and lucanthone [Miracil D, 1-(β-*NN*-diethylaminoethylamino)-4-methylthiaxanthone, **2**].

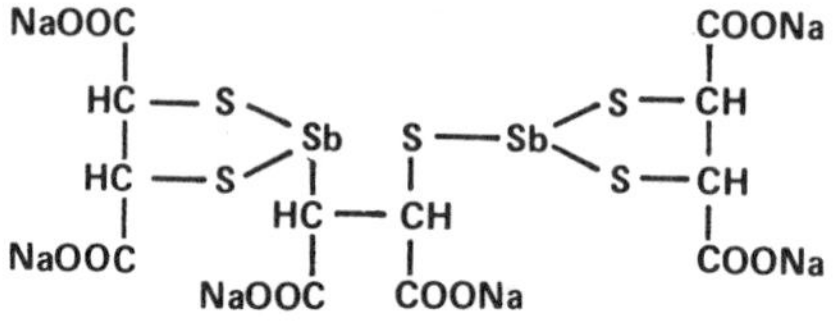

Stibocaptate

1

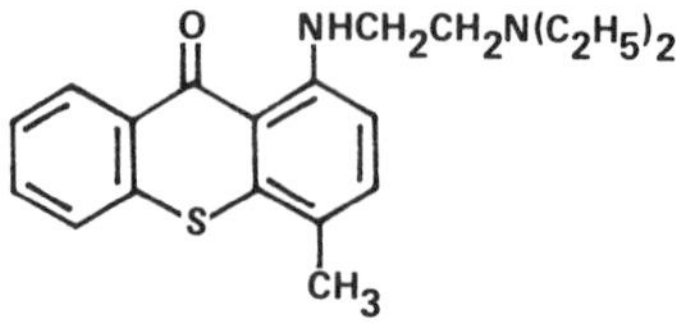

Lucanthone

2

These drugs suffered from serious disadvantages, which have been reviewed recently.[6] In summary, stibocaptate represented an improvement over tartar emetic (potassium antimonyltartrate — the first schistosomicidal agent to be used clinically, in 1918), but it produced marked toxic symptoms; repeated intravenous or intramuscular injections, administered by trained personnel, were also necessary. Lucanthone, the first metal-free schistosomicidal drug, also

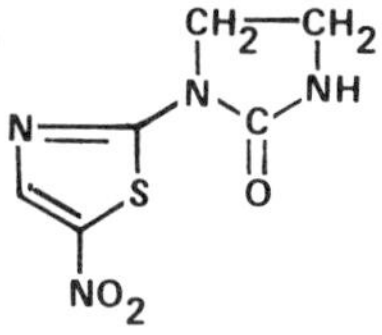

Niridazole

3

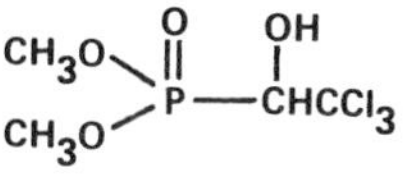

Metrifonate

4

produced unpleasant side effects (anorexia, vomiting, hallucinations, dizziness, yellow staining of the skin and mucosae, etc.) and several daily oral doses were required.

Niridazole [Ambilhar, 1-(5-nitro-2-thiazoyl)-2-imidazolidone, **3**] was introduced subsequently,[8] but treatment of several days duration was found to be necessary, and in some cases it was associated with serious neuropsychiatric side effects, which precluded its use for mass chemotherapy.[6] The cholinesterase inhibitor metrifonate (Dipterex, *O,O*-dimethyl 2,2,2-trichloro-1-hydroxyethylphosphonate, **4**), had found application in the treatment of *S. haematobium* infections, but there were conflicting opinions concerning its efficacy and there was some concern about side effects.[4] A clear need, therefore, existed for a nontoxic, highly effective drug, ideally taken in a single dose, and preferably by mouth, that would render it suitable for programs of mass treatment. The ideal drug would also be effective against all three species of schistosome — lucanthone was ineffective against *S. japonicum* — and active against all stages of schistosomes in mammalian hosts; low cost was also a prerequisite.

3. THE MIRASAN SERIES

Of the several approaches used in the project, one was concerned with a series of compounds, the mirasan series (**5**) first described in 1956 by Mauss et al.[9] These substituted *para*-toluidines were derived from the earlier miracils, which were substituted xanthones and thiaxanthones (**6**) of which **2** was the most active representative.[10]

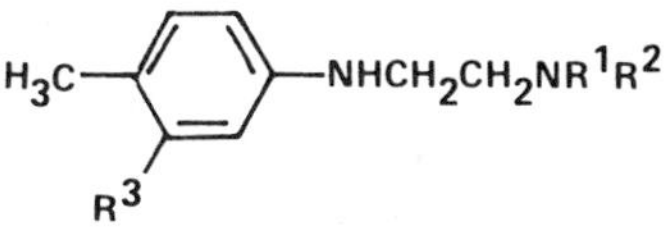

R^1, R^2 = H, alkyl

R^3 = electronegative substituent

5

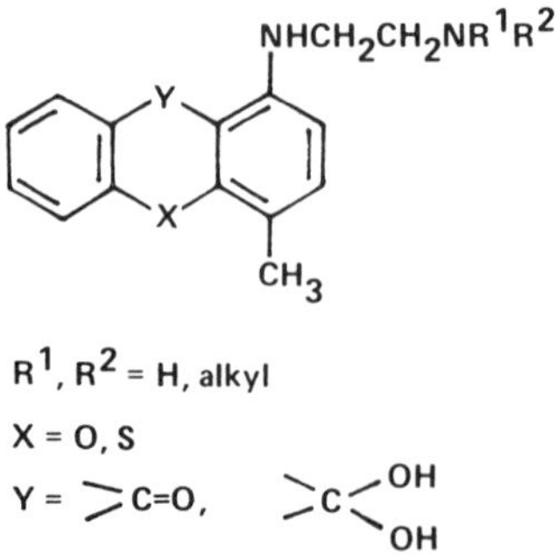

$$NHCH_2CH_2NR^1R^2$$

$$R^1, R^2 = H, alkyl$$

$$X = O, S$$

$$Y = \,>\!C=O, \quad >\!C\!<^{OH}_{OH}$$

6

The two structural features essential for activity and common to **5** and **6** were a methyl group *para* to a substituted aminoethylamino side chain and an electronegative substituent *ortho* to the methyl group. The significance of this requirement was to emerge in later years and is recounted below.

In series **5**, the most interesting member was mirasan (2-chloro-4-β-*NN*-diethylaminoethylaminotoluene, **7**), which is more active in mice than any member of series **6**. However, in contrast to certain members of series **6**, mirasan (**7**) was inactive in monkey and lacked efficacy in man.[11]

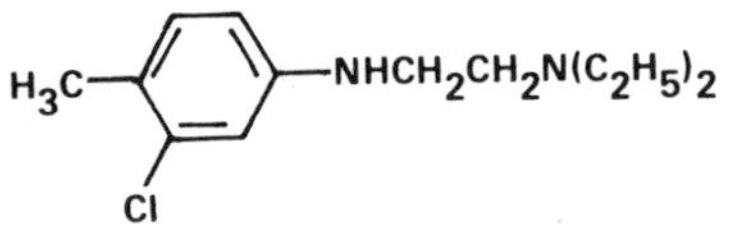

Mirasan

7

4. SOME THOUGHTS ON MOLECULAR CONFORMATION

Over the years, several workers have modified the structure of **7** in an attempt to improve the activity and overcome its therapeutic deficiency (see reference 5). Even though no agent of clinical interest emerged, three analogues (see Table 1) were of particular interest to us from a stereochemical standpoint.

First, the piperazine derivative *N*-(3-chloro-4-methylphenyl)piperazine (**8**) was active[11] and was approximately twice as effective as **7** in *S. mansoni* infected mice.[12] This activity showed that the flexible side chain of **7** could be constrained to good effect and also indicated a favored spatial relationship of the nitrogen atoms proximal and distal to the benzene ring.

Table 1
Activity of Mirasan Congeners

No.	Structure	Host species		
		Mouse	Monkey	Man
7	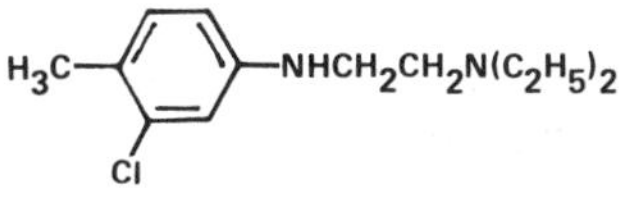 H₃C⟨⟩—NHCH₂CH₂N(C₂H₅)₂, Cl	+	−	−
8	H₃C⟨⟩—N(piperazine)NH, Cl	+ +	−	−
9	H₃C⟨⟩—NHCH₂CH₂N(C₂H₅)₂, CH₃, Cl, CH₃	+ +	−	−
10	H₃C, Cl—(tetrahydroquinoline)N, CH₂CH₂N(C₂H₅)₂	+	+	±

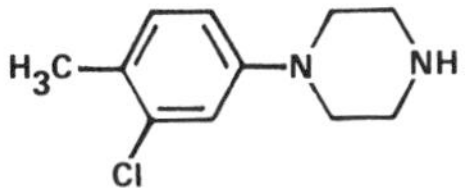

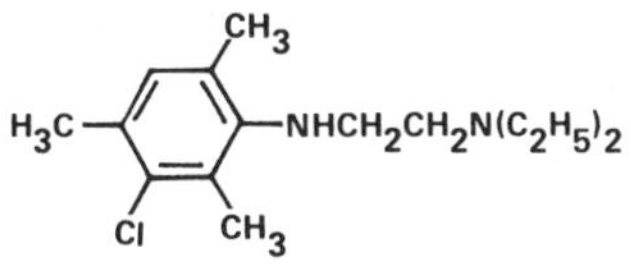

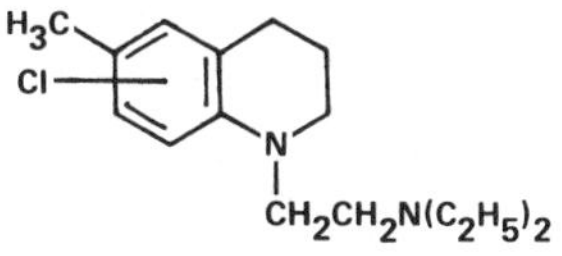

Cl = 5 and 7

Second, S. 616 (2-chloro-4-β-NN-diethylaminoethylaminomesitylene, **9**), showed improved activity compared with **7**.[11,12] In this structure, free rotation of the basic side chain is considerably hindered by the flanking methyl group.

Finally, a group of 1-substituted tetrahydroquinolines, typified by 5 (and 7)-chloro-6-methyl-1-(NN-diethylaminoethyl)-1,2,3,4,-tetrahydroquinoline (**10**), in which free rotation of the "original" side chain of **7** is prevented, was reported active in mice,[9] and although no convincing activity was shown against schistosomal infections in man, interestingly, efficacy was demonstrated in monkey.[11]

These observations offered considerable encouragement to us and we concluded that there may be other ways in which the molecular structure within the "mirasan class" could be modified to produce enhanced activity that would be of clinical use. Could we carry out a suitable constraint of the molecular conformation and "hold" the basic side chain, thereby facilitating the necessary drug-receptor interaction in the schistosome? Alternatively, if one considers the problem in metabolic terms, the effect of elaborating the structure could be to protect the molecule against loss of the essential side chain by biodegradation within the host; no metabolism studies had been reported for the mirasans or their analogues, but efficacy was obviously very host species dependent and indicated the possible importance of metabolic handling.

With these thoughts in mind, we considered the cyclic analogues, **11a, 11b, 12a,** and **12b** as possible types of target compound.

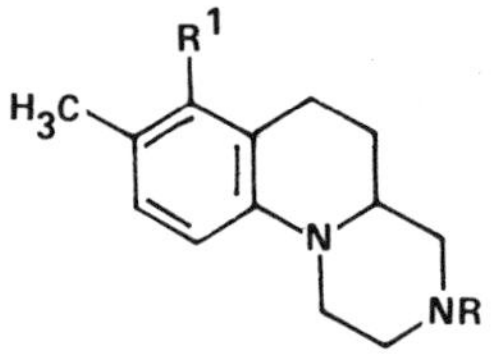

R = H, alkyl; R^1 = Cl, NO$_2$

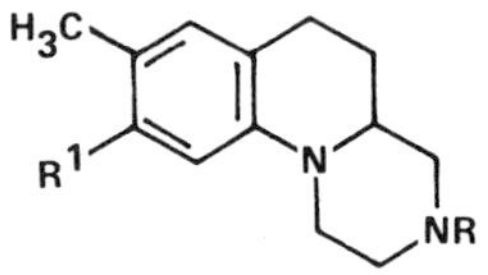

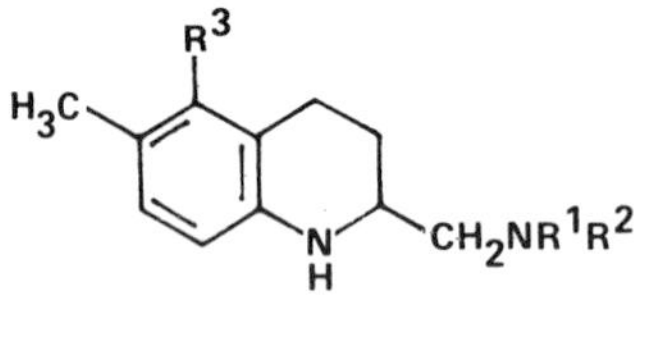

11a   11b

R^1, R^2 = H, alkyl; R^3 = Cl, NO$_2$

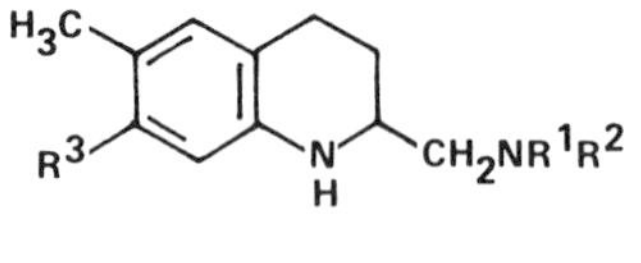

12a   12b

5. BIOLOGICAL SCREENING METHODS

Synthesized compounds were submitted for primary screening in mice infected with *S. mansoni*. Initial doses were usually 100 mg/kg, administered orally in one daily dose for 4 consecutive days, and activity was assessed[14] by the hepatic shift method (the movement of adult worms from the mesenteric plexus to the intrahepatic vessels) 24 hours after the final dose. In the case of active compounds, the assessment was repeated with the dose reduced, often to a single

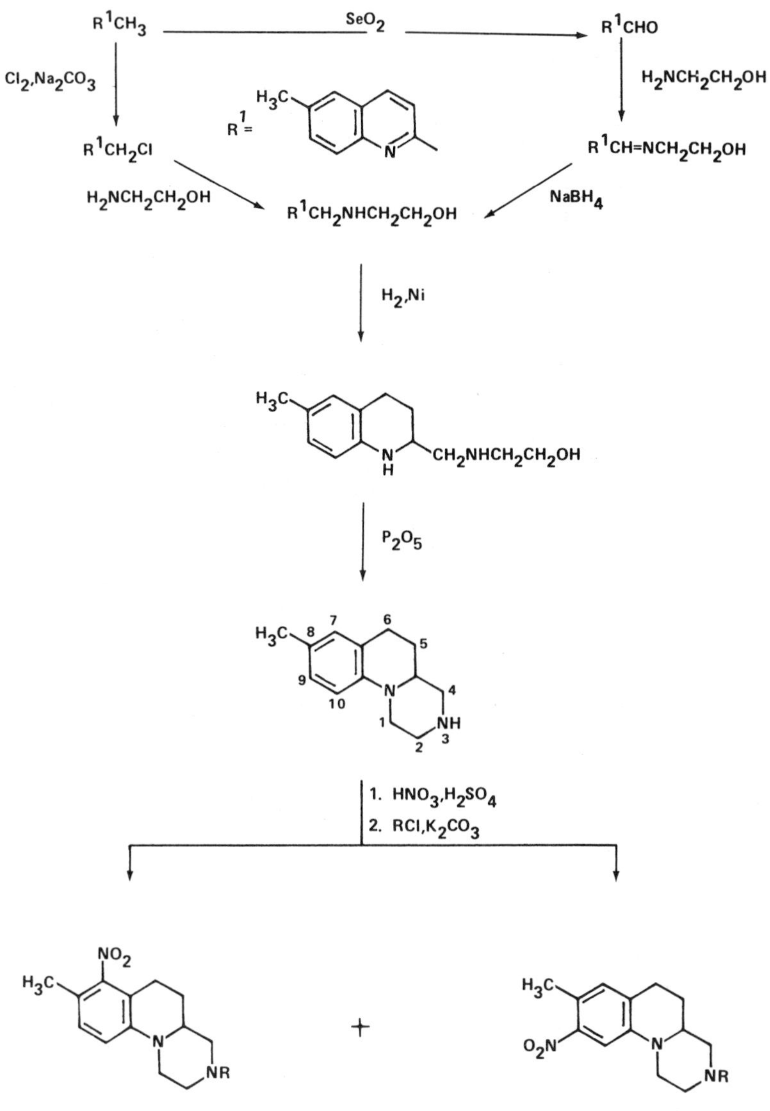
R^1CH_3
SeO_2
R^1CHO
Cl_2, Na_2CO_3
$H_2NCH_2CH_2OH$
H_3C
$R^1 =$
N
R^1CH_2Cl
$R^1CH{=}NCH_2CH_2OH$
$H_2NCH_2CH_2OH$
$NaBH_4$
$R^1CH_2NHCH_2CH_2OH$
H_2, Ni
H_3C
N
H
$CH_2NHCH_2CH_2OH$
P_2O_5
H_3C
8 7 6 5 4 3 2 1 10 9
N
NH
1. HNO_3, H_2SO_4
2. RCl, K_2CO_3
NO_2
H_3C
N
NR
+
H_3C
O_2N
N
NR

13

14

Scheme 1. Route to 7- and 9-nitro tricyclic compounds.

dose for very active compounds, and in some instances a dose-response curve was obtained to assess the ED_{50}, that is, the dose required to shift 50% of the mesenteric population to the liver.

Secondary evaluation was undertaken in monkeys infected with the same strain of *S. mansoni* employed for rodents. Fecal egg output (initially 5000-10,000/24 hours) was determined[15] daily before and after treatment, and efficacy was judged by the reduction in egg load. Treatment was claimed as curative when the count fell to zero and remained so for several weeks.

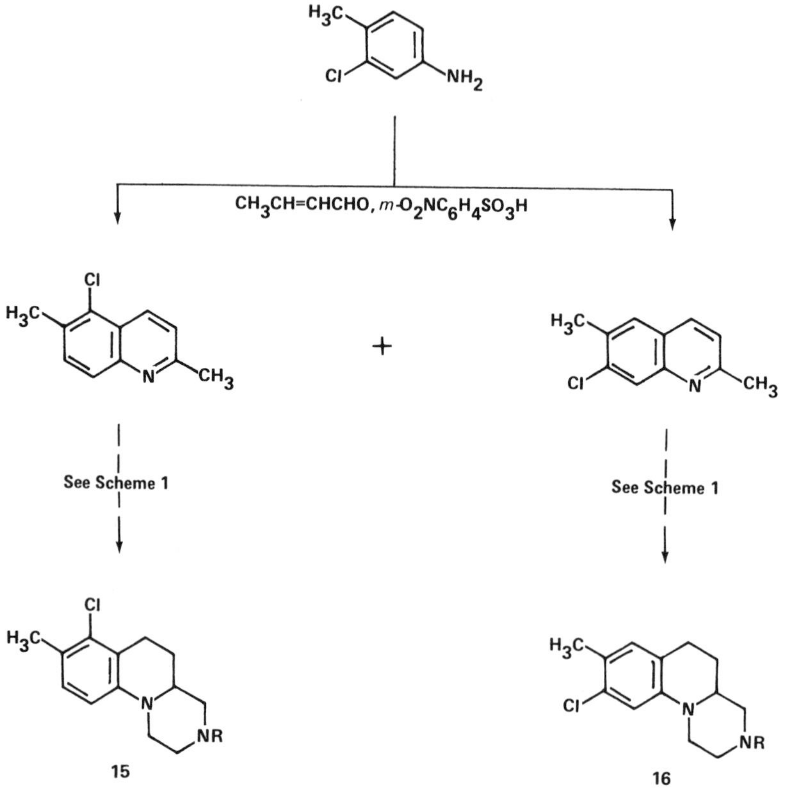

$$CH_3CH=CHCHO, m\text{-}O_2NC_6H_4SO_3H$$

15   +   16

Scheme 2. Route to 7- and 9-chloro tricyclic compounds.

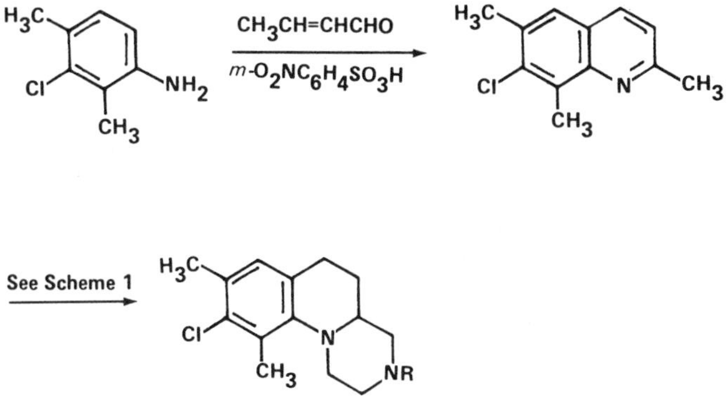

17

Scheme 3. Route to 9-chloro-10-methyl tricyclic compounds.

6. 2,3,4,4a,5,5-HEXAHYDRO-1*H*-PYRAZINO[1,2-*a*]QUINOLINES (11a AND 11b)

6.1 Summary of the Chemistry

The parent tricyclic ring system was prepared by Baxter and Richards[13] using a novel synthetic route that showed advantages over existing published methods. A route to nitro derivatives is shown in Scheme 1; the nitration step yielded mixtures of the 7- and 9-nitro derivatives (the 9-isomer predominating), giving rise to **13** and **14** respectively.

For the chloro derivatives (Scheme 2), functionalization of the quinoline 2-methyl group and final cyclization were carried out as for the nitro series (Scheme 1); the 9-chloro compounds (**16**) were more accessible since 7-chloro-2,6-dimethylquinoline was the major isomer of the initial Doebner-Miller reaction. No such isomer problem occurred during preparation of the 9-chloro-10-methyl tricyclic series (**17**) (Scheme 3).

Compounds were prepared and tested either as the free base or more generally as the hydrochloride or maleate salts.

6.2 Schistosomicidal Activity in Mice

Our expectation of good schistosomicidal activity for this group of compounds was realized (Table 2), and structure-activity relationships have been described in detail elsewhere.[13] Overall, the activity within the 9-chloro series (**16** and **17**) was higher than that of the 9-nitro series (**14**) (Table 2 gives activity ratings for **16** and **17** at one quarter the dose for **14**); this finding was in keeping with the known higher activity of the chloro analogues within the mirasan series.[9]

Table 2
2,3,4,4a,5,6-Hexahydro-1*H*-pyrazino[1,2-*a*]quinolines Relative Oral Activities[a] against *S. mansoni* in Mice

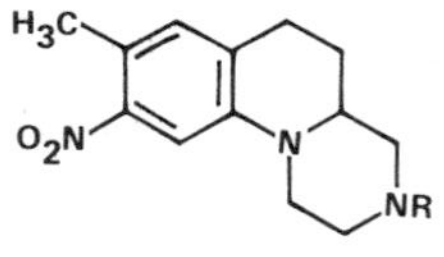

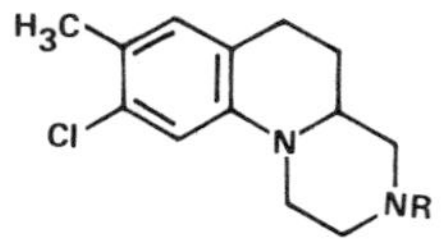

R	14 Cmpd. no.	50 mg/kg x 1	16 Cmpd. no.	12.5 mg/kg x 1	17 Cmpd. no.	12.5 mg/kg x 1
H	**18**	+ +	**35**	+ +	**52**	+ + +
CH$_3$	**19**	+	**36**	+ +	**53**	+ +
C$_2$H$_5$	**20**	+ +	**37**	+	**54**	+ +
(CH$_2$)$_2$CH$_3$	**21**	+ + +	**38**	+	**55**	+ +
(CH$_2$)$_3$CH$_3$	**22**	+ +	**39**	−	**56**	−
(CH$_2$)$_4$CH$_3$	**23**	+	**40**	−	**57**	−
(CH$_2$)$_5$CH$_3$	**24**	−	**41**	−	**58**	−
CH(CH$_3$)$_2$	**25**	+ + +	**42**	+	**59**	+ +

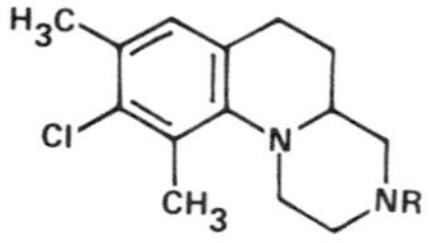

$CH_2CH(CH_3)_2$	26	–	43	–	60	–
$CH_2CH=CH_2$	27	+ + +	44	+	61	+ +
CH_2COCH_3	28	+ + +	45	+	62	+ +
$CH_2C_6H_5$	29	–	46	–	63	–
CH_2CH_2OH	30	–	47	–	64	+ +
$(CH_2)_6O$-⟨benzene⟩-$C(CH_3)_3$ 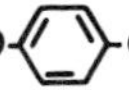	31	–	48	–	65	–
$COCH_3$	32	–	49	–	66	–
$SO_2C_6H_5$	33	–	50	–	67	–
$CSNHC_6H_5$	34	–	51	–	68	–

[a] Activity rating indicates hepatic shift at single oral dose (base equivalent) + + + , >60%; + + , 30-60%, + , <30%; – , nil; in the case of nil rated compounds, activity was sometimes displayed at higher dose levels.

267

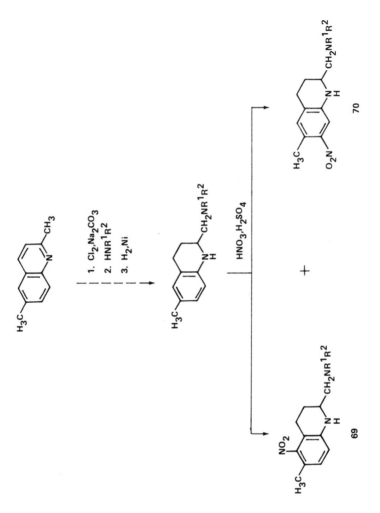

Scheme 4. Route to 5- and 7-nitro quinoline compounds.

Although they were less chemically accessible, several members of the isomeric 7-nitro and 7-chloro series, 13 and 15, respectively, were tested. High activity was displayed and the overall activity pattern was similar to that of the 9-series.

Of all compounds tested in the general class, the most active was the 9-chloro derivative 52 (Table 2), which produced a 99% hepatic shift in *S. mansoni* infected mice at a single oral dose of about 20 mg/kg. For a similar response, the mirasan dose would be 163 mg/kg,[17] and this was a clear indication to us of the potency-enhancing effect of constrained molecular conformation.

6.3 Schistosomicidal Activity in Monkey

A prime objective in the evaluation program was to establish whether our compounds displayed worthwhile antischistosome activity in monkey, since this would provide a further indication of possible efficacy in man.

Several members of the tricyclic group were tested and very satisfyingly proved to be highly effective in reducing fecal egg counts, even after administration of a single dose. Chloro compounds were again more active than nitro compounds, but there were occasional inconsistencies within a series, based on the mouse results; for example, compound 59 (Table 2) appeared to be somewhat more effective than 52 (the most potent in mice), that is, 59 at a single oral dose of 50 mg/kg produced egg count reductions similar to those of 52 at 70 mg/kg.

Preliminary toxicology was undertaken on selected tricyclic compounds in parallel with members of the tetrahydroquinoline class 12a and 12b, described below.

7. 2-AMINOMETHYL-1,2,3,4-TETRAHYDROQUINOLINES (12a AND 12b)

7.1 Summary of the Chemistry

Of the various synthetic routes studied by Baxter and Richards[18] the best general method for preparing nitro derivatives in the tetrahydroisoquinoline series is shown in Scheme 4; the final nitration gave mixtures of 5- and 7-isomers, 69 and 70 respectively, with the 7-nitro (70) as the major product.

Chloro compounds (71 and 72) were synthesized as indicated in Scheme 5 and synthesis of various other analogues of this general type have been fully reported.[18]

Compounds, occasionally isolated as the free base but more usually as the hydrochloride or maleate salts, were tested in the primary and secondary screens described above.

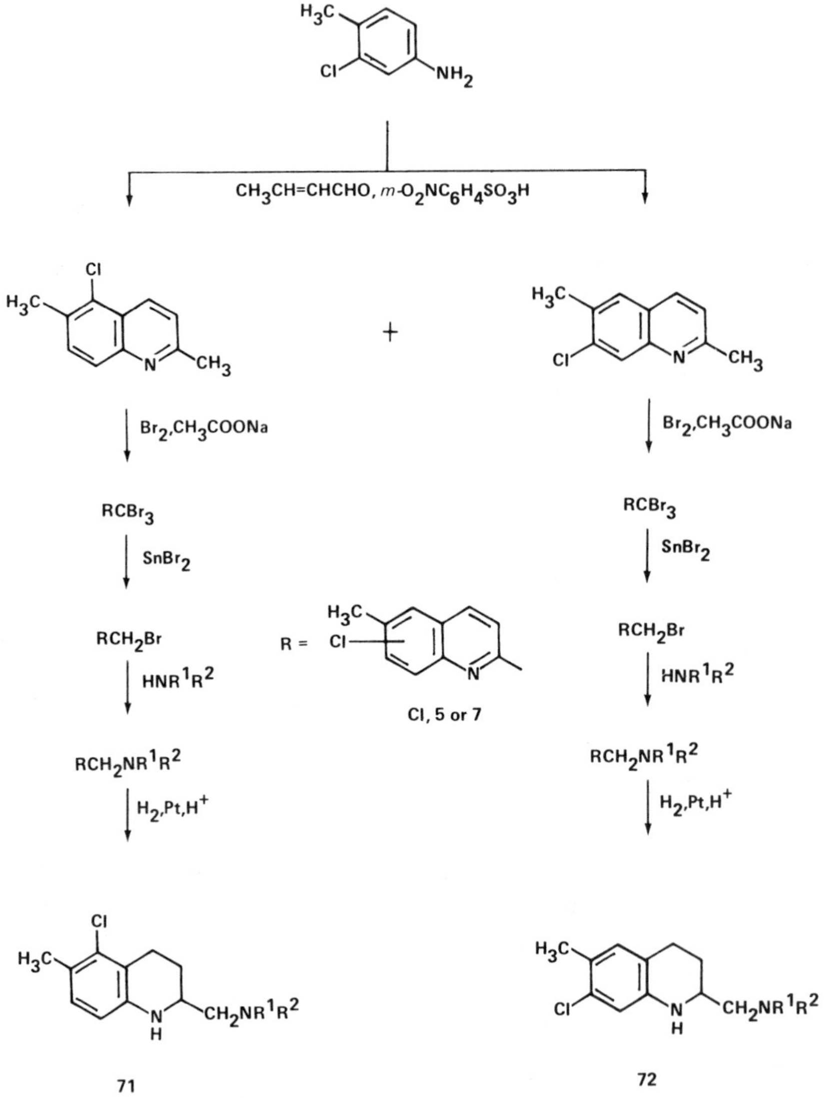

Scheme 5. Route to 5- and 7-chloro quinoline compounds.

7.2 Schistosomicidal Activity in Mice

Good antischistosome activity was shown by several members of the tetra-hydroquinoline class[18,19] and may be summarized as follows:

1. In keeping with the requirements for the mirasans, **75** and **76**, which lacked an electronegative substituent *ortho* to the methyl group, were in-

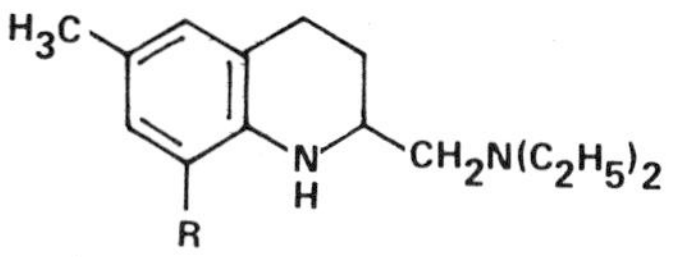

    75 R = H
    76 R = Br

active. Furthermore, in contrast to the high activity usually displayed by 7-substituted derivatives of type **70** and **72**, the isomeric compounds **69** and **71**, with an electronegative substituent in the 5-position, were inactive, which suggested that a critical steric factor was operative in this region of the molecule. This lack of activity was in sharp contrast to that found with the tricyclic class (cf. activity of **13** and **15**).

2. The activity order for the 7-substituent was NO_2 > CN > F > Cl > Br (see compounds **87, 96, 97, 98** and **99** in Table 3), whereas in the mirasan series the order is reversed that is, halogen > CN > NO_2, and an explanation based on lipophilicity has been suggested.[18]

3. Predictably, compounds **77** and **78** were inactive, since they lacked the essential 6-methyl group (see below).

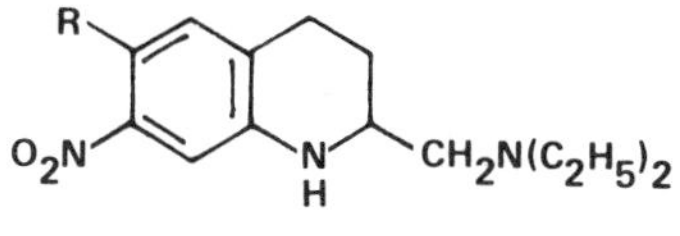

    77 R = H
    78 R = C₂H₅

4. Introduction of a lower alkyl group onto the heteronitrogen resulted in retention of activity (see **93**), whereas loss of basic character, by acylation, led to inactivity (see **94**).

Table 3
2-Aminomethyl-1,2,3,4-tetrahydroquinolines
Relative Oral Activities[a] against S. *mansoni* in Mice

Compound no.	R^1	R^2	R^3	R^4	25 mg/kg x 4
79	H	H	NO_2	H	−
80	CH_3	CH_3	NO_2	H	−
81	C_2H_5	C_2H_5	NO_2	H	+ +
82	C_3H_7	C_3H_7	NO_2	H	−
83	H	CH_3	NO_2	H	−
84	H	C_2H_5	NO_2	H	+ + +
85	H	C_3H_7	NO_2	H	+ +
86	H	C_4H_9	NO_2	H	−
87	H	$CH(CH_3)_2$	NO_2	H	+ + + +
88	H	$C(CH_3)_3$	NO_2	H	+ + +
89	H	$CH(CH_3)C_2H_5$	NO_2	H	+ +
90	H	$CH_2C(CH_3)_3$	NO_2	H	−
91	H	$CH_2C_6H_5$	NO_2	H	−
92	H	$CH_2C_6H_{11}$	NO_2	H	−
93	C_2H_5	C_2H_5	NO_2	CH_3	+
94	C_2H_5	C_2H_5	NO_2	$COCH_3$	−
95	$COCH_3$	$CH(CH_3)_2$	NO_2	H	−
96	H	$CH(CH_3)_2$	CN	H	+ +
97	H	$CH(CH_3)_2$	F	H	+ +
98	H	$CH(CH_3)_2$	Cl	H	+
99	H	$CH(CH_3)_2$	Br	H	+
100	H	C_2H_5	Cl	H	+
101	C_2H_5	C_2H_5	Cl	H	−

[a]Activity rating indicates hepatic shift after four single daily doses of 25 mg/kg (base equivalent), + + + +,>95%; + + +, 75-95%; + +, 50-75%; +,<50%; −, nil; in the case of nil rated compounds, activity was sometimes displayed at higher dose levels.

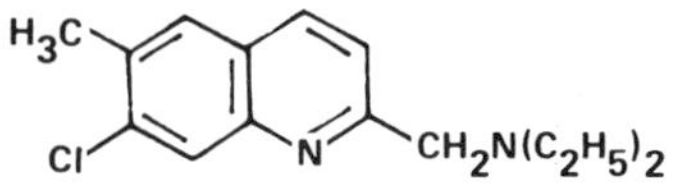

102

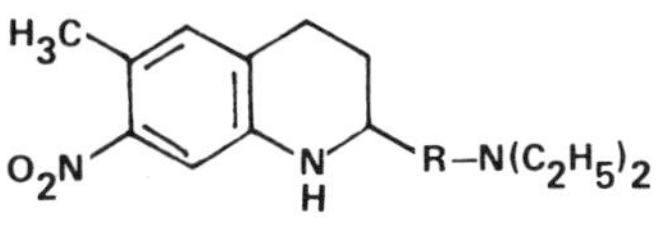

103 R = —CH$_2$CH$_2$—

104 R = —CH—
      |
      CH$_3$

5. The importance of the stereochemical and/or electronic nature of the heterocyclic ring was highlighted by the inactivity of the nonreduced chloroquinoline **102**.

6. Extension of the side chain by one CH$_2$ (**103**) reduced activity, a result that was in harmony with the finding[9] that in the mirasan series the N-N distance of the basic side chain is critical and activity is at a maximum with an ethylene linkage; inclusion of a methyl on the CH$_2$ side chain (**104**) also led to a reduction in activity.

7. Destruction of the basic nature of the terminal nitrogen by acylation (**95**) resulted in a complete loss of activity.

8. With respect to the effect of alkyl substituents on the terminal nitrogen, of the tertiary amines, **81** was the most active, whereas of the secondary amines bearing a straight alkyl chain, maximum activity was displayed by **84**; however, highest activity was possessed by compounds bearing an α-branched alkyl group that is, **87**, **88**, and **89**, which may be a reflection of their expected resistance to *in vivo* dealkylation to produce inactive **79**.

9. The size of the terminal substituent seemed to be an important factor, and possibly those compounds possessing a bulky group, for example, **90**, **91** and **92**, are incapable of being accommodated in a receptor "pocket" at this region.

10. Activity of 7-chloro compounds appeared to follow the same pattern displayed by the (more active) 7-nitro series. Thus, of the three 7-chloro compounds **98**, **100** and **101** (see Table 3) the isopropyl derivative **98** was the most active.

11. The chiral center at position 2 gave rise to optical isomerism within the series and all compounds were tested as racemic mixtures; in a few instances, *d*-α-bromocamphor-π-sulfonic acid was used to resolve the mixture and it was found that the *dextro* form was the more active isomer,[18] again a strong pointer to the stereochemical importance of the side chain. An optical resolution step would, of course, significantly increase the cost of a commercial product.

Table 4
Summary of Efficacy in Mouse and Monkey

No.	Structure	Curative single dose (mg/kg)[a] p.o. Mouse	Monkey
7	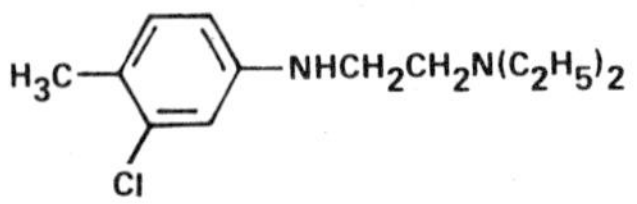 H₃C⟨benzene⟩Cl—NHCH₂CH₂N(C₂H₅)₂	163	Inactive
87	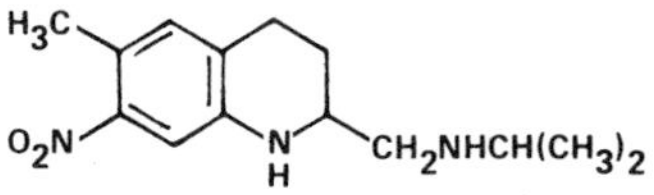 H₃C / O₂N tetrahydroquinoline N-H CH₂NHCH(CH₃)₂	65	50
52	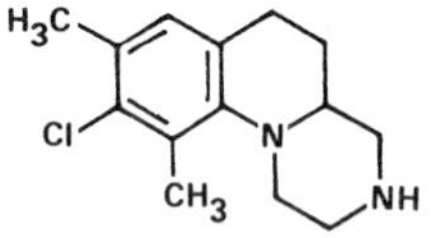 H₃C / Cl / CH₃ tricyclic ring NH	20	70

[a]Compound **7** given as hydrochloride; **87** as maleate; **52** as free base; all doses are quoted as base equivalents.

Within the whole group the most active compound tested (as the racemate) was **87**, 2-N-isopropylaminomethyl-6-methyl-7-nitro-1,2,3,4-tetrahydroquinoline, which was shown by Foster and Cheetham[17] to be curative against *S. mansoni* infections in mice treated with 17 mg/kg p.o. once daily for 5 consecutive days, or with a single dose of 65 mg/kg. Thus, based on a single dose ED$_{99}$ figure, **87**, which is less conformationally constrained than **52**, was about 3 times less potent, but nevertheless was approximately 2½ times more potent than mirasan (**7**) (Table 4).

7.3 Schistosomicidal Activity in Monkey

Several compounds from the tetrahydroquinoline group were (reassuringly) found to be active in monkey. Structure activity relationships roughly paralleled those in mice. Compound **87** was shown by Foster et al.[20] to be the most effective member of the series, complete cures being obtained with a single oral dose of 50 mg/kg (corresponding to 72 mg/kg of the maleate salt). Thus in monkey, efficacy was of the same order as that displayed by the most potent of the tricyclic class, described above (Table 4).

After full consideration of several factors, for example, data from extended biological tests and preliminary toxicity studies, and ease and projected cost of synthesis, **87** was selected as the candidate of choice for a development program leading to clinical evaluation. Later work showed that efficacy against *S. haematobium* and *S. japonicum* was lacking, but the world prevalence of schistosomiasis *mansoni* — an estimated 70 million sufferers[6] — fully warranted continued interest in the drug.

In the meantime, disclosures of Rosi et al.[12,21-23] on metabolism studies in the "mirasan area" stimulated further interest in our own group of compounds.

8. HYDROXYLATION STUDIES IN THE MIRASAN AREA

For some years it had been suspected that the schistosomicidal effect produced by the administration of lucanthone (**2**) was due to its conversion within the animal host to a biologically active metabolite, and various workers had tried to identify this product.[21,22,24] Rosi et al.[21,22] subjected **2** to the action of a range of microorganisms in the expectation that one of these would simulate the metabolic function of the host's enzymes and effect the desired conversion. Of the organisms studied, *Aspergillus sclerotiorum* most efficiently transformed the drug to a mixture of three new compounds, the major component being the 4-hydroxymethyl derivative (**105**), subsequently named hycanthone. Hycanthone (**105**) displayed high schistosomicidal action when administered *per se* to mice, was three to four times as potent as **2**, and proved to be the long-sought active metabolite of **2**.

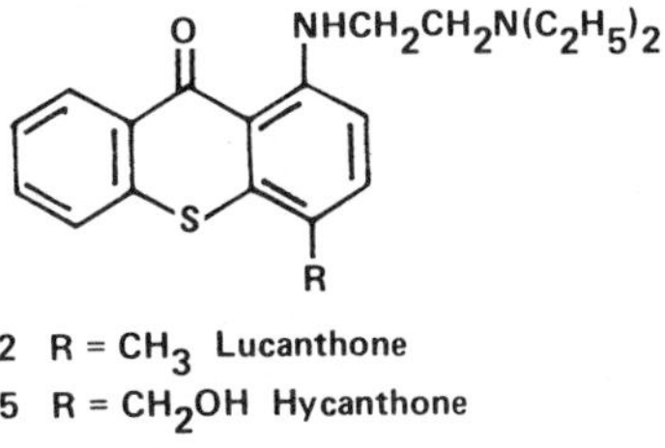

2   R = CH₃   Lucanthone
105   R = CH₂OH   Hycanthone

A process was developed for the large-scale manufacture of hycanthone from 2 utilizing the oxidative fermentation technique, and the drug is available clinically (Etrenol is the mesylate salt). Although 105 is effective against *S. mansoni* and *S. haematobium* when given intramuscularly at low dose (~ 3 mg/kg), hepatotoxicity is associated with its use.[6] The significance to man of the laboratory findings of teratogenic, mutagenic, and carcinogenic effects of 105 cannot be readily estimated.[6,7]

The foregoing metabolic studies clearly demonstrated the role of the all-essential methyl group in 2 and investigations were extended by Rosi et al.[12,23]

R—⟨benzene ring⟩—NHCH$_2$CH$_2$N(C$_2$H$_5$)$_2$

Cl

7   R = CH$_3$ Mirasan
106 R = CH$_2$OH

to mirasan (7) and its congeners. It was shown that in mice and hamsters metabolic conversion of the methyl group to the corresponding hydroxymethyl derivative did indeed occur — to give 106 in the case of mirasan — and that these derivatives were one- to sixfold more schistosomicidal than the parent in mice and two- to 33-fold more schistosomicidal in hamsters. Significantly, no such conversion of mirasan was reported to occur in monkey.

Against this background investigations were undertaken with our own series of compounds to determine whether the methyl group underwent *in vivo* hydroxylation.

9. IDENTIFICATION OF ACTIVE METABOLITES IN THE TETRAHYDROISOQUINOLINE SERIES (11b AND 12b)

Several of our compounds were used as substrates in a series of fermentation studies utilizing a strain of *A. sclerotiorum* Huber (No. 549.65) obtained from the Centralbureau voor Schimmelcultures, Baarn, Holland, to establish whether oxidation of the methyl group could be effected. Various products were obtained and, by means of preparative thin layer chromatography and NMR studies of the separated fractions, it was shown that hydroxymethyl derivatives were produced. Conditions were optimized to obtain good yields of these derivatives for biological evaluation.[25,26] All the hydroxymethyl compounds showed high activity in the mouse screen, by the oral or intramuscular route of administration, and the activity of any particular methyl compound was invariably enhanced as a result of hydroxylation. Structure-activity relationships roughly parallel those of the "parent" methyl compounds.

ACKNOWLEDGMENTS
The author wishes to acknowledge all colleagues for their contributions over the years to the oxamniquine program. This story could not have been told without their help.

REFERENCES

1. *Tropical Diseases Today — The Challenge and the Opportunity,* World Health Organization, Geneva, 1975.
2. P. Jordan and G. Webbe, *Human Schistosomiasis,* Heinemann, London, 1969.
3. O. D. Standen, *Experimental Chemotherapy,* Vol. 1, Academic Press, New York, 1963, p. 701.
4. L. M. Werbel, *Topics in Medicinal Chemistry,* Vol. 3, Interscience, New York, 1970, p. 125.
5. P. J. Islep, *Progress in Drug Research,* Vol. 17, Birkhauser-Verlag, Basel, 1973, p. 241.
6. N. Katz, *Advances in Pharmacology and Chemotherapy,* Vol. 14, Academic Press, New York, 1977, p. 1.
7. C. Wood, *Tropical Medicine — from Romance to Reality,* Academic Press, London, 1978.
8. P. Schmidt and M. Wilhelm, *Angew. Chem. Int. Ed. Engl.,* **10**, 857 (1966).
9. H. Mauss, H. Kolling, and R. Gonnert, *Med. Chem., Abhandl, Med. Chem. Forschungsstaetten Farbenfabriken, Bayer,* **5**, 185 (1956).
10. W. Kikuth, R. Gonnert, and H. Mauss, *Naturwissenschaften,* **33**, 253 (1946).
11. R. Gonnert, *Bull. World Health Organ.,* **25**, 702 (1961).
12. D. A. Berberian, E. W. Dennis, H. Freele, D. Rosi, T. R. Lewis, R. Lorenz, and S. Archer, *J. Med. Chem.,* **12**, 607 (1969).
13. C. A. R. Baxter and H. C. Richards, *J. Med. Chem.,* **15**, 351 (1972).
14. R. Foster, B. L. Cheetham, and E. T. Mesmer, *J. Trop. Med. Hyg.,* **71**, 139 (1968).
15. D. R. Bell, *Bull. World Health Organ.,* **29**, 525 (1963).
16. N. Katz, J. Pellegrino, C. A. Olivera, and A. S. Cunha, *J. Parasitol.,* **53**, 1229 (1967).
17. R. Foster and B. L. Cheetham, *Trans. R. Soc. Trop. Med. Hyg.,* **67**, 674 (1973).
18. C. A. R. Baxter and H. C. Richards, *J. Med. Chem.,* **14**, 1033 (1971).
19. H. C. Richards and R. Foster, *Nature,* **222**, 581 (1969).
20. R. Foster, B. Cheetham, D. F. King, and E. T. Mesmer, *Ann. Trop. Med. Parasitol.,* **65**, 59 (1971).
21. D. Rosi, G. Peruzzotti, E. W. Dennis, D. A. Berberian, H. Freele, and S. Archer, *Nature,* **208**, 1005 (1965).
22. D. Rosi, G. Peruzzotti, E. W. Dennis, D. A. Berberian, H. Freele, B. F. Tullar, and S. Archer, *J. Med. Chem.,* **10**, 867 (1967).
23. D. Rosi, T. R. Lewis, R. Lorenz, H. Freele, D. A. Berberian, and S. Archer, *J. Med. Chem.,* **10**, 877 (1967).
24. R. Strufe, *Med. Chem., Abhandl. Med. Chem. Forschungsstaetten Farbwerke Hoechst. A.G.,* **7**, 337 (1963).
25. Pfizer, South African Patent 68,03636 (1968); *Chem. Abstr.,* **71**, 30369 (1969).
26. Pfizer, German Patent 1,901,262; *Chem. Abstr.,* **72**, 21713 (1970).
27. R. Foster, B. L. Cheetham, and D. F. King, *Trans. R. Soc. Trop. Med. Hyg.,* **67**, 685 (1973).
28. B. Kaye and N. M. Woolhouse, *Xenobiotica,* **2**, 169 (1972).
29. N. M. Woolhouse and B. Kaye, *Parasitology,* **75**, 111 (1977).
30. B. Kaye and N. M. Woolhouse, *Ann. Trop. Med. Parasitol.,* **70**, 323 (1976).

31. B. Kaye, *Advances in Pharmacology and Therapeutics,* Vol. 10, Pergamon Press, New York, 1978, p. 41.
32. *The Selection of Essential Drugs,* Technical Report Series 165, World Health Organization, Geneva, 1977.

INDEX